NURSING MANAGEMENT SECRETS

NURSING MANAGEMENT SECRETS

Polly Gerber Zimmermann, RN, MS, MBA, CEN
Associate Professor
Department of Nursing
Harry S Truman College
Chicago, Illinois

HANLEY & BELFUS, INC. / Philadelphia
An Imprint of Elsevier

Publisher: HANLEY & BELFUS, INC.
                 Medical Publishers
                 210 South 13th Street
                 Philadelphia, PA 19107
                 (215) 546-7293; 800-962-1892
                 FAX (215) 790-9330
                 Web site: http://www.hanleyandbelfus.com

Disclaimer: This book is not intended to be prescriptive, but rather offers the collective wisdom of nursing managers. Although the information in this book has been carefully reviewed for accuracy, neither the authors nor the editor nor the publisher can accept any legal responsibility for any errors. Neither the publisher nor the editor makes any warranty, expressed or implied, with respect to the material contained herein. Case studies are profiled from the collective experiences of nurse managers. Names and other identifying information have been changed to protect anonymity.

Library of Congress Control Number: 2002102754

NURSING MANAGEMENT SECRETS

Permissions may be sought directly from Elsevier's Health Sciences Rights Department in Philadelphia, PA, USA: phone: (+1) 215 239 3804, fax: (+1) 215 239 3805, e-mail: healthpermissions@elsevier.com. You may also complete your request on-line via the Elsevier homepage (http://www.elsevier.com), by selecting 'Customer Support' and then 'Obtaining Permissions'.

ISBN-13: 978-1-56053-529-4
ISBN-10: 1-56053-529-6

Last digit is the print number: 9   8   7   6   5   4

CONTENTS

IV. DIRECTING AND CONTROLLING

V. MEETING STANDARDS

VI. RELATED TOPICS

CONTRIBUTORS

Mark Ambler, RN, BSN, CCRN
Unit Manager, Intensive Care Unit and Clinical Specialty Unit, Monongalia General Hospital, Morgantown, West Virginia

Nancy Bonalumi, RN, MS, CEN
Director, Emergency Services, Pinnacle Health Hospitals, Harrisburg, Pennsylvania

Karen Bry, RN, BA
Patient Care Committee Coordinator, Department of Quality Management, Hinsdale Hospital, Hinsdale, Illinois; formerly Director of Quality Management, St. Anthony Hospital, Chicago, Illinois

Vicki Sweet, RN, MS, CEN, CCRN
Clinical Educator, Emergency Department, St. Jude Medical Center, Fullerton, California; Associate Faculty, Saddleback College, Mission Viejo, California

Kathleen M. Ferriell, RN, MSN
Associate Administrative Officer, Norton Spring View Hospital Administration, Lebanon, Kentucky

Robin J. Gilbert, RN, BSN, CEN
Manager, Emergency Department, Central Maine Medical Center, Lewiston, Maine

Michelle Myers Glower, RN, MSN
Director, Medical Surgical Services, Alexian Brothers Health System, Hoffman Estates, Illinois; formerly Director, Emergency and Trauma Services, Elmhurst Hospital, Elmhurst, Illinois

Mary E. Fecht Gramley, PhD, RN, CEN
Assistant Professor, School of Nursing, George Williams College of Aurora University, Aurora, Illinois; Staff Nurse, Registry, Emergency Department, Delnor Community Hospital, Geneva, Illinois

Bernard Heilicser, DO, MS, FACEP
Director, Medical Ethics Program; Medical Director, South Cook County Emergency Medical Services System, Ingalls Hospital, Harvey, Illinois

Robert D. Herr, MD, MBA, FACEP, CMCE, CPE
Medical Director, Utilization Management, Puget Sound Regional Division, Group Health Cooperative; Attending Emergency Physician, Virginia Mason Hospital, Seattle, Washington

Camilla L. Jones, RN, BBA
Director, Emergency, Transfer, Forensic, and Chest Pain Services, Lewis-Gale Medical Center, Salem, Virginia

Laura A. Leigh, MBA, MSN, RN
Vice President, Patient Care Services and Chief Nurse Executive, Rehabilitation Institute of Chicago, Chicago, Illinois

Kathleen Lezon, RN
President, Healthcare Education Resources, Inc., Fort Pierce, Florida; Director of Operations, Emergency Medical Consultants, Inc., Port St. Lucie, Florida

Irene Louda, RN, BSN, MHA, CEN, CNA
Administrative Director, East Ohio Regional Hospital, Martins Ferry, Ohio; Ohio Valley Medical Center, Wheeling, West Virginia

Jo Manion, RN, PhD(c), CNAA, FAAN
President and Senior Consultant, Manion & Associates, Oviedo, Florida

Kirsten Johnson Moore, RN, MSN
Director, Emergency Nursing Services, St. Christopher's Hospital for Children, Philadelphia, Pennsylvania

James Noland, RN, MSN, CRNP
Clinical Education Specialist, Division of Pediatrics, Huntsville Hospital, Huntsville, Alabama

Barbara Pierce, RN, MN
Director, Emergency Services, Huntsville Hospital System, Huntsville, Alabama

Claire Raines, MA
Claire Raines Associates, Denver, Colorado

Laura J. Roepe, RN, MA, CEN
Senior Quality Systems Analyst, United States Surgical/Tyco Healthcare, North Haven, Connecticut; formerly Administrative Manager, Emergency Department, Norwalk Hospital, Norwalk, Connecticut

Teresa A. Savage, PhD, RN
Research Assistant Professor, Department of Maternal-Child Nursing, University of Illinois at Chicago, College of Nursing; Center for the Study of Disability Ethics, Rehabilitation Institute of Chicago, Chicago, Illinois

Susan Sim
Outcomes Case Manager, St. Anthony Hospital, Chicago, Illinois

Deborah S. Smith, RN, MS, MBA, CEN, CNAA
Assistant Administrator, Patient Services, OSF St. Joseph Medical Center, Bloomington, Illinois

Linda S. Smith, MS, DSN, RN
Assistant Professor, Oregon Health and Science University School of Nursing, Klamath Falls, Oregon

Susan K. Smith, BS, RNC, CNA
Staff Nurse, Emergency Department, Tyrone Hospital, Tyrone, Pennsylvania

Robert W. Stein III, BSN, MSHA, RN, CHE
President, LeNurse, Inc., St. Cloud, Florida; Charge Nurse, Emergency Department, Osceola Regional Medical Center, Kissimmee, Florida

John Vicik, MSIR, CEBS, SPHR
Director, Human Resources, Mather LifeWays, Evanston, Illinois

Steven A. Weinman, RN, BSN, CEN
Director, Office of Continuing Medical Education, Excerpta Medica, Inc., Hillsborough, New Jersey; Per Diem Instructor in Emergency Nursing, New York Presbyterian Hospital, Cornell Medical Center, New York, New York

Polly Gerber Zimmermann, RN, MS, MBA, CEN
Associate Professor, Department of Nursing, Harry S Truman College, Chicago, Illinois

PREFACE

I felt prepared when I assumed my first management role years ago. However, I soon realized that there were many things I didn't know and that many issues I thought I had a handle on were, in fact, constantly evolving. The advice I received back then was to avoid reinventing the wheel by networking and learning from others. That advice remains pertinent. Over the years, other people's resources, tips, and innovations have proven invaluable. Today, networking still helps me cope with our fast-paced health care environment.

Many people have generously shared their experiences with me, both on a personal level and through the *Journal of Emergency Nursing*'s Managers' Forum. My hope for this book is to pass on some of their wisdom. In that way, *Nursing Management Secrets* serves as another form of networking—to get information out there and to share experiences.

I am grateful to all those who have shared their experiences with me. In addition, I would like to thank Linda Scheetz, editor of the Nursing Secrets Series®, for providing me with this opportunity. Thanks also go to the publisher, Hanley & Belfus, Inc., for their support.

Polly Gerber Zimmermann, RN, MS, MBA, CEN

DEDICATION

To my husband, Rudi Zimmermann, for always loving, believing in, and supporting me

To my sister, Kelly Gerber Gerboth, for always being there for me

To my *Journal of Emergency Nursing* editor and friend, Gail Pisarcik Lenehan, for mentoring my writing and editing

PGZ

I. Management Role Differences

1. BEGINNING THE NEW ROLE

Laura J. Roepe, RN, MA, CEN

Beware of undertaking too much at the start. Be content with quite a little. Allow for accidents. Allow for human nature, especially your own.

—Arnold Bennett

1. How do I cope with my own fears about this new position?

The first step in being a successful manager is having self-confidence. This in turn helps you gain the trust and respect of staff and peers. Remind yourself that your having been hired for the position indicates that this trust and respect are already present in the hospital administrators.

2. What is the difference between being a staff RN and a manager?

- *Constant responsibility.* The manager has complete responsibility for the department all the time, 24 hours a day for 365 days a year. The staff member leaves work, and his or her responsibility is over when the shift ends. This never-ceasing responsibility is often cited as one of the more difficult aspects of a managerial role.
- *Availability.* You are essentially always on call. This can become less burdensome as the manager recognizes and develops staff members' leadership and problem-solving abilities.
- *Elusive completion.* A manager's work is never done, compared to a staff member whose tasks are technically finished at the end of the shift. A manager has to be comfortable with ongoing, open-ended work.
- *Leadership.* Staff members are accountable for their actions, but the manager is responsible for staff's actions. You must learn to accomplish things through other people instead of doing them yourself. You provide the direction and vision; they provide the ideas, means, and finished product. It is essential to become comfortable with directing and delegating.
- *Resource for problems.* Managers, unrealistically, are expected to know all the answers. The constant bombardment of questions and problems needing resolution can be a downside of the job. After all, who ever approaches the boss to say everything is perfect? On the other hand, it is challenging to have the additional resources and political power to create and implement some innovative solutions.
- *Public figurehead.* Managers are always on stage. Every word and opinion will be noted. "Venting" or blunt, sarcastic statements are never appropriate. The manager's representative presence is expected at key hospital functions even when it is something in which the manager has no personal interest (e.g., National Supply, Purchasing and Distribution Week celebration, retirement of a 30-year employee you don't know).

Some additional differences are listed in the following table.

Staff	Manager
Hourly wages	Yearly salary
Paid overtime	Compensation time
Policy follower	Policy maker
Patient caretaker	Staff caretaker
Shift accountability	24-hour responsibility

3. What will my official responsibilities be?

Manager job descriptions vary, but some aspects of nursing management are consistent. A sample job description for an Emergency Department Administrative Manager includes:

- Adhere to the Hospital X , Division of Nursing and Emergency Department policies and procedures.
- Function within the scope of professional practice as stated in the X State Nurse Practice Act.
- Comply with the Emergency Nurses' Association standards of practice.
- Assume responsibility for goal setting, prioritizing, and budgeting adequate personnel and supplies to meet patient care needs of the clinical area.
- Demonstrate fiscal accountability through prudent scheduling and monitoring of supply usage.
- Plan, provide, and evaluate the nursing care of patients within the clinical area by establishing and implementing standards of nursing care and practice.
- Develop and evaluate processes for monitoring care in collaboration with unit leadership and staff.
- Interview, hire, evaluate, transfer, and terminate (if needed) staff.
- Provide leadership and direction in developing and maintaining programs and systems to promote participative management.
- Plan and participate in the learning experiences of nursing personnel by coordinating the educational needs of the staff in conjunction with the Clinical Educator.
- Collaborate with Department Heads regarding problems and issues related to the clinical area.
- Maintain active membership in at least one professional nursing organization.

Job descriptions for manager-level and higher positions tend to be vague and open to various levels of interpretation, which is not necessarily a bad thing. They are often written this way to give the manager a chance to accomplish goals using whatever style is appropriate and comfortable. However, get a clear understanding of your boss' interpretation and expectations based on the job description you are provided.

4. Can a staff member successfully move into a management role within the same department?

Absolutely! The staff member who is promoted to management has the advantage of knowing the staff, the organization, and how the department functions. The most difficult part is the change in relationships with staff who may be social friends. A delicately balanced professional distance must be achieved. This is not to say your friendship should be abandoned, but avoid discussing work. Never negatively discuss another employee or hospital administrator.

Sometimes a newly promoted manager is accused of playing favorites. However, often the opposite is true, and friends tend to get put upon in the manager's attempts to avoid playing favorites.

Not everyone feels comfortable making this transition, and there is always the risk of losing a friend or two. Get experience in some management tasks, such as making the schedule or being in charge, while you are a staff member. It will allow you to begin feeling comfortable with the distinction between work roles and friendships.

5. What do I wear as a manager?

Dress codes and accepted clothing vary greatly by geographic region, facility, and even departments. For instance, hospitals in East Coast states tend to have more formal business attire than those in the midwestern or western states. Departments in the hospital without public or patient contact may be permitted to wear casual attire or even have "blue jeans Fridays."

The best advice is to observe, ask, and wear what is comfortable. Use your supervisor and peer's type of dress as an example. An old adage is to dress for the position immediately above yours.

It is, however, important to dress carefully. The manager's dress pattern helps convey expectations to the staff. A manager who always wears a suit is communicating "I will not participate in any patient care." A lab coat over a dress or slacks can indicate a willingness to help with patients if necessary. Scrubs definitely communicate "I am here to work beside you today."

Managers may find themselves in all three outfits during the course of a day or week. If patient care is an occasional part of the job expectation, it is wise to keep scrubs and sneakers ready in the office. Always have a lab coat available; many hospitals require it for any patient-contact work. Refer to Chapter 2, Management and Leadership Styles, for more discussion about what to wear.

6. How do I get started in my new position?

Map out a daily plan for the first week and a weekly plan for the first month. It will include learning your staff and your unit's routine, peers in the organization, and your supervisor's expectations. Some managers choose to come in for a few hours in the week before the official start day to meet a few people and get a tour and overview of the facility and department.

7. What should I do the first day?

- *Arrive at least 15 to 20 minutes prior to the start of the shift.* Make it a point to eventually meet all employees on every shift during the first week.
- *Introduce yourself to everyone.* This includes the nurses, assistants, secretaries, physicians, and housekeepers. Take the initiative and do not wait to be introduced. Shake everyone's hand and memorize names.
- *Take report with the staff.* This provides an overview of the unit and its normal routines. Be visible during change of shifts.
- *Review staffing with the charge nurse.* This gives the staff an opportunity to learn your views, as the new manager, on skill mix. It also ensures that standards, when applicable, are met.
- *Master the facility's layout.* Take a tour. Know how to find key departments. Just being able to find the cafeteria and restroom will boost your confidence.

8. What else should I strive to accomplish that first week?

- *Make it a point to be conspicuous in the department throughout the day.* Visibility to the staff says availability and interest. You can interact and begin to know the staff better and vice versa.
- *Continue introductions as new people enter the department.* Change of shift is a vital time. In the same theme, many managers recommend mastering the names of key players within the organization.
- *Take ownership of the office.* Arrange the furniture; put out personal items. A comfortable, familiar space will ease tensions for these first stressful days. The office layout and tone provides clues about your leadership style and expresses your personality.
- *Become comfortable with the reporting structure.* I recommend that a new manager meet with his or her supervisor at least twice a day for the first week. It does not always need to be a formal meeting; perhaps a structured morning meeting and then a casual wrap-up at the end of the day. The direct supervisor is best able to share the vital knowledge of the expectations for the manager role in the institution. Use this time to obtain direction, ask questions, and gain support during the transition period.
- *Learn key players.* Take the initiative to introduce yourself to people you will need to work with in the future, such as risk management, public relations, and pharmacy directors.

9. What is the most important thing to accomplish this first week?

Get out and get known. Colleagues will decide "who" you are in the first 60 days. Resist the temptation to hide in the office, because, in reality, there is probably a lot of initial work to do. One survey said a common reason managers fail in a new position is not building good re-lationships with peers and staff.

10. How should I handle the second week?

Use this time to learn the various unit positions, meet the institution's other managers, and remain in close contact with your supervisor.

- *Work clinically in the department with a preceptor.* This provides a means to learn the department routine, begin to assess the strengths and weaknesses of the staff, and let the staff see you in action.
- *Meet other managers.* There is no network or support system more vital to success than the other managers in the organization. Invite them to lunch. Some managers recom-mend the goal of talking in-depth with at least four different people.
- *Begin to learn who the senior administrators are in all departments.* Newly hired ad-ministration at a manager/director level will sometimes attend other departmental meet-ings for formal introductions.
- *Continue meeting with your boss.* You should continue this daily meeting until both you and your supervisor feel comfortable with each other. Be honest and keep communica-tion open. The supervisor's main objective is to see the new manager succeed and thrive.
- *Clarify expectations and performance.* Give and get feedback about management orienta-tion and the reaction of staff and peers. One of the main problems for new managers is often a confusion or uncertainty about what is expected. A suggestion is to ask your supervisor, "What will it look like (or will I have done) if I am wildly successful 6 months from now?"
- *Look through department resources and files.* Get a feel for what is there. Be slow to throw out old material. One new manager threw out all personnel information to have a "fresh start," only to learn later that some was needed for a pending hospital lawsuit.

11. I am not clinically competent in the area for which I was hired to manage. Won't the staff pick that up if I work with them?

If clinical competency is not required of the managers in the organization's structure, make sure the staff are aware of this immediately. It is still good advice to shadow the staff to learn their way of working and their concerns. Working directly with the staff lets you begin to see who the strong members and the informal leaders of the units are, as well as the real problems and successes of the unit.

However, if managerial clinical competence is important in the organization, prove yourself. The staff will gain respect and develop confidence from a calm, competent manager. Asking questions is fine, especially in a new department or organization. However, staff do expect the manager to have a knowledge of basic nursing practice, even if the manager is not an "expert."

12. Why is meeting other managers so important? Shouldn't all of my initial energies be directed toward my own department?

Every organization functions differently, so it is important to learn what makes a manager suc-cessful in your facility. All nursing units need to work together, so having a solid relationship with the other managers will eventually assist the staff in creating good relationships with each other.

A feeling of alienation is common if allies among other managers are not sought out. Besides, managers with similar backgrounds or functional units tend to have related concerns and needs. It is natural to become friends and even "cover" for each other during time off. Common examples of informal groupings include the critical care units (ICU, SCU, ED), the medical surgical units, and maternal/child/pediatric.

13. Tell me what I should do by the end of the third week.

Have a formal department staff meeting. By this time, most of the introductions have been made and everyone is becoming comfortable with the transition. The staff now need to know the values and expectations of their manager. At this meeting,

- *Do most of the talking.* Use it as a forum to share the vision and acceptable behaviors for the department.
- *Keep focused on the future.* Avoid allowing the staff to do the "but we've always done it this way" or "the person before you did..." whine.
- *Talk about your leadership style.* Each manager is unique, and describing your style and approach with the staff will allow them to adjust to the changes more easily. Explain your office policies, such as open door or hours.
- *Share the management job description.* This assists the staff in getting a clear picture of what upper administration is expecting of their new leader.

14. Is there anything I should avoid?

Most managers do not recommend excessive references to your former positions or facilities. Each institution is different. Constant mentioning of the previous job may be resented as a sign of your not wanting to understand *this* department. If you have a stellar program or idea to import, just say that you've seen it work well this way.

15. Suggestions for the following weeks?

- *Write your job responsibilities and priorities as you perceive them now.* Communicate and resolve any discrepancies from what you were told during the job interview and the current situation. People are hired to long-term and hoped-for goals, but there are usually short-term corrections and clarifications needed first.
- *Accomplish something concrete that's visible and makes sense.* Focus on something you know you'll do well that will be seen as a significant contribution in the eyes of your colleagues.
- *Keep a focus on adequate department staff and stock.* Although there are many possible goals, these two elements are essential for safe, effective patient care.
- *Keep a diary about your experiences and observations.* Include things that impress you as inefficient or possibilities for improvement. You may not choose to change it now. But unless deliberately noted, it will become "the way we do it here" by 6 months. However, also note what already works well. Even positive things can become extinct if they are not reinforced.
- *Do things in moderation.* There is a tendency to have an adrenaline surge those first few weeks and tackle everything. But not everyone is on your schedule. Think through decisions: it won't hurt to wait a little.

16. When can I start making changes?

Patience and timing are vital to making changes that will actually be embraced by the staff. Dangerous or unsafe practices affecting patient or staff safety or outcomes need to be changed immediately and without discussion. This is where you as the manager get to say, "It will be done this way, period." Be able to give a solid rationale if questioned, quoting standards, policies, and regulations. Examples include recapping sharps, verbal/physical abuse to staff or patients, inappropriate restraint use, or not adhering to sterile technique.

Changes to practices, equipment, and workflow that are not unsafe but just annoying or in need of improvement can begin to be made after 2 to 3 months. This time frame gives the manager a chance to thoroughly study the history of the problem and discuss it with the people it affects. This may entail meetings or work groups.

A slow transition allows staff control over their environment and practice. It gives them a sense of ownership. Examples include dress code, placement of supplies, documentation, or treatment regimens.

17. There are volumes of policy books. How important is it that I read them?

A manager does need to thoroughly know and use these books. Often staff expect the manager to be a walking policy reference source. Learning as much as you can about the unit can only bring more respect from staff and give you a sense of control.

You will have the opportunity to address and update these policies. This is a great opportunity to create an organized and thriving department. But it has to start with your knowing what is already there.

Some managers have found that an updated policy book is key in developing self-sufficiency in the staff. You start an effective habit when you can confidently direct staff with questions to the policy book.

18. I found old policy books in the office. Can I throw them out? I want staff to use only current information.

Check with your legal departments. Usually former policies must be stored for an extended period, such as 5 or 10 years, in case of lawsuits. Hospitals must produce the policies they were using at the time of the incident that is named in the suit.

19. Have I made a mistake accepting a management position? It sounds like there are so many difficulties.

Management is a great challenge with many rewards and learning experiences. The first months are thrilling, as well as a little bit frightening. Be confident, self-assured, and outgoing. Think through decisions. Get acquainted with your staff and allow the staff the same pleasure. Know that, in the end, the accomplishments and achievements will outshine any of the frustrations along the road.

BIBLIOGRAPHY

1. Bennis W: On Becoming a Leader. New York, Addison-Wesley, 1989.
2. Cook MJ:Effective Coaching. New York, McGraw-Hill, 1999.
3. Krieff A: Manager's Survival Guide: How to Avoid the 750 Most Common Mistakes in Dealing with People. Upper Saddle River, NJ, Prentice-Hall, 1996.
4. Marrelli TM: The Nurse Manager's Survival Guide. St. Louis, Mosby, 1993.

2. MANAGEMENT AND LEADERSHIP STYLES

Vicki Sweet, RN, MS, CEN, CCRN

In Aristotelian terms, the good leader must have ethos, pathos *and* logos. *The* ethos *is his moral character, the source of his ability to persuade. The* pathos *is his ability to touch feelings, to move people emotionally. The* logos *is his ability to give solid reasons for an action to move people intellectually.*

Mortimer Adler

1. Is there a difference between leadership and management?

Yes, there is, even though the terms are often used interchangeably. The term *management* implies supervision, control, or direction of a unit or group of employees. Managers plan, organize, and coordinate, often directing individual efforts toward the achievement of a common goal. A manager is a defined position within the institution. Managers have employees or staff who report to them through a defined structure.

Leadership, on the other hand, is often thought of as more inspirational or guidance-oriented as well as informal. Leaders have followers, supporters, or protégés and can influence others either through a formal structure or by informal relationships.

A manager is in a position of leadership, but he or she may not have leadership qualities. A leader does not necessarily have to be a manager. Supporters of a leader often follow willingly and with enthusiasm. This is not always so with managers who have no leadership skills. Managers may have organizational skills, whereas leaders may have personality and charisma.

As Stephen Covey put it in his book *The 7 Habits of Highly Effective People*, "Management is efficiency in climbing the ladder of success; leadership determines whether the ladder is leaning against the right wall."

2. So, is it desirable to have both management and leadership skills?

In a supervisory position, management and leadership overlap. A manager definitely needs well-developed management skills to run an organized, efficient unit or department. Leadership qualities can enhance your ability to manage successfully.

If you blend traits from both, your staff will be more motivated to strive for improvement. Going back to Stephen Covey's ladder, your having both skills will demonstrate to your staff that the ladder you have put out for them to climb will lead to success because where it has been placed makes sense, not only to the staff, but to upper management as well.

3. I've heard that you can learn management skills but that leadership is a quality that someone either has or doesn't. Is this true?

Certainly, the task-related skills of management can be learned. These could include scheduling, budgeting, or delegation and the legal issues of supervision.

Leadership, however, relies more on personality traits and "people skills." These can definitely be developed by gaining experience, having a mentor, or attending classes (e.g., coaching, team-leading).

With effort and discipline, many people do learn to be both an effective manager and a successful leader. Even though you may possess good organizational skills and are seen as a leader, it is important to remember that it is difficult to have all staff be satisfied all of the time.

4. How do I know if I am a manager, a leader, or both?

Good question. We've all probably known people in management positions who do not inspire their staff to follow them toward a common, defined goal. These "non-leaders" may know something is wrong, but they aren't able to identify the source of the problem.

Often, the solution lies in effective two-way communication, with emphasis on listening to your staff. For you to determine which qualities you have, exercise close self-scrutiny and accept advice and constructive criticism from others.

5. What are some leadership styles and when should they be used?

Trying to find a style that works for you can be a daunting task. Simply put, there are times when a firm, autocratic style is needed, especially when dealing with safety, regulatory, or policy issues. An autocratic style is used to obtain maximum control and there is little discussion needed.

Other times, your style may be collaborative or democratic, as when encouraging staff to actively participate in solving a problem as a group. Encouraging staff to be a part of the solution will gain support for the ultimate outcome. Many managers have a policy that staff may not bring a problem to them without also offering at least one possible solution as a basis for discussion.

Some managers adopt a style of minimal control, allowing staff the opportunity to make decisions and stepping in only when those decisions are contrary to safety, regulation, or policy. This works when there is a dedicated and highly motivated staff.

6. Should I adopt a single leadership "style" and stick with it?

Leadership style is a pattern of behavior and can vary depending on the situation. Many experts feel that you should have an overall philosophy of management but that the style of how you deal with different individuals might need to be situational.

For instance, suppose your philosophy is that staff members should try to deal with interpersonal issues one-on-one with their coworkers first before coming to you, the manager. This is well communicated and applied consistently. But you might use a different approach if Sandy comes to you in tears, rather than anger, saying that Richard was rude to her in front of a patient. Your usual style might need to change based on Sandy's personality, current frame of mind, and needs at the time.

7. What are some of the traits of a successful manager or leader?

A manager's success within the institution is often measured in concrete terms, such as his or her ability to get reports in on time, keep the department within budget constraints, or maintain staffing levels. The staff views a manager's success in terms of what the manager is able to do for them, such as provide performance evaluations on time, ensure that the unit is appropriately staffed and stocked, or intervene with problems. A great manager will be able to show success both up the institutional ladder and down.

Successful leaders have been described as motivating, empowering, mentoring, optimistic, and supportive. These are less tangible traits as compared with the more concrete characteristic management skills; yet they can inspire results as well as respect from upper management, peer groups, and subordinates. It is human nature for people to follow those whom they see as being able to provide them with what they want or need.

8. What are some other things that will make me a better leader?

- *Accept responsibility and accountability for your actions and decisions.* It will demonstrate your integrity. Managers who constantly blame mistakes on others are not well respected.
- *Have clear goals and communicate them.* It will make it easier for staff to follow your lead. When the goals are confusing or contradictory, staff may decide that you don't know where you are going and therefore won't follow.
- *Recognize staff for jobs well done.* The gratitude should always be sincere and should be equal to the task performed or goal accomplished. Strive to acknowledge the positive more often than criticizing the negative.

9. You've mentioned inspiration and motivation as desired traits. Can you elaborate?

The ability to inspire or motivate is really one of the core personality traits needed to be successful when managing people. A manager can make policies, set goals, or create compliance standards, but if the staff is not motivated to follow, it will be an uphill battle. Motivation is that inner quality that causes people to achieve set goals. People who are successful at motivating will be optimistic, demonstrating an outward positive attitude. Successful managers will have almost a "cheerleader" quality. Optimism and a positive outlook can be as contagious as pessimism and negativity. Which would you rather catch?

10. How can I learn to be a better manager? A better leader?

If you have the luxury of taking outside courses, do so. Many hospitals provide new and experienced managers with educational opportunities. Often, it is an expectation that these courses be completed soon after attaining a management position. Management and leadership courses are also available via the Internet or local community colleges.

Another way is to observe the interactions of others that you admire. Make an appointment and "pick the brain" of successful managers. Learn how they have been able to survive and succeed in their career, however short or long it may be. New managers can provide insight about their transition into their role. More seasoned managers can base their advice on years of experience.

11. I feel inadequate to manage my department. What should I do about this feeling?

Many managers who are new in the role often feel ill-equipped to handle their new job responsibilities. Surely someone else has all the answers, they think. It is a common human emotion, especially in new roles. Pope John the 23rd said, "It often happens that I wake at night and begin to think about a serious problem and decide I must tell the Pope about it. Then I wake up completely and remember that I am the Pope."

One idea might be to schedule weekly meetings with your immediate supervisor to review decisions and issues that have come up. The meeting can be a simple as an informal debriefing session or may be a more formal review of decisions. Bouncing ideas off a more experienced manager can validate your decisions and bolster your confidence. If you have supervisors who report to you, regular interaction with them can also have reinforcing value as you discuss issues and concerns as a group.

12. Many of my staff have worked in the unit much longer than I have. How do I handle that?

When such a situation exists, you may need to "prove" your ability as their manager or supervisor. Some staff may
  • *Challenge you to make decisions.* They may have a difficult time believing that you might now actually enforce those rules that you questioned as a staff nurse.
  • *Simply sit back and observe.*
  • *Validate your decisions with other managers.*

For example, one new manager had to counsel a 20-year staff nurse who made a clinical error. The manager, who had been in the position only a few months, had worked in the unit as an aide while she went to nursing school. The seasoned RN refused to agree that there had been an error in clinical judgment. She had a hard time believing that this "younger" nurse could know more than she did. She discussed it with a manager from another unit.

You need to make your decisions carefully, fairly, and consistently. Support the policies and philosophy of the institution, but balance that with the needs and perceptions of the staff. At first, you may need to do more preparation and research before making a decision. Eventually your staff should see your dedication to being their manager and will let up in their testing.

13. Now that I'm in a position of leadership in the department, I want to make some changes. So many of the staff have a "we've always done it this way" attitude. What should I do?

To make a smooth transition to something new, the staff must buy in to the idea. Your "cheerleading" qualities will be very important when you want to change something. Let the staff know that you welcome their thoughts, suggestions, and concerns. Show them how the proposed change can benefit both the functioning of the unit and the individual staff member. Collect data to support the need for change and share your information with staff so that your decision does not appear to be arbitrary.

An oft-quoted phrase is that "sacred cows make the best burgers." One of the best ways to get people to show up for a staff meeting is to announce that you are considering change of one of the "sacred" systems of the unit. Once people show up to see what you are going to do, you can encourage open discussion of the issues. People might be very interested in participating to protect "their way" but may actually end up championing the process.

14. I have to enforce a policy that I don't agree with. How do I communicate the information to my staff without letting my personal opinions show through?

As part of the management team, one of your roles is to support the policies, procedures, and values of your institution. It is important that you help them to understand the importance of the policy and to see how it fits in with institutional philosophy. You may question the history of the policy privately with your own manager to get an idea of how the policy came about. But, if you publicly criticize the policy, your staff, whether they agree with you or not, may tend to not follow the rules. Your unit, as well as the institution, might suffer. A sense of trust will be lost. If you truly believe the policy is not a good one, you'll need to work through channels to make the changes that you feel are important. See also Chapter 25, Coaching and Disciplining.

15. How should I dress?

Your decision about dress should be guided by the practice in the facility. If the culture is that managers dress in street clothes with a lab coat, then you should follow suit. Your street clothes should be comfortable and on the conservative side.

If you work in an environment where you feel you should "dress like a nurse," have some discussions with your immediate supervisor to find out the history and see if there is opportunity to make a change. Be sure to have a good rationale for your request, not just that "scrubs are more comfortable."

The advantage to dressing like the staff is that you can jump in to help provide patient care, reinforcing that you are still, first and foremost, a nurse. This enhances your credibility. The manager who can work side by side with a staff nurse is often respected.

16. My director/administrator wants me here 8–5, Monday through Friday. I'd like to occasionally come in on off-shifts. How can I accomplish this?

Explain the benefits of being able to interact with all of your staff members during their work periods. Do make sure, however, that your director knows that you are committed to attending required meetings and meeting all deadlines. Then plan your off-shift time around those meetings and deadlines. The extra effort you expend to develop relationships with all shifts will have a positive affect. Increased visibility builds a sense of trust and mutual respect.

When you do show up on the off-shift, make sure that you are available to the staff and are not just making a token appearance. Think about how the night shift feels when the manager breezes in at 5:00 AM, cheerfully says hello, pours a cup of coffee, and then disappears into his office, never to be seen again. Take some time with the staff so that you will have an opportunity to get to know individual staff members and gain an understanding of that particular shift's issues. You are demonstrating that you are concerned about the unit 24 hours a day, 7 days a week.

17. Some staff are my good friends. How do I avoid the illusion of favoritism?

It is very important for the manager to maintain unit standards by treating each person, no matter what the personal relationship, with fairness. One manager used the concept of hats. When needing to counsel or discipline her good friend, she would approach her, saying, "Kathy, I have my serious manager hat on." That was the signal that the interaction would be strictly as manager-employee. Outside of work, the manager hat was off and the friendship flourished.

The manager was cautious not to participate in unit gossip outside of the facility and never betrayed personnel issues, even though there might be times when it would be tempting to share stories. Her extra precautions to separate friendship and management were seen by her staff as both fair and consistent. In addition, her friend was now her ally in the unit.

18. I have so many new responsibilities as a manager, yet there are days when my staff need me to be with them on the unit. How do I balance this?

Just like being a triage nurse in the emergency department, a manager must be able to prioritize tasks for the good of the department. If a manager is able, the simple act of putting down a report and helping to transport a patient to another unit can have a tremendously positive effect on a harried, overworked staff. Stepping out of the office to intercede with an angry family member or frustrated physician clearly demonstrates the manager's support of his or her staff.

Conversely, there are times when the manager cannot be available to the staff. There also may be times that the manager feels that the staff need to solve their own problems. Stepping in to rescue them may be detrimental to their professional growth. You might stand next to them and provide encouragement as they problem-solve, but you would allow them to do it themselves. With experience, a manager can definitely learn when to be flexible for the good of the unit or the facility.

19. I've heard the word *empowerment*. What exactly does it mean and how do I do it?

Empowerment means that you are entrusting others with the power to do certain things. Empowerment can have the effect of improving efficiency because staff feel that they have the authority to make decisions without having to wait for someone else's permission. Additionally, staff report increased job satisfaction because they may feel more autonomy and more involvement in the unit management. They feel a sense of importance and appreciate the manager's trust in their ability.

When empowering staff, it is important to remember to keep open communication, provide them with necessary information and resources, and give support for the decisions they make. It can be demoralizing to have the manager regularly reverse decisions made by staff.

20. I had a manager who seemed to listen but did not hear. He told us what we wanted to hear, but then behaved in a contradictory manner. How can I avoid this?

The obvious answer is to listen carefully and to act as you promise to act. Many managers become adept at seeming to listen, but they may actually be thinking about other issues or projects. Strive to be present in the moment.

These managers need to be reminded that communication is a two-way process. It is often said that the reason we have two ears and one mouth is so that we listen twice as much as we talk. Actively listen and process the information before responding. Because we think much faster than we speak, it is easy to think ahead and misinterpret.

Make notes during conversations. You keep focused on the issues at hand and also have a record of the conversation. Many managers will send a follow-up memo to reinforce the issues and outcomes.

21. I've heard that a good manager grooms his or her replacement. Is this really a good idea?

By delegating some of the responsibilities of unit management, you are in effect beginning to prepare others to step in to your position. The manager who helps others learn the workings of the unit is often more respected than the manager who keeps everything secret. Staff may view those managers as lacking confidence in them or as having something to hide. Another advantage is you have someone who can assist covering for you when you are gone.

22. Being a manager is pretty complex and a lot of hard work. Why should I do it?

There are the obvious perks—promotion, salary, title. It can also be very rewarding, especially when you blend those management and leadership traits successfully for your unit to exceed its goals.

Managers have power. They have the power to control the unit according to the policies of the institution. They also have a benevolent power to reward. Power can help make changes for the better.

BIBLIOGRAPHY

1. Covey SR: The 7 Habits of Highly Effective People. New York, Simon & Schuster, 1989.
2. Hein EC, Nicholson MJ (eds): Contemporary Leadership Behavior, 4th ed. Philadelphia, Lippincott, 1994.
3. Peters T: A Passion for Excellence. New York, Random House, 1985.

3. OFFICE MANAGEMENT

Polly Gerber Zimmermann, RN, MS, MBA, CEN

Do what you can, with what you have, where you are.

Theodore Roosevelt

1. I've never had an office before. How do I go about setting it up?

What is important is to make your office work for you. Some basics include the following:
- File system (generally letter size is recommended)
- Contact telephone index card file (e.g., Rolodex)
- A storage source (binder, file) for each regular, important paper report you will receive (e.g., meeting minutes, budget variance reports)
- An "in" box to put things in until you will process them

In addition to the obvious supplies (paper, pens, tape, stapler), I have reference books, such as JCAHO standards, a medical dictionary, and a regular dictionary. Don't overlook the importance of adding decorative touches to make it bright and cheery.

2. List what I should ask myself about each piece of paper I handle as a manager.

Consultant Barbara Hemphill recommends asking these questions:
- Do I really need to keep this?
- Where should I keep it?
- How long should I keep it?
- How can I find it?

Hemphill further recommends developing and maintaining a system that will handle every incoming sheet of paper. Everything can fit into one of seven places: "to sort" tray (for papers you haven't looked at yet), wastebasket, calendar, "to do" list, phone index card file/phone book, action file, and reference file.

3. What will help make my file system more effective?

- *Keep it simple, easy, and manageable.* Start with major areas of responsibility, such as administration and projects. Most people can fit their work's paperwork within 5 major categories.
- *Create working subject files within each area.* For instance, there could be a file for each committee, regulatory agency, project, equipment contracts, or resume submittals for an open position. The important part is to have a place for everything.

4. Is this exactly what you do?

Not really. I, like most managers, keep modifying and customizing these basic concepts so they work best for me as my responsibilities change. Allow several months to truly try a system to determine whether it will work for you.

I've added a birthday list (i.e., a monthly list by day of people's birthday's I want to remember), a follow-up list (i.e., things I'm waiting for such as a refund or a response), and a folder for important papers for upcoming external events (e.g., a meeting's plane ticket or registration verification). I use all color-coded files for each project and a unique color for important, special files. I further divide my daily list into e-mail messages, phone calls, letters and memos to write, and people to see/topics to discuss.

Another person's system is to have a manila envelope for each day; the manager carries this with him. Things to deliver or be picked up go inside. In each one of the four corners, he writes people to see, places to go, set appointments, and mandatory things to accomplish. Another manager has an index card for each person or area she deals with (e.g., Vice President, pharmacy committee, scheduling concerns). When a related topic arises, she notes it on the appropriate index card so that in each meeting she has a running list of appropriate items.

5. List some tips for better filing. I have trouble retrieving something once I've filed it away.

Consultant Odette Pollar offers this advice:
- File papers in the broadest possible category.
- Head file names with a noun in the key subject area. Avoid labeling a file with a number, date, or adjective.
- File any articles you want to save by the subject they discuss.
- Avoid nonspecific file labels such as "articles," "general," or "pending."
- Keep extra file folders close at hand. Make it easy to create that new file while you are holding those papers.
- Place the most recent document in the front of the file.
- Resist the temptation to copy a paper and place it in multiple, related files. Put it in the category most likely to come to mind.
- Do not feel compelled to file repetitive information or items other people simply insist you take.
- Maintain your filing system. Purge files frequently of excess information or out-of-date items to keep your system useful, rather than a paper trap.

6. I keep ending up with piles of papers on my desk, but I think that works for me. Isn't that OK?

It is estimated that the average manager has at least 36 hours of backlogged paperwork around their desk. And it is enticing to "vertically file" papers on the top of the desk. I think it provides the false illusion that you are dealing with them. However, the most important paperwork does not magically sort itself to the top. At a minimum, keep two-thirds of your desk clear for working.

Stacked paperwork actually represents delayed decisions that add clutter and consume more time to resort. Consultant Hemphill finds that people who have difficulty making decisions about the paperwork usually either lack information or fear failure.

A neat-appearing office gives the impression you are organized and competent to staff and patients' families. Besides, it is demoralizing to walk into a mess in the morning.

7. Share some tips that will help prevent me from creating piles of papers.

Common advice includes:
- *Handle each piece of paper once.* If you have to have a "slush pile," then deal with it regularly.
- *Have a place for everything so everything can be in its place.* I like file folders, with my pending topics kept in one area. Other managers use binders or folding accordion files.
- *Allot time to deal with paperwork.* One of my problems was trying to do paperwork just "sprinkled on top" of everything else, which was never enough time. Planning 30 minutes a day specifically to deal with the paperwork keeps it from overtaking you.
- *Consider whether you need to keep that paper before filing it.* Liberally use the "circular file" (aka wastebasket). The best timesaver is not saving and filing the paper in the first place. E-mail is an efficient way to store and deal with matters that would create paper piles.

8. How do you manage a contact file?

Some type of card file is the most common. Any brand or style works, as long as it allows easy replacement when the current card is outdated.

I use a 3 × 5 index card for each person. This give me enough room to write details, such as the project we worked on together, driving directions, or even something important to them in the person's private life (e.g., new grandchild, love of sailing). It's a wonderful way to jog the memory.

Make it a priority to keep this file updated. An old address or phone number gives the false illusion that you can reach someone but, in fact, is pretty useless.

One tendency is to dial the fax number by mistake. I now either color code the fax number or write it out with different spacing, such as:

Phone xxx-xxxx
XXX-XXXX FAX

9. Do you recommend also using the contact file for employees?

Yes, I keep a card for every employee I supervise. In addition to their contact information, I make notations through the year on their positive contributions. This goes beyond obvious major projects to things more easily forgotten, such as the time someone was exceptional with a difficult family or stayed late to help cover an emergency. That way I avoid the common pitfall of having the annual evaluations only reflect the past 3 weeks. And I keep one on myself for my own self-evaluation!

10. It seems as if the ways of communication just keep increasing. How do I decide what to do first?

The general rule of thumb is to answer them in this order: telephone, e-mail, interdepartmental mail, and U.S. mail because they usually represent the order of urgency with which someone will choose to contact you.

11. How do I effectively use e-mail?

More than 23 million workers are connected by e-mail networks. It is often the preferred method of communication for nonemergency matters, but it can take time.

I do the e-mail in blocks, removing the alert that a new message arrives. I quickly scan the name of the senders to sort it initially into "important" (anything from my boss) and "later" (conference notices, ads, complaints). One CEO checks her e-mail only 3 times a day: first thing in the morning, once during lunch, and then again before going home.

Another tip is to use your company e-mail address only for work-related e-mails. Distractions are avoided by having all personal messages (and junk e-mail) go to a separate account (at home or work).

12. List some basic guidelines for using e-mail.
- *Don't type in all capitals.* (IT IS CONSIDERED SHOUTING!)
- *Remember grammar and spelling.* Use the same care you would for a written memo. Don't let the speed lull you into thinking the errors are not glaring.
- *It is not necessary to reply to every message.* This is especially true when your response is simply "I agree" or other polite, but unnecessary, comments. Save your replies for requests for clarification or sharing additional information.
- *Always enter something on the "Subject" line.* Carefully worded subject lines are invaluable for clueing the recipients in about the urgency of the message and for helping them find the message again.
- *Don't put anything in an e-mail that you don't want to be accountable for.* The informality and convenience can make you forget that it still could be detrimental if the wrong people saw these thoughts. And office e-mail is corporate property; chances are one in three that someone is routinely screening it.
- *Don't use e-mail for things that need to be said in person.* This includes personnel discipline, sensitive matters, or evaluations.
- *If the matter is urgent, call in person.* Similarly, personal contact is warranted as a response if there is an ongoing lack of resolution through e-mail or rude or inappropriate remarks.

- *Most managers recommend treating e-mail like paper and handling each message only once.* I leave a message about a pending topic in my e-mail file as my tickler that the issue has not been resolved. I then have the data there to resend to the person later if the subject has not been dealt with.
- *Notify everyone if your e-mail address changes.* You wouldn't think of moving homes without a forwarding address. People will be unable to reach you if you don't send out a notice about your new change.

13. Describe what a listserve is.

Internet mailing lists are a quick and free source of a "community" with whom to share ideas of common interest. You feel connected and it is comforting to know your management problems are not unique. You can just read, respond, or post a message or inquiry on a new topic. To join, you send a message to the list administrator. Save the "welcoming" response e-mail, as it includes the rules, how to post, and how to unsubscribe.

14. Tell me about the types of listserves.

There are two types: discussion and announcement. Discussion lists sends you an e-mail whenever any member posts a message. Any opinion, information, or advice is allowed as long as it stays on the topic and is polite.

An announcement listserve is most often from a company, industry, or news agency. It contains breaking news or information on changes, such as a new drug gaining FDA approval. Two sources I've found helpful are Frew Consulting Group's legal advice regarding government regulations (medlaw.com) and Shelley Cohen's Health Resources Unlimited's weekly manager tips (*http://www.hru.net; educate@hru.net*).

Ask peers what listserves they find helpful. You can also search for topics of interest through *www.Isoft.com/catalist.html* (over 43,000 lists), *www.intellihealth.com/IH/ihtlH* (medical- and dental-related mailing lists), *www.liszt.com, www.paml.net* (publicly accessible mailing lists), or *http://groups.yahoo.com*. In addition, many professional associations have "chat rooms."

15. Any tips for more effective use of a listserve?

- Choose carefully whether to reply only to the sender or to the whole group.
- If you have something that is a different angle to add to the discussion, it is helpful to change the "subject" line slightly to indicate that it is a reply to the previous message but also a new thought.
- Just taking what you want from the listserve and "running" is rude. Proper etiquette indicates you should also occasionally participate and help other subscribers to pay back the benefits you received.

16. How do I set up my voice mail?

Managing voice mail is important today since more than 75% of the business calls go directly into it. Some tips include:

- *Keep the voice tone of your message upbeat.* Look in a mirror and smile while you record it.
- *Allow more than 1 minute for your callers to leave a message.* Otherwise the only message they leave is "call me back."
- *Consider your phone mail as you would an in-box.* Handle each call once and do not let them pile up.
- *Try calling your department once a month and ask for yourself.* It's a good test to verify that the process is working.

17. List tips for leaving effective voice mail messages.

- *Leave your full name and something to jog the memory about how the person knows you.* When I get a first-name-only caller, the delay to mentally figure out whom I am listening to distracts me from hearing the message.

- *Provide your phone number each call.* I have picked up messages away from my central rolodex and not been able to call the person back.
- *Repeat your phone number twice, often saying it the second time a little differently.* For instance, the first time I say "one-zero-four-eight," the second time "ten-forty-eight." This way the receiver does not have to replay the whole message to verify the number.
- *Deliberately slow down when articulating key numbers.* Often callers rush through the area code or some other aspect they are familiar with.
- *Repeat your name and purpose again at the end.* Hearers are often distracted at the beginning.
- *Indicate when you will be available if you expect the person to call back.* This can help eliminate "phone tag." Give several options.

18. Name some aids to writing good letters and memos.

These are some basic writing guidelines:

- *Use action words rather than passive voice.* When you read "it was decided," you are left with the question "Who?"
- *Avoid the "ations," such as "utilization" or "authorization."* They seem abstract and impersonal. Say, for example, "The committee implemented or will implement."
- *Keep sentences under 20 words and include only one idea per sentence.* Your words lose power if the reader has to reread the sentence to understand it.
- *Use short paragraphs to lead the readers.* Paragraphs should not exceed eight to ten lines in a memo or five to six lines in a letter.
- *Be certain your pronouns are clearly defined.* Who are "they"?
- *Establish a clear point of view.* Use a consistent tone and arrange the material logically.

19. Any other tips for improving my writing correspondence?

Rules I apply include the following:

- *Keep the letter to one page with rare exceptions.* The message will be more likely read and received if it is succinct.
- *Limit revisions to three times.* You can always improve writing, but I decide it will be "good enough" after a maximum third reread.
- *Always include full contact information on each letter.* This includes name, title, address, phone/fax number, and e-mail address. This makes it easy for the person to respond to you.
- *Keep the business signature neat.* A hurried scrawl on official matters can be interpreted as egotistic or sloppy. Slowing down your writing by only 15% improves legibility.

20. I think I am right-brained, and I can't seem to get my office organized. Any tips?

A popular idea grew in the 1960s from Roger Sperry's work that one side of the brain is dominant for most people. The left brain dominates thought, and these people are supposedly better at logical thinking and linear reasoning. Right-brained thinkers are supposed to be better visually, at solving spatial problems, and at reasoning intuitively. In other words, the left side is logical, the right side creative.

However, this is being challenged. Some studies suggest that this independence is not so prominent. The left side probably processes details while the right side is the "big picture" thinker. Still, most people feel more comfortable being either analytical or operating from their gut. Most time-management tools are designed for an analytical, left-brained process, but with some individualization you can easily accommodate them to a more creative flair.

21. How do you make black-and-white time management tools more usable for right-brained people?

Author Lee Silber recommends that right-brained people use the following tools:

- *Color.* Color-code appointment entries to differentiate their importance.
- *Pictures.* Instead of words, find pictures that represent a goal or activity.

- *Wall calendar.* Right-brained people sometimes forget to look at their personal planner. It's hard to ignore a big, color-coded wall calendar with pictures.
- *Tickler file.* Place it prominently, put all loose notes in a dated slot. Force yourself to check it daily for 2 weeks until it becomes a habit.

Silber also recommends trying to make work more of a game. Creative thinkers are bored with just having a list of things to do. He suggests writing tasks on slips of paper, mixing the papers up, and then drawing as often as necessary to get all of the tasks done.

22. How can I protect material I feel is confidential, such as our patient fees or supplier discount list?

All ideas begin in the category of public domain, which means they do not belong to anyone. Information that gives your hospital an advantage over others can be considered a trade secret. Once these ideas are put to use, the owners have the right to protect them against infringement from others. Use a confidential stamp on the information, limit distribution, and attach a directive cover that states, "for internal use only."

23. I developed a new form. Can I copyright it?

Something produced as part of your job responsibilities or while on the job is most likely classified as a "work made for hire." In these cases, the employer is considered the corporate copyright owner. However, you could publish an article describing the form and its use, which then gives you some of the credit.

24. How do I copyright something created on my own time?

There is still a rumor that you need to mail yourself any created written work to unofficially "register" the copyright and prevent someone from stealing it. This is unnecessary under U.S. copyright law.

Copyright law protects your work as soon as you create it or when it is fixed in a copy. If you are worried about future lawsuits over your work, save your initial notes and drafts. This will assist you in claiming initial ownership of anything you wrote.

However, practically speaking, you can be exposed to "innocent infringement." A person who, in good faith, thought it was in public domain because there was no notice on the work, can copy it and not be held liable for damages. The way to prevent this is to place an appropriate notice, such as the word "copyright," its abbreviation, or the symbol (©) with the copyright owner's name and the year when the work was first published. Sources of copyright information are the U.S. Copyright Office's web site (*http://lcweb.loc.gov/copyright*), the American Society of Journalists and Authors (*www.asja.org*), and the National Writers Union (*www.nwu.org*).

25. I found a form in a journal article I'd like to use. Can my department just copy it and start using it?

It is necessary to contact the article's publisher (the copyright owner) and request permission with a description of the intended use. When written permission for use is granted, keep a copy and follow the publisher's instructions for acknowledging this permission. It is a professional courtesy to also contact and inform the author about your project. Often, permission to use something obtained on the Internet includes the stipulation that you provide a link to the source.

26. Can I use something I find on the Internet without permission?

You do not need permission to list an Internet site, similar to being able to list a reference journal citation. However, use of the contents usually requires permission. An exception is government sites, such as OSHA. These sites are considered public domain.

27. Any other ideas about office organization?

I personally use the following guidelines:

- *Have one date book.* I use the same one for work and personal commitments. It gives me one central location from which to organize my time and prevent accidental conflicts.

- *People first.* Paperwork projects have an allure because they seem permanent, but in reality they can become useless with one administrative decision. But the effect you have on people can last a lifetime.
- *Carry a portfolio with you.* It sends the subtle subconscious message that you are "working" and it gives you a place to write things down as you think of them.
- *Write things down immediately.* It keeps you from forgetting. And, as Francis Bacon said, those (thoughts) that come unsought for are commonly the most valuable. Keep your loose scrap paper of a consistent size to lessen accidental misplacement.
- *Make your boss look good.* Regardless of what mature people should be like, it is only human nature to like those who shed a positive light on you. In the end, it helps everyone.
- *Make it easy for others to respond to you.* Not only do you get quicker responses, but people enjoy working with you.
- *Be generous with your appreciation and gratitude.* It is politically astute. But more important, it is the right thing to do.

28. Do you have recommended references that will help me in this area?
- Richard Carlson: *Don't Sweat the Small Stuff at Work.* New York, Hyperion, 1998.
- Stephen R. Covey: *The Seven Habits of Highly Effective People.* New York, Simon & Schuster, 1989.
- Barbara Hemphill: *Taming the Paper Tiger at Work.* Washington, DC, Kiplinger Washington Editors, 1998.
- Richard Moran: *Fear No Yellow Stickies.* New York, Fireside, 1998.
- Richard Moran: *Cancel the Meetings, Keep the Doughnuts, and Other New Morsels of Business Wisdom.* New York, Harper-Collins, 1995.
- Odette Pollar: *365 Ways to Simplify Your Work Life.* Chicago, Dearborn Financial Publishing, 1996.

BIBLIOGRAPHY

1. Beardsley D: Don't manage time, manage yourself. Fast Company 14:64–68, 1998.
2. Davis JH: Managers Ask and Answer: Permission to use. J Emerg Nurs 24(1):78, 1998.
3. Dear Writer. The Writer 114(3): 9, 2001.
4. Hendrickson N: You've got mail. The Writer 114(8):18–19, 2001.
5. Moran R: Managers Forum: Use of voice mail. J Emerg Nurs 26(6):608, 2000.
6. Moran R: Managers Forum: Business wisdom. J Emerg Nurs 25(6):546, 1999.
7. Pollar O: Manager's Forum: Filing. J Emerg Nurs 25(1):45, 1999.
8. Staton T: In your right mind? Am Way Nov. 1:150–158, 2000.
9. Zimmermann PG: Managers Forum: E-mail. J Emerg Nurs 26(4):370–371, 2000.
10. Zimmermann PG: Managers Forum: Managing the flow of paperwork. J Emerg Nurs 24(2):181–182, 1998.

4. TIME MANAGEMENT

Polly Gerber Zimmermann, RN, MS, MBA, CEN

> *You can do anything—but not everything.*
>
> David Allen

1. What are the essentials to managing my time.

- *Planning, including priorities.* Without this, you begin managing by crisis. Focus on the important, not just the urgent.
- *Understanding of the expected amount of time.* This includes time for planning and completing your individual responsibilities. A common mistake is not to initially allow adequate time, especially when the learning curve is steep.
- *Include the "big hairy goals."* Unless deliberate attention is given to more visionary aspects, they will fall by the wayside.

2. I feel overwhelmed with all I have to do. Why can't I get "caught up"?

Productivity expert David Allen indicates that the typical business person experiences 170 interruptions per day and faces a backlog of 200 to 300 hours of incomplete work. In other words, there will always be "too much to do," especially in today's environment of so much possibility.

Allen believes that this phenomenon is a result of a basic need to be acknowledged with meaningful work. In an attempt to achieve that goal, we all keep letting more and more stuff enter our lives.

Realizing that is the first step. Controlling our aspirations will simplify things. Learning to set boundaries, or to say no, is usually incredibly difficult. Author/speaker Loretta LaRoche humorously suggests we watch how often we use the words "have to" or "must." It sets us up for excessive "musterbating."

3. I feel I have set realistic expectations. What else will help?

Allen teaches that the second step is realizing we have a deep need to finish what we start. Much of the stress we feel doesn't come from having too much to do, but from not finishing all the "open" input (e-mail, phone messages, reports, conversations) that entered our lives. That clutters our minds with vague promises and unreasonable expectations regarding what we *should* be doing.

4. Tell me more about this concept.

Allen's point is that everything that isn't where it should be is an incomplete task that becomes a distraction. He says productivity and satisfaction come from completion. Allen uses the example that people feel best about themselves right before they go on a vacation because they've cleared up all the "to do piles," even if this clearing up involved reassigning tasks to be completed after the vacation. He advocates doing this on a weekly rather than a yearly basis.

Allen recommends, when confronted with an action item that can be completed within 2 minutes, to just do it immediately. Reduce the rest to the next simplest step and then capture those steps on a series of specialized "to do" lists.

That does not mean you finish them then. But you now know where to start when you have the time, energy, or resources to tackle them. This allows you to focus your creative energy on what you are doing, not on trying to remember everything you could be doing. We only have so much energy and every "open" thing takes some of it.

5. What lists are good to maintain?

Allen advocates maintaining lists through which you've completely covered your life. Once a week, process every loose paper, note, previous calendar dates, or miscellaneous scribbling into an appropriate action item or list.

His lists include the following:

Projects—commitments that cannot be completed in one sitting. What is the status of each project?

Next Actions—the next sequential step for each active project

Waiting For (or *Pending, Support*)—next actions someone else must take to move a project forward

Calendar—time- or day-specific deadlines, appointments, and actions

Maybe/Someday—discretionary items, personal dreams.

6. There still are too many action items to do. How do I complete the most important ones?

Today no one gets extended, uninterrupted periods of time to accomplish things. Instead, we must learn to be productive in the 5 or 15 minutes we have between meetings or phone calls.

You can't always be doing the most important thing. But Allen advocates that knowing you are being productive during all the time that you have, even if it was just to water the plants in a 2- minute break, improves your overall approach. It is not working harder, but better. For more information, read David Allen's book, *Getting Things Done: The Art of Stress-Free Productivity*.

7. Any other ideas?

- *Delegate.* Is there anything you do that can be given away to others? Limit others' informal delegation to you. When someone says "What about...?", don't take it on. Learn to answer, "That is a good question. Let me know what you find out."
- *Pick your battles; learn acceptance of some situations.* Many use the Serenity Prayer as a perspective: "Lord, grant me the Serenity to accept the things I cannot change, the Courage to change the things I can, and the Wisdom to know the difference."
- *Let things go.* If I haven't gotten to some project for more than 6 months, it probably wasn't that important. Or if I believe it is, then I must decide specifically what else I will give up to make time for it.

8. My problem is that I have my plans, but staff social visits keep interrupting me.

This assumes that the interruptions are not significant issues but rather repetitive socialization or rambling venting. Consider your office arrangement. Position your desk so your back faces the door so you aren't tempted to look up every time someone walks by. Better yet, close the door. That discourages casual conversation.

Avoid allowing your office to become an unofficial social hangout. I only have a table with chairs and my desk and chair, rather than extra chairs for lounging. It sets a tone that there will be a purposeful conversation.

9. How should I handle a long-winded visitor?

Learn to control the conversation. If the person is rambling, break in and say, "I'm sorry, but I'm not getting your point. What do you want me to understand?"

Stand up and interrupt yourself with, "Oh look at the time, I have something I have to do (even if it is only to leave the room)." It does not seem rude as long as you interrupt while *you* are speaking.

Another trick is to limit people to a scheduled visit. Tell them not now, but "around 10:00 AM I will have some free time. Why don't you see me then?" The person won't bother if they just wanted to chat.

10. A lot of times I'm dependent on the contribution of others. Name some practical suggestions for this situation.

- *Use deadlines.* Most people produce related to a deadline, often right before it. It develops an increased sense of commitment. Effective deadlines are often between 2 and 4 weeks. Many find this also works for themselves when procrastinating. Either set a deadline or tell yourself, "I really have to do this, NOW."
- *Create a sense of urgency.* Nothing is more deadly for getting results than to say "whenever you get a chance."
- *Determine what, if any, steps will need completed sequentially in your projects.* Otherwise it is like trying to birth a baby in 1 month by having nine pregnant women.
- *Realize the enemy of "good" is "perfect."* You need to make intelligent choices for the best at this time.
- *Limit the amount of time spent at required official functions.* What matters to people is *who* shows up. How long you stay is rarely recognized. Try leaving the next "open house" sooner.
- *Put the ball in their court.* Nurses tend to quickly offer help for someone else's need. This automatic response can commit a lot of time for something that may not even be that important to the requesting person. Instead, tell the person to contact you later (or better yet, to use other resources) for that information. Then it is up to them to decide if they want it enough to spend *their* time.
- *Use post-action reports for every major recurring function you worked with.* Right after the event, write down what was done and suggestions to make the planning easier next time. You'll have a record of a prepared starting point for the next year rather than trying to create it from memory.

11. Sometimes my projects are held up because someone else doesn't do their part. Now what can I do?

- *Avoid a confrontation, especially initially.* Ask, "What do you think is preventing completion of this project?" It lessens the tendency to have a defensive reaction. There may be some minor hurdle you can help overcome.
- *Consistent, regular pleasant persistence.* The squeaky wheel gets oiled.
- *Recognize others' patterns of behaviors.* Most people handle new material in the same way they did the past. For instance, one individual loses 25% of what I give her, so I always give it to her early and keep a copy.
- *Indicate an absolute abdication deadline.* I will indicate a future deadline from which I will proceed. Depending on the task, that may be turning it in without their part, assuming agreement with what I do, or approaching the administrative overseer for a replacement. Phrase it as doing "a favor because the person obviously has too much to do at this point."

It's human nature not to want to lose face, and this prospect will sometimes spark action. Other times, it is not important to them and they don't care if things move forward without them. Sometimes, they are even relieved.

12. I feel stressed from the demands on my time. What can I do?

The job probably isn't going to change. All you can control is your response to it. Author/speaker Loretta LaRoche champions the use of humor. She recommends making a generous "things *not* to do" list—that is, everything you already accomplished. Include every item, such as called my mother, stocked toilet paper at home, or got dressed. You'll appreciate all you actually *do* accomplish, a regular "house of fulfillment."

Author Richard Carlson offers attitude-changing thoughts such as avoiding the phrase "I have to go to work," staying focused in the present, and not becoming stressed by the predictable. Commonly used solutions also include exercise (especially that which uses large muscle groups) and taking breaks.

13. I frequently hear about taking a break. I don't have time to do that.

Take your scheduled breaks (coffee, lunch) rather than working through them. That keeps you refreshed and productive. Go outside, or at least walk down some halls.

Moran suggests 2-minute vacations to smell the flowers or look at the clouds. Many advocate learning to back off and be quiet. Just sit and do nothing for 10 minutes a day.

When you retreat from the routine, you can gain a new perspective. It is hard to continually respond appropriately and effectively when you are constantly in the chaos.

14. What is balance between work and personal life?

How do you honestly answer the question, "What do you do for *fun*?" It should cause you to re-evaluate things if you can't quickly answer something outside your field.

Psychologist Ilene Philipson has identified a current unhealthy trend of people transferring all of their unmet needs to the workplace. In a different era, these needs would be expected to be also met by family, religion, and community life. We all still need multiple anchors for affirmation.

One study found that 24% of workers were chronically angry because the employer didn't fulfill their expected "psychological contract." But rather than finding new sources of fulfillment outside of work, or even expressing their anger, they responding by becoming more lethargic and unproductive at their job.

15. Talk about the signs that indicate a proper balance in your life.

A common internal signal that things are amiss is a sense that you lost your zest for this type of work. But the reaction many people have to that feeling is to work harder, rather than do something recreational that will recharge the batteries.

Psychologist Ilene Philipson offers three key warning signs:

1. *You rarely miss work, even if ill.* You skip your vacations and you choose work over a family commitment. If you constantly give more than 100% of yourself to your job, you have nothing left for friendships, family, or yourself.

2. *What you enjoy most about your job is the praise you receive.* Although people with this problem state they "love" their job, it is actually a love of the praise and recognition they receive than the work itself. Praise is nice, but never a guarantee. You need to be able to feel internal gratification from a job well done.

3. *Your closest friends are your work colleagues.* Work has politics and competition. When your entire support network is at work, you lack a balanced source for emotional support to deal with job-related difficulties. Work relationships should be collegial, but not your only human connections.

16. List some things I can do to maintain balance.

- *Take a hard look at your motivation.* Understand why you are overworking. Are you escaping, is it a habit, do you seek your life's purpose, or do you enjoy the financial reward? Once you pinpoint what motivates you, you'll be better at driving your own life.
- *Limit hours.* There are emergencies, of course, but watch for a pattern of excess evening and weekend work. And, besides, the quickest way to give yourself a raise on a salaried position is to stop working so many hours.
- *Regular participation in an outside interest.* Make yourself keep a scheduled appointment to do something, whether it is a dance class or a walk in the park.
- *Use your vacation time for a vacation.* Do something besides attend a nursing conference in another city.
- *Fence off areas of your life from work.* With today's multiple, portable communication options, there is a blurring of the boundaries between work and home. Everyone needs time and space that is separate. Establish some ritual, such as changing clothes, that signals you are now "home."

17. List some references that will help me in this area.
- Richard Carlson: *Don't Sweat the Small Stuff at Work.* New York, Hyperion, 1998.
- Stephen R. Covey: *The Seven Habits of Highly Effective People.* New York, Simon & Schuster, 1989.
- Loretta LaRoche: *Relax—You May Only Have A Few Minutes Left. Using the Power of Humor to Overcome Stress in Your Life and Work.* New York, Villard Books (Random House), 1998.

BIBLIOGRAPHY

1. Beardsley D: Don't manage time, manage yourself. Fast Company 14:64–68, 1998.
2. Carlson R: Don't Sweat the Small Stuff at Work. New York, Hyperion, 1998.
3. Hammond KH: You can do anything—but not everything. Fast Company 35:208–214, 2000.
4. Kruger P: Betrayed by work. Fast Company 29:182–196, 1999.
5. LaRoche L: Relax—You May Only Have a Few Minutes Left. Using the Power of Humor to Overcome Stress in Your Life and Work. New York, Villard (Random House), 1998.
6. Moran R: Managers Forum: Business wisdom. J Emerg Nurs 25(6):546, 1999.

5. MANAGING MEETINGS

Polly Gerber Zimmermann, RN, MS, MBA, CEN

To say the right things at the right time, keep still most of the time.

John W. Roper

1. Meetings often seem to be nonproductive. How do I plan an effective meeting?

Determine first if a meeting is even necessary. Of the 24 million business meetings held every year, one-third are considered worthless or irrelevant.

Meetings serve many different purposes, including generating ideas, narrowing down a field of options by information gathering and analysis, committing to a decision, and simply sharing information. Knowing the purpose of the meeting is an essential beginning.

Both you and the attendees should understand the purpose. An agenda distributed ahead of time will help. Otherwise, you could be asking for final decisions on budget priorities for the department while others believe that it is appropriate to explore new ideas, as if it were a brainstorming session.

Tailor your nonverbal behavior to match the meeting's purpose. Stand up or sit at the head of the table for decisions but sit at the side if seeking collaboration.

2. What should I include on the agenda?

JCAHO looks for key areas related to high risk, high volume, or past events. You want to prove you have been bringing these important issues to staff's attention. Many managers automatically include them on every staff meeting's agenda.

For department staff meetings, most managers include information-sharing reports of significant events or incidents, current and upcoming events, and new actual or considered changes in the department or institution. You could also include some more visionary topics, such as customer satisfaction skills, or appreciation, such as recognizing extra efforts.

3. How often should I schedule staff meetings?

Have some type of regular schedule—most managers do either monthly or bimonthly. Having a regular available forum will lessen the need for other time-consuming forms of communication.

4. Discuss considerations about the timing of meetings.

Experienced meeting planners share these tips:
- *Avoid scheduling a meeting first thing Monday morning.* They are not as effective as ones later in the week.
- *Start on time.* People straggle in when they know the meeting typically starts late.
- *Keep the meeting to an appropriate length.* They never should last more than 90 minutes. One trick is to have everyone stand during a brief meeting. People are motivated to keep the subject matter moving when not settled in comfortable chairs.

5. Describe things I can do that will help make my meeting more effective.

- *Stick to the agenda.* Sometimes it is helpful to post a time limit for each subject on the agenda.
- *Plan your beginning introductory sentences on a topic.* It will eliminate the deadly hemming and hawing as you transition into a new area.
- *State your point upfront.* Today's society has programmed people to listen in "sound bits." Avoid long historical lead-ins.

- *Keep your comments to a maximum of three bullet points.* People tend to not pay attention or remember beyond that.
- *Specifically review the meeting process itself.* Some recommend setting aside 5 minutes at the end of every meeting. Ask how the meeting itself went and possible changes that could be made. Sample questions include "What did we do in this meeting that worked well?" or "What do we not want to repeat?"

6. **How should I handle it when I have to deliver difficult information?**
   Experts suggest the following steps:
   - *Identify the problem clearly.* Keep the focus on the message and not the messenger.
   - *Face your own fear ahead of time, and get over it.* Do not let your fear prevent you from dealing with the issue.
   - *Get the message out.* Be tactful, but do not waste time with beating around the bush. Being indirect just creates tension. Within the first minute, you should be into your message.
   - *Think about your listeners' prejudices and shape the script accordingly.* Too often we focus on our perspective rather than the receivers. We say "hit the bottom line" (which is good), but the staff may hear "do more work" (which is bad).
   - *Consider nonthreatening techniques, such as scenario analysis.* Present a hypothetical situation in the third person. It can help make your points apparent without being threatening, since the discussion is about somebody else, not us. Subtlety can make hard truth more palpable. Avoid blunt questions that put people on the spot.
   - *Consider mixing in some passion.* Bad news is often delivered calmly, quietly, and analytically. However, sometimes it pays to mix in some emotion to grab people's attention or stir their feelings.
   - *Allow reaction time.* Make your point; then stop. You have probably spent weeks thinking about this, but it may be like a bomb for those who just heard it.
   - *Keep the conversation going.* Delivering a tough message often changes relationships. To make it for the better, continue regular contact and stay on the message.
   - *Listen at least 1 minute longer than you think it necessary.* People do not want to feel cut off when dealing with unfavorable topics.

7. **Our interdepartmental meetings always include large groups that seem to become inert. What can we do?**
   Some organizations have a culture in which everyone even remotely involved is included on the meeting's "invitation list." This can result in key players being absent (they assume their presence is not essential) or wasted time for the group to update those who aren't involved.

   This was the problem at one hospital in planning the yearly disaster drill. It had 25 members; the cafeteria manager even came! We solved it by verifying the availability of the five main players, and then selecting a representative for other departments. Those less involved were sent minutes with the name of a contact person if more information was needed.

8. **I chair an interdepartmental group in which the attendees don't regularly work together. What can help make this type of meeting more effective?**
   Consultants recommend paying attention to the social side. Sometimes it is necessary to have 5 minutes of open time at the beginning just to encourage people, especially those not ordinarily working together, to relate to each other. Providing light snacks seems to aid the conversation's flow, even though most attendees don't eat any.

   Consultant Begeman recommends including kinetic items in the room, such as a squeeze ball or Slinkies. Toys are a great stress reliever. He found it involved the whole person and seemed to bring out more creativity. One business I worked in had a well-anticipated "playtime" for 5 minutes every Friday. For additional ideas, try the 3M Meeting Network website, www.mmm.com/meetings/.

9. My group constantly gets sidetracked into good, but not related, topics. Any suggestions?

Officially "park" distracting ideas or comments. Some use a flip chart placed at the side of the room as a "parking lot." When an unrelated topic comes up, it is written down there as an acknowledgment. There is the understanding that it can be dealt with, if appropriate, at another time.

Another trick is to set limits. Announce at the beginning that only 10 minutes or 10 questions (whichever comes first) will be allowed for this topic. Participants tend to restrict themselves when they know there is a limit.

One business I worked for allowed any member to say out loud "ADD" (Attention Deficit Disorder) to signal a need to bring the discussion back in focus. Another company makes participants pay 25 cents for every comment made during discussion sessions. They found comments were more developed with less automatic, reactive criticism. And, as the story goes, when one member threw down his credit card and began to speak, everyone paid attention!

10. My problem is the opposite. When we have brainstorming, no one says anything.

- *Try phrasing the concept broadly.* Rather than asking for a response on "How can we stop negative talk in the presence of patients?" ask "What would make this a better environment for caregiving?"
- *Find some merit in every idea.* Initially respond to every idea with interest, not criticism. And even if you realize it will never work, always say what you like about the idea first.
- *Have all ideas or comments recorded.* With this technique, people feel "heard." But avoid the use of a flip chart to record ideas during the gathering stage. Independent observers have noted that participation lessens when the flip chart begins to fill.
- *Allow for some confusion.* Part of the creative process is initially feeling unsure. Let rumors and spontaneity flow.

11. Any other ideas?

A concept used in nursing schools, championed by Deborah Ulrich, PhD, RN, and Kellie Glendon, MSN, RNC, of Miami University, involves cooperative learning through unfolding case studies. Provide a scenario, such as no empty beds in the hospital, discharges are pending, and ED and OR are holding patients.

Participants have 1 minute to think about it and then "pair and share"—go into groups of two to share their thoughts about it with each other. Having pairs with members from different areas, either a specialty or institution, can help enlarge the perspective.

Another variation is to have a round table in which each person, one at a time, writes down one thought about the situation, reads it aloud, and then passes it to the next participant. Go around the table at least twice.

In both situations the ideas grow as people feed off one another's input. And, the quiet members are more likely to participate.

12. It seems to take so long for our group to reach a consensus or decision. Any suggestions?

Use multiple media. People can read five times faster than they speak or hear. There are computer programs that allow participants to anonymously place their comments on a group screen. But a less expensive version is to have participants write comments on self-stick notes and place them on a wall in grouped categories. Often a group consensus is reached quickly.

At one meeting, participants were asked to write down their biggest barrier to success in their job. The facilitator then read the thoughts out loud. It was apparent that most were dealing with one of the same three themes. Time was then spent on those problems.

13. My day is spent in meetings that others plan. Name some tips to make them more worthwhile.

- *Meetings always seem to last 50% longer than you think they will.* Plan accordingly.
- *Always arrive 5 minutes early or on time.* You appear collected, rather than rushed and disheveled. It sets the tone that you are trustworthy and considerate.
- *Sit at the table rather than in the back along the wall.* You'll be more involved in the process.
- *Vary whom you sit beside at group meetings.* Resist the comfort of always sitting next to the same people. Use this opportunity to expand your horizons and network within the organization.
- *Always take your scheduler/day planner.* This prevents time-consuming rescheduling delays from unknown conflicts.
- *Go prepared, even if others don't.* You want the reputation of being reliable and responsible. And always finish strong: people remember the ending.
- *Jot notes as others speak.* It signals that it was heard and considered. Besides it helps you pay attention. The tendency is to nod your head to indicate you are paying attention, but most interpret that as agreement.

14. Talk about how I can have more impact when I offer input at a meeting?

- *Minimize your movement when entering and sitting down.* Women tend to fidget (adjusting clothing, jewelry), which lends to a less powerful appearance in a business situation.
- *Sit leaning slightly forward.* The body language indicates interest.
- *Keep voice intonation low when suggesting an idea.* Women tend to raise their voices at the end of the sentence. However, a lower tone is perceived as more credible.
- *Present your ideas confidently and decisively.* Never torpedo your thought with a belittling qualifiers such as "I'm not sure but...."
- *Float the idea ahead of time.* Talking to a few members of the group ahead of time will prepare you for what the group's response might be. In addition, you may win some allies, who will then quickly chime in with their support at the meeting.
- *Tailor the length to your listeners' position.* Be more direct when communicating upward, more expansive with explanation when communicating to a peer or subordinate.
- *Slow your speech down if your information involves change.* Speaking too fast can lead people to think you are covering up other details.
- *Do not feel obligated to have a comment on every issue.* Sometimes it is best to say nothing.

15. I never know how much to put into the minutes. What should I include?

First, be sure to have staff meeting minutes (and make nonattenders responsible for reading them). JCAHO surveyors will often review them.

Focus on three categories of information: decisions reached, action items that people need to follow-up on, and open issues. This confirmation of expected action is essential. After a lengthy discussion, the exact final decision or participation may be unclear. In one study, observers from Anderson Consultants found a 20% discrepancy between what was said and what was actually written in the minutes. Some deal with this by have a distinct action list distributed afterwards (e.g., what is to be accomplished by who by what time.)

16. How can I have the right resources for the right meeting? Often I realize that papers I need are back in the office.

I keep a three-ring binder for each committee or project I participate in; some use a spiral notebook per group. Then all notes and minutes are in one tidy source. I also have a tote bag for each group. I put material related to upcoming topics or even just something I need to give to someone on the committee in the appropriate bag. With my bag and notebook at the meeting, I have memory joggers for new issues as well as past material.

17. What is a staff "retreat" and how is it used?

A staff retreat is a time away from work to deliberately clarify universal departmental goals, purpose, or mission. It can be a productive and unifying experience. As a new manager, I had one with all levels of personnel (unit secretary, assistants, RNs, MDs) for team-building. We ended up with an agreement on acceptable behaviors that supported our reason for existence. It then became easier to enforce certain changes because it had been a group decision, not mine alone.

18. Are there other versions of "retreats"?

Yes. The point is to allow for reflection, something we tend to not do. One CEO schedules quarterly "fireside chats." His goal is to set up a cozy, relaxed atmosphere in which tough issues can be talked about in an informal setting. He purposely opens a homemade cardboard picture of a fireplace and pulls up two chairs at the beginning, because people clam up if the atmosphere is deadly earnest. He then ask questions to help people open up. Examples are "How can we make our work more fun?" or "How can you become more productive?" It not only gets a pulse of the collective mood but also helps identify important issues.

Another CEO calls for a 10-minute "time out" before a major decision is finalized. He has the group's members purposefully just sit there and reflect on the decision and implications before moving on.

19. I feel that during our idea sessions, staff tends to say what is "politically correct." How can we get "out of the box" candor?

Separate process and power. For this type of meeting, have the facilitator be someone other than you or anyone else who has the final say. We used someone from pastoral care; others found that psychiatric clinicians were well versed in handling group sharing. And don't sit toward the front where everyone can watch your nonverbal behavior.

Consider who should attend. I deliberately did not have our Vice President attend, a non-nurse who many felt did not understand patient care issues. I then went to him with a report of the group's experience afterwards.

I find it helpful to be personally vulnerable early on. For instance, I admitted there were days when I just dreaded having to take care of patients who were hostile. Not an extraordinary revelation, but others are more willing to take a risk and be honest after they see you do it first.

20. I'm a participant in the hospital's plan to hire a consultant. Any advice?

First, clearly define the desired results so the right type of consultant is chosen. Do you want a process redesign? Or are you just looking for cost-cutting? In that case, your organization already knows how to do that.

Ask for the right information as you interview potential consultants. Just because they have names of other companies they have worked with does not mean the approach will be appropriate for your organization's unique needs or culture. One hospital spent more than $1 million to receive a standardized formula solution that did not work for their unique, inner-city, multicultural population.

21. What questions are good to ask consultants during the selection interviewing process?

- *What is your theoretical basis?* You want to know if they use system analysis or quality statistical data. They should be founded in theory rather than hunches or a "cookie cutter" recipe.
- *What are your values?* Make them answer first so they do not just agree with what you already told them. Their intrinsic operating patterns must align with your institution's emphasis.

- *What would you do differently (or what did you learn) in your last job?* You want individuals who are constantly growing because their personal essence will affect their outcomes.
- *Who will be doing the on-site work?* Many times the individual who markets the work is not the same person who will be on location. Ask also to interview those individuals. In one experience, the consultant who "sold" the job emphasized openness and flexibility, but the person who would be on location used the phrase "my bias is that we will..." 18 times during his interview.

22. I have an interview with a reporter about our new program. Any tips?

Nurses need to be comfortable being visible and marketing their benefits. Journalists complain that many nurses have a fear of the media, with a corresponding "protect" rather than "promote" response.

Plan ahead what points you want the journalist to take away from the interview. Otherwise it can be as Earl Bush (press aide to Chicago's Mayor Richard Daley, Sr.) said, "[You reporters] should have printed what he meant, not what he said."

- *Return any phone calls promptly.* Journalists have tight deadlines.
- *Always have available and offer to send/fax materials.* This includes information on your program or innovation, as well any supportive research studies. The reporter will usually not take the time to look up an article.
- *Assume the interviewer knows nothing.* Journalists' expertise is writing, not your specialty. That is why you are being interviewed. Give the essential basics in a nutshell.
- *Provide specifics.* It is not enough to say vague global statements, such as government cutbacks have affected patient care. Give details, data, and dates.
- *Repeat several main, preplanned points.* Make sure the reporter hears what you think is essential.
- *Provide illustrative "people stories" or analogy.* Everyone loves, and remembers, a good story.
- *Do not give an opinion on hypothetical situations.* Sometimes a journalist will attempt to lead you into a "gray" area you don't want to address by asking "What if...." Simply respond that you do not address hypothetical situations. Don't let the reporter's expectant silence or repeated question pressure you into answering something you don't want to.

BIBLIOGRAPHY

1. Begeman M: Managers Forum: Meetings. J Emerg Nurs 26(1):63–64, 2000.
2. Gordon S: Managers Ask and Answer: Marketing yourself. J Emerg Nurs 24(1):77–78, 1998.
3. Imperato G: You have to start meeting like this! Fast Company 23:204–210, 1999.
4. Matson E: Managers Ask and Answer. J Emerg Nurs 23(6):642–643, 1997.
5. Moran R: Managers Forum: Business wisdom. J Emerg Nurs 25(6):546, 1999.
6. Schwarz J: Managers Ask and Answer: Hiring a consultant. J Emerg Nurs 23(5):635–636, 1997.
7. Warshaw M: Managers Forum: Breaking bad news. J Emerg Nurs 25(3):224–225, 1999.

II. *Planning and Organizing*

6. FITTING WITHIN THE ORGANIZATION

Robin J. Gilbert, RN, BSN, CEN

An empowered organization is one in which individuals have the knowledge, skill, desire, and opportunity to personally succeed in a way that leads to collective organizational success.

Stephen R. Covey

1. Why should I care about the bigger picture? Shouldn't all of my focus be on my unit?
Understanding what your organization is all about will help you in managing and guiding your area's involvement in this institution's business.

2. What is strategic planning?
Strategic planning is selecting and organizing the institution's business to keep it healthy in spite of unexpected upsets from within the industry or competitors. It usually considers 3 to 5 years in the future.

The process involves an external assessment to examine opportunities and potential threats and an internal assessment to identify its strengths and weaknesses. These relate to the organization's mission to give direction, set goals, and improve communication and services. See also the chapter on Managing Business Strategy.

3. Explain organizational culture.
Every organization has a culture, a system of shared meaning that distinguishes it from other organizations. This is a combination of the key assumptions, customary values, language (terms), and behaviors of the members of an organization. These "norms"—specific thinking and behaviors—often must be learned by new employees before they are truly accepted as part of the organization. It is important to consider whether you have a good cultural fit (e.g., congruence with the organization's values and style) with the employing institution.

4. How does organizational culture manifest itself?
Manifestations of culture include the following:
- *Style of communication* (formal/informal, oral/written, group announcements/individual)
- *How change occurs* (behind-the-scenes politics, group discussion, senior power moves)
- *Reward criteria* (performance, seniority, favoritism)

For instance, in one hospital physician preference is the ultimate deciding factor, whereas in another hospital research literature (from any discipline) is considered the most important factor.

5. What are types of cultures and management styles?
William Schneider (1994) describes four core cultures:
- *Control:* authoritative, conservative, impersonal, tough-minded, realistic, systematic, task-driven, objective, prescriptive. The manager is the more autocratic leader.
- *Collaborative:* adaptive, collegial, democratic, informal, participative, personal, relational, supportive, and trusting. The manager is a coach.

- *Competence:* challenging, efficient, emotionless, formal, impersonal, intense, objective, rational, and task-driven. The manager is an assertive, visionary standard setter who recruits the most competent people and seeks to have them stretch.
- *Cultivation:* attentive, emotional, enabling, humanistic, nurturing, people-driven, personal, promotive, relaxed. The manager is a catalyst, cultivator, empowerer, inspirer, and promoter.

6. What is a toxic organization?

Toxic organizations have some elements of dysfunctional leadership, such as excessive control, a constant state of crisis, or blaming people rather than fixing problems. One sign is an abnormally high, rapid turnover in employees, especially among those in leadership positions.

7. What is the difference between mission, purpose, and vision?

An organizational mission statement reflects the organization's core value. It gives direction for goals and objectives. A purpose is the reason for an organization's existence. The terms *mission* and *purpose* are often used interchangeably.

The vision of an organization depicts where the organization wants to go and what it will look like when it gets there. It is an image of the desired future.

An organization creates an institutional mission statement and/or vision from which individual departments then create their own mission statement and implementation.

8. Why do organizations have a mission statement?

The mission statement provides a primary focus. It assists decision making, program creation, and departmental function. The best ones are limited in focus (purpose) and have a visionary motivation.

For example, the organization may state that part of the mission is to provide preventative education in the community. The emergency department (ED), as a manifestation of that vision, may provide Don't Drink and Drive lectures at the local schools.

9. How does a department develop a mission statement?

Specific steps that should be considered include the following:

1. *Identify who the customers are.* Customers may include patients, staff, physicians, and/or the community.

2. *Identify the major role this department will take.* For instance, a labor and delivery department may identify healthy, client-involved childbirth as their major function and then establish prenatal education as a part of that role. An education department may identify staff teaching, training, and competency assessment as their major functions.

3. *Identify the relationships between cost, benefit, and quality.* A patient care area's mission statement must commit to both cost effectiveness and quality of care.

4. *Identify the department's responsibility in meeting strategic objectives.* This makes a promise to the organization that the department is part of the team.

10. Tell me more about an institution's philosophy.

A philosophy is a statement of values and beliefs that direct an organization in its attempt to achieve its mission. When developing a philosophy as a manager, it is important to consider the historical background, education, theory, practice, research, and nursing role in the overall organization. For instance, a teaching medical complex affiliated with a major research university might have a different emphasis in patient care (e.g., pursuit of cutting-edge technology solutions) than a small, community, religious-owned hospital within a retirement community (e.g., strengthen an individual's spiritual and emotional support).

11. How are goals and objectives reflective of the mission statement?

Goals relate a desired outcome. From them objectives for achieving the mission and philosophy are developed. Goals are central to the entire management process. Objectives are specific statements that will be evident when the goal is accomplished. Objectives must be achievable, measurable, and outcome-oriented and have a target date.

For instance, the goal may be to promote patient self-management. An objective for that could be starting a monthly diabetes support group or hiring a certified diabetes educator. More detailed action steps are then created to achieve that objective, such as verifying room availability or creating a job description.

12. Describe the relationship between the institution's mission statement and individual jobs.

The mission plays an important role when the manager develops a job description, performance evaluation tool, or disciplinary actions. Professional responsibilities in a job description should be tied to the core mission of the organization.

The performance evaluation tool is then taken from the job description. It helps determine what areas to evaluate, such as customer satisfaction, clinical competence, attendance reliability, research participation, and community involvement. Both the description and the evaluation should reflect what is considered vital to the success of the department and organization.

If this process is followed, it is then easy in disciplinary actions to show the individual that his or her values, performance, or commitment have diverged from those of the organization.

13. How do I accomplish goals and objectives?

Policies and procedures make goals and objectives operational.

14. Explain the difference between a policy and a procedure.

Policies explain how goals will be achieved. They should be clear, concise statements that establish areas of authority. For instance, the hospital's policy related to public information might be that requests for information from the media will be handled by the nursing supervisor or public relations department.

Regulating organizations, such as the Joint Commission for Accreditation of Healthcare Organizations, look for institution-wide consistency between departmental policies for the same issue. For example, all areas must have the same requirements for administration of conscious sedation or application of restraints.

Procedures give more specific guides to action. They operationalize a policy. Procedures can be intradepartmental or interdepartmental and tend to not affect the overall organization to the same extent as a policy. Examples could be the steps to administer blood or to store a patient's valuables. Liability is limited as long as the nurse adheres to the institution's policy. Procedures should be consistent with professional standards of practice.

15. How do I review a policy to see that it will accomplish what it was intended to accomplish?

Use these questions to guide your review of the policy:
- Is there a need for this policy?
- Is the policy relevant to this organization and staff?
- Is the policy consistent with the nursing service philosophy?
- Does the policy create any inequities between hospital staff or patients?
- Is the policy reasonable?
- Is the policy clearly written so anyone unfamiliar with the information can understand it?
- Is the information accurate?
- Is the policy complete?

16. What information should be included in a procedure?

Typical content for a procedure includes the following:
- Equipment and material necessary
- Correct sequence of steps
- Contraindications

- Rationale for each intervention
- Current clinical nursing references, if applicable

17. What are unwritten rules?

Every work setting has informal, unwritten assumed "the way we do things here" that usually governs minor departmental functions—for instance, who makes the coffee or one physician's unique preference regarding his patients' dressing change.

The clearer these types of expectations can be communicated, the easier it is for everyone. It can be difficult for new employees to figure out these "local" customs. One unit had employees even create an orientation booklet of unwritten rules. Unwritten rules should be consistent with institutional policy.

18. Describe the trend for organizational structure.

The trends for organizational structures are changing from hierarchical to a flatter organization with multidisciplinary, cross-functional teams. As a result, it is believed that there are fewer boundaries and more free access to communication. The employees benefit by increasing their ownership, empowerment, and accountability. This helps to develop future managers. The ability to work in a team is a critical skill in a flatter structure.

19. What strategies do I need to succeed in an environment of organizational change?

Tips include:
- Focus on what the organization can become
- Create an open atmosphere where questions can be asked.
- Don't deny problems; welcome criticism as an opportunity to improve.
- Make employee feel that their achievements are important to the organization.
- Maintain career-developing programs for yourself and staff.

For more ideas, see the chapter on Managing Change.

BIBLIOGRAPHY

1. Abruzzese RS: Nursing Staff Development: Strategies for Success, 2nd ed. St. Louis, Mosby, 1996.
2. Berlandi JL: Organizational ethics and managers. Surg Serv Manage 5:20–21, 1999.
3. Coccia C: Avoiding a "toxic" organization. Nurse Manager 29:32–33, 1998.
4. Peters TJ, Waterman RH: In Search of Excellence: Lessons from America's Best Run Companies. New York, Harper & Row, 1982.
5. Scheider WE: The Reengineering Alternative: A Plan for Making Your Current Culture Work. Burr Ridge, IL, Irwin, 1994.
6. Sluetal MR: Review of literature. Climate, culture, context, or work environment? Organizational factors that influence nursing practice. Semin Nurse Managers 8:2–4, 2000.
7. Tomey AM: Guide to Nursing Management and Leadership, 6th ed. St. Louis, Mosby, 2000.

7. MANAGING CHANGE

Michelle Myers Glower, RN, MSN

One of the greatest pains to human nature is the pain of a new idea.

Walter Bagehot

1. How can I avoid change?

You can't. In today's turbulent health care environment, change is inevitable, and not all change is bad. Covey, Merrill, and Merrill's (1994) definition of insanity is "to keep doing the same things and expect different results."

In the past we looked for loyalty in employees; we now look for flexibility and those who are not possessed by the way things have always been done. It is people's response that is key to succeeding in managing change.

2. Can I control change?

Not really. Common advice is to try to be a part of it. But there are no guarantees. At one organization I assumed I would not be a part of the reorganization because I was part of the planning team. But in the end, they restructured me out of my position. Therefore, it is important to recognize that changes exist, so you are not caught unawares like a deer in the headlights.

3. What is change theory?

Lewin's (1951) theory of change with three stages is considered the classic, with Lippitt's (1958) theory providing seven phases to illustrate the process. They are as follows:

Unfreezing (motivation to create change occurs)
  • Diagnosis of the problem
  • Assessment of the motivation and capacity for change
  • Assessment of the change agent's motivation and resources
Moving (the actual change with new responses developed)
  • Selecting progressive change objectives
  • Choosing the appropriate role of the change agent.
Refreezing (change is integrated and stabilized)
  • Maintenance of the change once it has been started
  • Termination of the relationship between the change agent and changed system

4. How is change implemented?

  • *Design the change.* Understand what the purpose of it is, why it is necessary, and that it is workable. This often includes the gathering of data.
  • *Plan the implementation.* Identify and plan how to strengthen driving forces and lessen restraining forces.
  • *Implement the change.* Pace the change depending on the change's magnitude and complexity as well as the current stress level of the people involved.
  • *Integrate the change.* Verify that the change is now well incorporated into everyday operations and accepted. Change sticks when, instead of being the new way to do something, it becomes "the way we do things around here."

5. What other forces affect change?

Besides the role of the change agent, there are always driving forces (facilitate the change) and restraining forces (impede the change). The manager often plays the role of a change agent to bring about positive changes. Being aware of, and dealing with, what is working for and against the change will help the change process succeed.

6. Why do employees resist change?

Resistance to change tends to come from technical concerns, psychosocial needs, or a threat to a person's position and power. Employees are usually comfortable with the status quo because they feel safe, like living in a cozy cottage. It is viewed as a means of having control. When change occurs to people or something they perceive as secure, they begin to ask, "Am I next?" or "What about me?" Change is often more difficult when it is not expected.

7. Describe the ways in which staff can resist change.

Active resistance can include attacking the idea, refusing to change, arguing against the change, and/or organizing resistance of the other people. Passive approaches use avoidance, such as avoiding discussion about the change, ignoring the change, refusing to commit to the change, or verbally agreeing with the change but not actually adapting it.

Often active resistance seems more troublesome. But the indirect passive resistance can be actually more difficult to recognize and to deal with in the long run. Try to regard staff speaking out about concerns as a positive thing. Then, at least, you are aware of what the issues are.

8. How do I lower my staff's resistance to change?

Universal strategies to lower people's resistance include any of the following four approaches:
- Information dissemination
- Disconfirmation of currently held beliefs
- Providing for their psychological comfort
- Require that the change be made

9. Talk about why some staff has trouble with a change.

Change is like dying for some; and they need to go through the grieving. Bridges (1994) suggest the following in getting staff to let go.
- Realize that not all staff grieve at the same time or in the same numbers, so be patient.
- Address the loss when the employee is stuck in the denial phase for more than a few days, before the negativity spreads.
- Identify who's losing what.
- Don't be surprised at "overreaction."
- Acknowledge the losses openly and sympathetically.
- Expect and accept signs of grieving.
- Compensate for the losses.
- Give honest information over and over.
- Treat the past with respect.

When we had a major change in our department, I addressed all of the above by having several staff meetings specifically on the loss they are experiencing. My experience has taught me that being honest and straightforward toward your staff builds credibility and trust. It may be difficult to get staff to buy into your change process if trust doesn't exist.

10. What emotional reactions should I expect from staff toward change?

The gamut can be seen from crying and aggressively communicating that they need no change to offering their assistance with changes that they have longed for. It is normal for staff to *overreact*. You are moving them out of a "comfort zone."

In addition, change involves a loss of the familiar. You may be seeing a reaction to one or more losses from their past that occurred without the chance to grieve, rather than a reaction based totally on this current change.

11. How do I handle these emotions?

Allow time. Be patient while staff has a chance to adjust, and you will usually eventually see responses become more rational and participative.

12. How do I answer employees' questions about how this change will affect them?

Employees ask this question out of fear of the unknown. There is often a growing fear that the change will bring a situation that is worse than what currently exists. Many have a tendency to focus on what could go wrong, rather than on the positive results than can come if everything goes right.

Johnson (1998) describes a reward process when you get past your fear so that you may enjoy the adventure. That reward can come with opportunities for improvement or growth. Without taking the leap, you won't know what the reward will be.

Compare it to something personal you have experienced. I like to use marriage. If you want to be married you have to date, and maybe kiss, a few frogs. I guess that's why it is called "taking the plunge."

13. Share some other suggestions or principles about making change more acceptable.

- Ensure that the need for change is justified, even if there is not agreement. Change for the sake of change is never justified.
- Diffuse anxiety by having those involved create the vision for change.
- Recognize the competency and skill of the people involved. Express that you value everyone's contributions.
- Work from a previously established set of impersonal principles. Point out the similarities between the old and the new.
- Change is best received when it follows other successes rather than failures.
- Space events so that there is adjustment to one change before another is introduced.
- Realize that people new to the organization tend to react to change more comfortably than people with longevity in the system. (The latter have more vested interests.)
- Choose change agents with psychological sensitivity to serve as a bridge to other participants.
- Focus attention on the future, not the past. Try to guarantee some personal benefits—things should get better, not worse.
- Provide a climate of acceptance in which some mistakes can be made without negative consequences for the individual.
- Accept some aspects of the proposed change that may need adjustment. Encourage open expression of concerns. Be ready to compromise once everyone is clear on the things that are nonnegotiable.
- Never withhold information as a source of power.

14. Some are worried that patient care will be affected by the changes.

Patient care should always be enhanced when change occurs, not deteriorated. Monitor your patient satisfaction scores before and after; pay particular attention to the comments. Monitor patient outcomes. Reassure staff that if you notice a negative trend toward a particular issue, you are willing to consider reverting to the way it was prior to the change.

15. What can I do as a new manager to prevent everyone from leaving like a herd of cattle to avoid a change?

Recognize upfront that it is normal for some staff to leave with a management change. They may have been thinking about it anyway or may not feel the new direction is for them. As a new manager, I did lose some staff, but was left with a solid team. And a stable staff is key in an ever-changing environment. See also the chapter on new beginnings.

16. Are there different categories within the staff?

Hall describes the phenomenon of staff members being in one of four categories.

1. Those who thrive on change and embrace it
2. Those who like proven change
3. Those who resist change unless it is necessary

4. Those who will not change. These persons tend to be the ones who have used their 10 years of clinical work to obtain 1 year of experience repeated 10 times.

Appeal to the first group. They will respond enthusiastically and then pull in the second group. At this point, you have about 50% of the group so many in the third group will start to go along. You are now in a position to clearly indicate that "We are doing it this way." Those who cannot buy into this change may want to consider moving on.

The fourth group will always be with you. They may never completely change. But do not count on them leaving on their own, as that would be a change for them. However, do not be consumed with converting them; you already have the majority.

17. How do I include staff in change?

Johnson (1998) states, "After you change what you believe, you change what you do." Help staff understand the "why" of the change. Make sure they see "the big picture" and know what they are doing. Actually, many of the staff want an opportunity to be involved. They want to have influence over how their work gets done.

On the other hand, as the manager, you must be willing to risk trusting the employees. They need to feel that you have confidence and trust their thinking. Provide assurance of administrative support and freedom to act without the constant need for approvals. This makes for a committed staff.

18. What steps will build a trusting relationship with the staff?

Trust is important. In one survey, it was listed as one of the two most important indicators for employee retention.

- *Maintain open communications.* To help staff with the change I have many open discussions, honestly answer questions, and freely admit when I don't know. Do not lie. It will come back to haunt you.
- *Have one-on-one discussions with each employee.* Though this takes time, it reaches the quiet ones, who can become slowly disgruntled. These sessions allow them to privately ask questions and voice their concerns. It signals that you consider each employee important.
- *Ask staff to identify needed resources.* Staff usually have a clear picture of what resources they need to make their environment more workable, such as new equipment or reimbursed continuing education. However, make them prioritize their wish list.
- *Do what you say you are going to do.* Staff will remember and monitor your promises.

19. Whom should I seek to put on my leadership team? Do I want people with whom I am most comfortable ?

Trofino (1997) suggests using teams that want to seek out new opportunities to ensure what she describes as "cross-fertilization of ideas." This helps to reduce barriers to change and progress. Build a leadership team from long-term employees who see change as necessary.

Selecting my team involved hiring people who are not like myself, so there are role models for diversity. If everyone were like me, how could we generate new ideas? You need various methods of communication and different styles for interacting with others and energy flow. Having diversity will help you speak the language for all of the personality types within your staff.

20. What can I use to promote understanding among the leadership team, e.g. the clinical coordinators?

Consider using a personality inventory. I found the Myers-Briggs Type Indicator (MBTI) personality inventory four scales to be very helpful in describing and understanding our differences and likenesses. The Myers-Briggs personality types include the following:

- Extravert/introvert refers to how a person is energized.
- Sensing/intuition refers to what a person pays attention to.

• Thinking/feeling refers to how a person decides.
• Judging/perceiving refers to the lifestyle the person adopts.

21. What are the possible benefits from using the MBTI?
  • Appreciate others so as to make constructive use of individual differences
  • Perceive approaching problems in different ways
  • Understand how we can work together as a group even though we are different
  • Communicate more effectively with each other and employees
  • Improve teamwork
  • Adapt to differences in management style
  • Promote conflict resolution

22. How did you use the MBTI with your leadership team?
I had a behavioral health facilitator assist the group. We defined the effects of preferences in work situations and preferred methods of communication among us. This allowed everyone to see that we were all at different places in our lives, with different preferred methods of communicating. Our facilitator helped us understand how to problem-solve using each person's different preferences. From this, we used it to manage change on an ongoing basis.

23. Are there other ways to build a strong team?
Team-building exercises assist the team in identifying that is alright to be in "different places" with regard to our ideas and approaches to problem-solving. Use exercises such as the Subarctic Survival, Square Wheels, Stuck Truck, and Gilligan's Island to develop and strengthen staff's problem-solving and team-building skills.

24. What are other ways to have staff buy in to change?
  • *Use the staff's own priority list to guide your decisions.* Then they will feel "heard." I purchase equipment in their order because I assume they know best what is needed.
  • *Develop a shared governance, such as a Nursing Practice Council (NPC).* This is a group of leadership and staff who initiate ideas for change in the department. As a result, staff has autonomy and becomes a part of unit decisions. People respond better to change that affects them when they feel some control.
  • *Develop your own customer service team.* I made this group responsible for reviewing quarterly customer service scores, and where the opportunities of improvements are. Staff who excel are recognized.
  • *Have staff read the book,* Who Moved My Cheese. It is a short, quickly read book that illustrates many aspects about change.
  • *Color-code (type-indicate) all staff.* The Myers-Briggs Type Indicator is based on behavior. In a similar theme, color coding is based on motive, or inner drive. It uses four colors to represent main motive: red—power, blue—intimacy, white—peace, and yellow—fun (Hartman, 1998; LeFevre 2000). It is less expensive and involved than using MBTI, however. My use of staff color-coding created a sensitivity and awareness about others personalities to help staff manage themselves and others.

25. How do I keep staff informed of ongoing progress?
Communication is key. Use the hospital e-mail and staff meetings. Have all committees make monthly progress reports. A newsletter keeps staff updated with current happenings in the department and hospital. But I've found that, most important, the staff wants to see you involved.

26. How can I achieve compliance with the planned changes?
You want commitment, not compliance. Compliance is going along with forced-upon change. Commitment means you will do it even when the boss is not present. Everyone wants that. However, it takes much longer to accomplish because some personal behavioral change is required.

27. How do I achieve commitment?
   • *Listen to your employees and give credence to their legitimate issues.* One study found that 7 of 10 employees said they would not speak up. It seems that if they have been discounted before, they will not take the same risk again.
   • *Be consistent, with adequate explanations.* Another study found that employees would rather follow a leader they didn't agree with than someone who kept changing for the sake of change.
   • *Capture their emotions for the same visionary outcomes.* It is hard in today's turbulent health care environment because we all tend to be individualistic. But when someone's heart is engaged, they will stay the course even when there are difficulties or positive alternatives. Most nurses went into the profession to help people, a simple but captivating motive to call upon.

28. Some of the staff ideas involve monies that the budget does not have. Are there other sources?
   Besides hospital budgets, there are available monies from outside sources (e.g., state trauma fund, contingency hospital fund, women's auxiliary guild), self-funding, and donations. For instance, administration purchased a fish tank for our waiting room but staff, including the local paramedics and hospital physicians, bought the fish.
   It is sometimes the easiest to find funding for items related to pediatric illness. The Starlight Children's Foundation is an international nonprofit organization that will provide a free *Mobile Entertainment Fun Center* (a cabinet on wheels with Nintendo, VCR, and TV) for pediatric patient populations (*www.starlight-chicago.org*). Others have received toy donations by writing directly to various toy manufacturers. Ask the nursing instructor or the student nurses on your unit if they have any duplicate, unused reference books.

29. How do you improve morale in the department?
   I give staff thank-you notes through e-mails, their mailboxes, and recognition certificates from my computer. Some managers offer candy kisses. Keeping a bowl of candy often brings staff into your office to talk. Some managers send staff to a professional conference through a drawing of eligible employees (e.g., employed greater than 1 year, no disciplinary action). See also the chapter on motivating and empowering.

30. Tell me how to handle negativity that brings down the unit's atmosphere.
   You will always have chronic complainers because these individuals want attention and this lets them be on stage, so to speak. Involve them in the very thing they are complaining about. They will either need to improve the situation or stop complaining, because now they are an inherent part of it.
   If you have a truly toxic saboteur, you may need to get more drastic. Allowing such a person to continue gives them a negative power. One manager had a staff member who constantly put down any topic brought up in staff meetings by muttering negative comments out loud. After a period of time, the manager directly confronted the employee about this behavior. She warned her that she would "take her on" in the next meeting by putting her in front of the group and directly dealing with her negativity. As a result, the person stopped her negative behavior.

31. How can I keep prepared for unexpected career changes?
   • Always keep an updated curriculum vitae (CV).
   • Keep current with what surrounding hospitals are doing.
   • Network within the organization and profession.
   • Know and understand your institution's organizational culture.
   • Participate in your professional nursing organization.
   • Read anything pertaining to change.
   For more information, see Chapter 39, Managing Your Career.

BIBLIOGRAPHY

1. Bridges W: Managing Transitions Making the Most of Change. Boston, Addison Wesley, 1991.
2. Covey S, Merrill RA, Merrill R: First Things First. New York, Fireside Simon & Schuster, 1994.
3. Hall G: Managers Forum: Instituting change. J Emerg Nurs 24:591–592, 1998.
4. Hartman T: The Color Code. New York, Simon & Schuster, 1998.
5. Hirsh S, Kummerow J: Introduction to Type in Organizations, 2nd ed. Palo Alto, CA, Consulting Psychologist Press, 1990.
6. Joel LA, Kelly LY: The Nursing Experience: Trends, Challenges, and Transitions, 4th ed. New York, McGraw-Hill, 2002.
7. Johnson S: Who Moved My Cheese. New York, G.P. Putnam's Sons, 1999.
8. LeFevre AR: Don't worry, be happy! Harmonize diversity through personality sensitivity. Nursing Spectrum Career Fitness Online. Available at http://nsweb.nursingspectrum.com/ce236.htm. Accessed August 2000.
9. Lewin K: Field Theory in Social Science. New York, Harper & Row, 1951.
10. Lippitt R, et al: The Dynamics of Planned Change. New York, Harcourt & Brace, 1958.
11. Tappen RM, Weiss SA, Whitehead KD: Essentials of Nursing Leadership and Management, 2nd ed. Philadelphia, F.A. Davis, 2001.

8. MANAGING BUDGETS

Deborah S. Smith, RN, MS, MBA, CEN, CNAA

Get your facts first, and then you can distort them as much as you please.

Mark Twain

1. What is a budget?

A budget is a written plan of expected expenses and revenues over a defined period of time. Budgets are used by managers as a means of expressing in quantitative terms the resources for which they are responsible.

2. How long is a budget cycle?

Budgeting cycles are usually set for 12 months, or a fiscal year, which may or may not coincide with the calendar year. A budget on a continuous basis, a perpetual budget, is done monthly so that 12 months of future budget data are always available.

3. Are there different types of budgets?

Indeed, there are many types and categories of budgets. Budgets can be defined by the following:
- The scope of the operation that they cover (project budget, product line budget, departmental budget, organizational budget)
- Their purpose (supply budget, personnel budget, statistical budget, capital expense budget)
- The time frame that is covered (monthly budget, annual budget, long-term budget)

4. What is the difference between incremental budgeting and zero-based budgeting?

An incremental budget's baseline is the previous year's expenditures. Managers start with what they spent last year, and then add to it based on new programs or inflation.

In contrast, zero-based budgeting starts at zero each year. Every dollar needs to be justified. It prevents automatic continuation, but it is more time consuming.

5. Which budgets will I, as a manager, need to know about?

Managers need to have an understanding of the overall budgeting process of the organization. Many of the underlying principles of budgets are the same, so it's a matter of building from there once you understand the basics. Those budgets for which managers would most likely have responsibilities for developing and monitoring include the operating budget and the capital budget.

6. Describe what an operating budget is.

An operating budget typically plans for the revenues and expenses of a department or service for the coming year. Preparation and control of the operating budget is likely to be where managers spend a significant portion of their time relative to financial management. Operating budgets usually consist of up to four components:
- The statistical (or volume) budget
- The revenue budget
- The labor (or salary and wage) budget
- The supply and expense budget

Through these four budget elements, managers can detail their department operations with some degree of accuracy.

7. What is a capital expense budget?

A capital expense budget projects the planned costs of major purchases. Items in a capital budget are defined in terms of their dollar value and a long-term investment. Capital purchases can also be referred to as long-term investments, capital investments, capital assets, or capital acquisitions. The money used to purchase long-term investments is often referred to as capital. Examples of capital expense items may be a magnetic resonance imager, defibrillator, or a patient bed.

8. How much does an item have to cost to be considered a capital expense item?

Capital acquisitions are often quite expensive, but the high cost alone is not a required element for it to be classified and treated as a capital asset. What defines a capital expense is that the item has a lifetime beyond its year of purchase. However, the purchase of a coffee pot, for example, which has the useful life of more than 1 year is not likely to be treated as a capital purchase because tracking depreciation on multiple small items like this would be extremely time consuming.

Most organizations set a minimum dollar amount for an item to be considered a capital expense. This figure may be set at any amount, but common minimums are $500, $1000, or $5000.

9. Why is the capital budget considered separately from the operating budget?

The capital budget is considered separately from the operating budget because of the multiyear nature of the purchases. In any one year, the organization earns only a portion of the revenues that the capital asset may generate of its useful lifetime. Similarly, the capital expenses are depreciated over the purchased item's anticipated lifetime.

10. What is a statistical budget?

A statistical (or volume) budget is measured in terms of units of service based on the type of activities or service that the department is engaged in. For patient care areas, this is typically measured in patient days, outpatient visits, surgery hours or cases, childbirth deliveries, and so on. In non-patient care areas, units of service also vary. For example, dietary services may measure meals served or housekeeping might use square feet cleaned. It is important to have as accurate a statistical budget as possible, because this forms the basis for calculating revenue, expense, and labor budgets.

11. How is a statistical budget developed?

Usually the number of units of service can be attained from your information services or chief financial officer (CFO). However, take into consideration the types of activities you are measuring and whether the volume measurement is homogeneous. A patient acuity measurement system may give insight into the number of various patient types that are cared for. The workload associated with caring for diverse patient types may vary. This variation needs to be accounted for in all phases of budget planning.

Once a total volume has been identified, that volume must be dispersed over the course of the year. Take into consideration historical trends and the type of department for which you are preparing the budget. For instance, in a pediatric unit, the number of patient days may be higher during the respiratory infection season, and an emergency department in a summer resort area will have its visits affected by tourists. Make sure, when you are spreading out your total volume over the course of the year, that these factors are taken into consideration. See also the chapters on scheduling and staff budgets.

12. Is a revenue budget prepared the same way?

The revenue budget is a factor of two items, the expected revenue based on charges and the statistical budget previously prepared. To calculate revenue from operations, simply multiply your projected volume for a month by the projected revenue per unit (e.g., visit, delivery). Take into consideration any anticipated increase in charges for the upcoming year.

Although most of your revenue will come from the provision of service-related activities, you may have "special revenue" or nonoperating revenue from sources such as special programs or services provided by your department. One emergency department funded their educational programs from the profits of their own vending machines. These may or may not be related to the statistical volume and should be calculated separately.

13. Will all charges be collected and credited to my department?

Not all of the services provided are paid for in full by all payors in today's health care reimbursement system. The revenue budget should therefore include estimates of deduction from full charges of account for things like bad debt (unpaid bills) and payor discounts. In many instances, this will be done on an organizational basis and may not be reflected in your departmental budget.

Your total expected revenue budget is referred to as your total operating revenues. This amount, less your deductions, equals your net operating revenues.

14. What does the salary and wage budget involve?

The salary and wage, or personnel budget, is usually the largest portion of a departmental expense. You need to know what your personnel complement will look like before you can begin to itemize the expenses that may be associated. Calculation of your personnel budget requires knowing the number of staff you need, the staffing mix, and productivity. You may have RNs, LPNs, technicians, nursing assistants, secretaries, clerks, educators, and others as a part of your budget. Will all personnel providing care be employees or will some be contracted services through an agency? Are the majority of the staff full-time or part-time? How much staff education and training should be planned? What is variable, as opposed to fixed, staffing? These and other questions must be answered prior to proceeding.

When calculating your salary and wage budget, make sure to take into account variables such as shift differential, bonuses, anticipated overtime, sick time, relief coverage for family medical leaves, and so on. Once a grand total has been obtained, it should be apportioned over the year in alignment with the projected volume. See also the chapter on staffing budgets.

15. Explain what a supply and expense budget is.

The supply and expense budget includes many different and varied items, such as medical supplies, office supplies, or education and training costs. The first thing to do is to either obtain a chart of accounts from your organization or to develop one yourself. Calculation of these expenses are derived from past utilization as well as projected additional consumption. Expenses, such as medical supplies, linen, and forms, are driven by the volume of patients you care for. The non–volume-driven expenses, such as education, professional organizational membership dues, books, and maintenance contracts, can be controlled through careful planning during the budget development process.

16. How do I prepare a supply and expense budget?

Beginning with the volume-sensitive accounts, determine what your costs were per unit of service (e.g., patient day, outpatient visit) for the previous year and for the year-to-date for each item. Multiply the projected volume by the cost per unit of service and divide this on a monthly basis, aligned with your projected volume.

Take into consideration any fluctuations in the timing of purchases. For instance, supplies ordered weekly from a central storeroom will affect the budget differently than special order, infrequently-used items that must be purchased in a required volume.

Some judgment calls will need to be made to determine what cost you will predict for the coming year. Consider things such as the following:
- New physicians who will request special supplies or equipment
- New procedures that will be performed in your service area
- Facility issues such as replacing worn furnishings

17. What about inflation?

The cost of hospital supplies continues to escalate each year. Your materials management or purchasing department should be helpful to you in predicting inflation factors. It is a wise idea to check with your pharmacy director on anticipated increases in drug prices.

18. Are non–volume-sensitive accounts done the same way?

The planning phase is similar. Once again, start by looking at historical trends. If your costs are incurred reasonably evenly throughout the year, take the average monthly approach. If all seminars and meetings, for example, take place during certain months of the year, then the money needs to be budgeted in those months. Some items, such as journals, nonmandatory educational funds, and replacement of nonessential departmental supplies, are often budgeted for the end of the budget year. In the case in which there are budget cutbacks, these funds may not be spent to help in meeting budgetary projections.

19. I saw items like "floor rental" on the budget. What is that all about?

Every institution has some essential fixed costs that do not vary by the volume nor are they a direct cost, that is, attributable to a specific source. Common examples include electricity, heating, or environmental services.

Since these items benefit all hospital cost centers, institutions often use an equitable way to divide up the responsibility for this type of expense. (A cost center is the smallest functional unit for which cost control and accountability can be assigned.) Physical space is a common criterion, for instance, so much per square foot.

Because the unit (cost center) cannot function without these types of items, it is a fair inclusion in the budget. It is a cost consideration for doing your unit's business. However, it is an indirect expense that you cannot, and are not expected to, control at a unit level.

20. What steps are included in the preparation of a capital budget?

First, generate a list of proposed needs for your department. If existing capital assets are aging and have required frequent service, they may need to be replaced. New technology may be available, which would improve productivity or the quality of care. Plans may include the addition of new services or expansion of an existing service, requiring additional capital equipment.

Once the list is together, prioritize it. A useful tool in ranking is labeling each item as urgent, needed, or desirable.

- Urgent items are those required to meet licensing or accrediting needs or those that have an impact on the safety or health of patients or employees.
- Needed items result in cost savings, represent new or additional market share, or replace old or obsolete equipment.
- Desirable items are those that *could* result in the improvement of patient care or employee relations.

21. Identify the information needed to submit an item for consideration as a capital expense.

Information that is routinely asked in preparing a capital budget request includes the following:

- A description of the item
- Its estimated lifespan
- The net price
- How it has been prioritized
- A description of the function or purpose of the proposed purchase
- Alternatives considered other than purchasing this item to meet the need
- The risks and consequences if the item is not purchased
- The regulatory/code requirements that would rank something as urgent
- How the item links with the organizations' strategic plan

The final step might include the item's impact on patient care, patient satisfaction, operating efficiency, enhancement of market share or revenue, and physician satisfaction.

22. Are there any other factors I should consider?

Don't overlook the impact that the proposed purchase may have on other departments within the organization. For instance, if you are proposing the addition of a new computer software system, make sure that the information systems department can provide the necessary support for installation and training. Include costs for these, as well as any wiring and hardware costs, in the proposal.

Some purchases may require renovation or remodeling. Don't plan on buying something until you know where you're going to put it. The renovation costs are usually included as a component of the capital request.

23. I don't think the unit needs any new equipment this year. Should I just pass on requesting capital budget monies this year?

You may wish to request an item now that you don't need for another 2–3 years just to get it exposure. The time from your initial proposals to the end of the implementation can be as long as 2 years, and unexpected needs can arise. It is usually easier to get approved funds redirected toward a different item midcycle than to obtain new capital funds.

24. What determines whether a capital purchase request is approved?

Capital budgets are generally considered on an organization-wide basis in light of the cash available to spend. An investment that seems to make a lot of sense to a manager may have to be put off for a year or even indefinitely simply because the organization does not have enough cash to make the purchase. In light of other requests, the organizational priority for the item you are requesting might not make the cut.

Even if your organization has the cash, it may choose not to acquire an item because of its financial evaluation. A key financial evaluation wisely used is the "payoff approach." The number of years it would take for the profits from a capital expenditure to repay the initial case outlay is calculated. The less time it takes to recover the initial investment, the better the project. Certainly there are items for which there would be no profits generated but are still needed, such as a wheelchair, and these would be considered separately.

25. Explain what *book value* and *depreciation* are.

When a capital item is purchased, its useful life is determined and then it is depreciated yearly until there is no "book value" left. For example, a new patient transport stretcher costs $7000 and is expected to last 7 years. With straight line depreciation, the $7000 is spread over the 7 years or depreciated at the amount of $1000 per year. At the end of the seventh year, the stretcher would be "fully depreciated" and have no remaining book value. If in year 5 the stretcher were sold, it would have a remaining book value of $2000, and this would have to be taken into account in the sale of the item.

26. What is a budget variance?

Even with the best planning, things happen that were not anticipated and can cause a variation to the planned budget. Determining the how and why of a variance requires careful analysis. The objective of examining budget variance is not only to determine why the variance occurred but also how to plan better in the future.

27. How are budget variances examined?

Start by comparing the actual expenses of each line item in a budget report to what was budgeted for the month and on a cumulative year-to-date basis. For the analysis to provide a true benefit, it must be done in a timely manner. Budget variance investigations done several months after the fact are of less benefit than those done at the end of every month. Information about the most recent month's performance should be used to improve performance for the remaining months of the year.

When determining which budget variances need additional attention, focus your efforts on those with a significant variation. Your organization may have defined guidelines, such as a variance that is both a 10% difference from the original budget and a dollar amount greater than $200. Line items exceeding this guideline should be more thoroughly investigated.

28. What if unit volume exceeded the budget in any given month?

Looking at variances on a unit-of-service basis is helpful in examining both revenue and expenses. Of course costs are going to increase if you had budgeted 500 patient days in March and instead had 600.

But still determine whether the costs per patient day were elevated. If they remained within what was budgeted on a patient-day basis, there is likely justification for the increased expense. The same principle should then be applied to revenue per patient-day as well.

29. Are salary and wage (personnel) budget variances examined the same way?

Essentially yes, although there are additional factors to examine. Again, look at the amount of the variance compared to that budgeted amount for the month and on a year-to-date basis. Determine what personnel costs were per unit of service basis. Don't forget to include the costs of any contractual or agency staff, which may be included in a separate line item.

30. What are other contributing factors to salary and wage budget variances?

Other contributing factors include increases in personnel expenses (productivity, costs, and volume). Productivity can be examined by looking at the hours worked by all staff on an hours-of-service basis to determine whether there is a variance. Costs can be affected by paying higher hourly rates than what were budgeted for, either through overtime or through use of contracted personnel. Increases or decreases in volume will affect the total dollar amounts spent on salaries.

Additional variances may occur from a higher-than-anticipated ratio of total paid hours to total worked hours. Medical leaves, increased orientation costs, staff education hours, vacations, and sick time all contribute to nonproductive paid hours and add to the total salary costs. A variance will occur when these items were not accurately anticipated in budget planning. Also see Chapter 9, Staffing Budgets.

31. As long as I meet my projections, will I be safe from any budget cuts?

At any point in the budget planning, preparation, or implementation cycle, budgets may need to be altered because of unanticipated financial situations within an organization. Your unit is like one ship in the fleet; sometimes sacrifice is required by all. However, you may be required to make fewer cuts if you show that your department is cost-effective.

32. What is the best way to cut the budget?

Expenditures not essential to patient care and the day-to-day operations of the department are those that are the easiest to target for reductions. Easy targets may be meetings and travel to outside conferences and seminars. Required staff educational courses are less expendable.

When examining a budget for reductions, keep in mind that minimal savings can usually be attained through across-the-board reductions in the supply and expense budget. Remember the Pareto principle. It states that about 80% of the problems are the result of about 20% of the causes. Sometimes targeting a key aspect can have a large impact. For instance, some departments with high access to multiple groups of outsiders find that taking theft precautions (such as locking cabinets or bolting some equipment) can make a significant difference.

The most significant savings occur where the greatest expenditures are, which is usually in the personnel budget. Keep a tight control over staffing and productivity throughout the year and there will be less need for reductions in this area. This includes examining staffing mix on an annual basis to determine whether you are providing the best quality of care with the most efficient complement of staff.

And finally, if the organization is experiencing a cash flow problem, anticipate a slow-down in capital spending.

33. Is there an objective way to account for the charity work we do?

Most hospitals are not-for-profit institutions That distinction means it is financed by funds that come form several sources, but the providers of these funds do not have any owner-ship. Profits generated are frequently funneled back into the organization for expansion or capital acquisitions. There is a trend to ask not-for-profit organizations to quantify their com-munity benefit and thereby justify their tax-exempt status.

Obviously, monetary charity is tracked at a senior financial level, such as emergency surgery for a homeless individual or a bad debt. But, in addition, any departmental direct or indirect dollars spent for community benefit projects that do not have a financial return can be tracked.

For example, calculate the fair market value of a room's rental space if used for an Alcoholic Anonymous meeting or for a community education class on "safe sitters." Itemize and document nursing time and supplies for any community projects such as a Teddy Bear Clinic or a medical tent at a 5K charity run. Following this process will enable you to express charity budget expenditures in financial terms and provide a better comparison between projects.

34. Any tips on making the budgeting process easier?
- Spend the budgeted monies as needed to maintain departmental operations. If you do not spend a category, such as educational monies, it may be viewed as unnecessary and targeted for reduction in the following year by the CFO.
- Contact your CFO on a friendly, regular basis throughout the year, not just when you need something.
- Round out final figures. During initial calculations, it is helpful to know that an item listed thousands of times costs $.69 versus $.99. But the CFO is working with millions of dollars and doesn't need to know the total was $996.83. Just indicate $1000.
- Meet the given deadlines. Make life easy for the CFO.
- The more data, standards, and examples you have to back up your budget figures, the better. As they say, "In God we trust, all others bring data."

BIBLIOGRAPHY

1. Finkler SA, Kovner CT: Financial Management for Nurse Managers and Executives. Philadelphia, W.B. Saunders, 1993.
2. Gray L: Managers Ask and Answer. J Emerg Nurs 23(5):477–478, 1997.
3. Huber D: Leadership and Nursing Care Management, 2nd ed. Philadelphia, W.B. Saunders, 2000, pp 274–299.
4. Marquis BL, Huston CJ: Management Decision Making for Nurses, 3rd ed. Philadelphia, Lippincott Williams & Wilkins, 1998.

9. STAFFING BUDGETS

Susan K. Smith, BS, RNC, CNA, *and*
Polly Gerber Zimmermann, RN, MS, MBA, CEN

Do not put your faith in what statistics say until you have carefully considered what they do not say.

William W. Watt

1. Why are staffing budgets important to a nurse manager?

Staffing budgets, also known as personnel budgets, are the largest and most time-consuming part of your unit's budget. Nationwide, nursing represents 28% of total hospital full-time-equivalent positions (FTEs). Of these, registered nurses (RNs) make up 60% of the nursing department employees. Hospitals report budgeting 13.7% of their nursing budget for unlicensed assistive personnel (UAP). An accurate budget works with you to provide quality care.

2. Describe my managerial responsibilities regarding the staffing budget.

The end result of a properly prepared and accurate budget is a nursing staff budgeted to ensure adequate and safe nursing coverage for all patients on the unit 24 hours a day, 7 days a week, and 52 weeks a year. Your responsibilities include the following:
- Creating a cost-effective, adequate staffing plan using historical data and future predictions
- Anticipating coverage needs for all scheduled absences
- Making ongoing adjustments to staffing based on daily changes in acuity, census, or volume
- Justifying variances that occur

3. List the stages of the budgeting process.

1. Data collection stage
   - Determine activity level, such as average daily census (ADC)
   - Select skill mix needed
   - Identify types of supplemental staff to be utilized
2. Development stage
   - Calculate nursing care hours (NCH)
   - Calculate staffing pattern
   - Calculate FTE's needed or staffing requirements
   - Calculate and factor in any anticipated use of external sources, such as agency or travelers
   - Calculate and factor in the nonproductive time (holiday, vacation, sick, education)
   - Calculate and factor in anticipated overtime
3. Implementation stage
4. Evaluation stage with justification of variances

4. What is "activity"?

Staffing is usually based on some activity standard, usually identified by the finance department. For example, a nursing unit may use patient days, a clinic may use visits per month, or a surgical area may use number of cases. Some also include a patient classification system that accounts for varying patient acuity.

A commonly used standard is the ADC, or the average number of patients cared for per day during a specified period of time, usually a year.

5. How do I find the average daily census?

Find this number by using the following equation:

$$ADC = \frac{\text{Sum of daily census for 1 year}}{365 \text{ days in year}}$$

For example, if your nursing unit expects 11,349 patient days over the next year, your ADC would be:

$$\frac{11,349}{365} = 31.1 \text{ patients per day}$$

The finance department sometimes provides you with the anticipated number of patients for the upcoming fiscal year. For an in-patient unit, you can also take your occupancy percentage times the number of beds on the unit to determine the number (90% occupancy × 30 beds = 27 patients per day).

6. I manage an emergency department with monthly variances. Is there a way to plan for staffing for a varying volume?

A version of a moving ahead average (MAA) has worked for many managers in this type of situation. The MAA is a time-series analysis that is sensitive to monthly trends and more accurate than actualization.

$$\text{Forecast (f)} = (3M1 + 2M2 + 1M3)/6$$

where M1 = prior month's data, M2 = 2 months ago data, and M3 = 3 months ago data.

Example: monthly emergency department (ED) visits
January = 1800   April = 1550
February = 1750   May = 1600
March = 1650   June = 1700
July's projection = 5100 (1700 × 3) + 3200 (2 × 1600) + 1550 (1 × 1550)/6 = 1642

7. Are there standards for staffing levels?

There is no universal standard, but various professional organizations have developed their own position statements. For instance, the American Academy of Emergency Medicine's (AAEM) Position Statement (passed on 2/22/01) for Emergency Physician-to Patient ED ratio states that the ED physician staffing ratio in a comprehensive, moderate acuity ED should not exceed 2.5 patients per physician per hour (rate of influx means how many patients on average arrive in the ED in any given hour). This number was derived from a time study. They also assert that the minimum guideline for emergency nurse-to-patient ratio should be 1:3 or based on the rate of patient influx such that the rate of 1.25 patients per hour is not exceeded. (*http://www.aaem.org/positionstatements/nursetopatient.html*). Check with your professional association.

8. We have "bedded" out-patients in our unit, an out-patient surgical floor. How do other institutions account for them?

Institutions use one of four methods to account for resources needed of "bedded" outpatients. (These are distinguished from a short-term out-patient, such as an individual requiring only a simple blood specimen.) These methods are
• Adjusted in-patient day financial calculation
• Number of hours all patients were in a bed totaled with 24 hours = 1 in-patient
• Standard percentage, e.g., 1 out-patient = ½ in-patient
• Equal equivalent, e.g., 1 out-patient = 1 in-patient.

9. What about "held" patients, such as an ED holding an admitted patient while waiting for an available bed on an in-patient unit.

When there is a pattern of a large number of patients waiting for long periods of time, additional hours of care equivalent to in-patient hours per patient day should be allocated to the emergency department. See Chapter 10, Interacting within Management, for an example of one formula to accurately allocate this time.

This problem is predicted to become worse because hospital occupancy is increasing. The average reported hospital bed occupancy nationwide is 74.1% of available beds; 5 years ago it was only 60% with many hospitals at 50% occupancy.

10. What is the difference between staff distribution and skill mix?

Staff distribution is the determination of the number of personnel allocated per shift. For instance, of the total number of staff, you may want 45% of them on days, 35% of them on evenings, and 20% on nights to most closely correlate with the unit's activity flow.

Skill mix is the percentage of RNs to other clinical staff members. The goal is to plan the best mix of staff to provide good patient care and cost-effective use of the skill levels. For instance, a unit may have 70% RN and 30% nursing assistants. Skill mix does not usually does not include clerical staff, supportive services (housekeeping, laboratory, respiratory) or station filled positions, such as an administrative nursing manager who does not take a patient assignment.

The term *skill mix* is generally used for overall staff hires, but the concept can be adjusted for each shift as acuity and census change. For example, a surgical floor has a decreased census during the week of Christmas. An RN has call out sick for the 3 to 11 shift, and substituting an LPN for that RN could help control costs.

In one survey, 83% of the responding hospitals have position control systems in place. It should list out the number of full-time and part-time employees by skill mix in each department.

11. Is it best to use as many unlicensed assistive personnel (UAP) as possible to save money?

There have been cost-cutting trends to excessively replace RNs with UAP. The term UAP refers to over 50 different job titles of workers who are not highly skilled or otherwise credentialed.

It is obviously not effective use of the RN staff to do custodial tasks, such as stocking supplies. But studies show that excessive RN replacement by UAP for direct patient care has a negative effect on quality. This has been particularly evident as studies were refined to include preventable complications, unit variances, and the distinction between RN hours involved in direct patient care from the institution's total RN hours (including administration).

12. Can you give some examples of these research findings?

- Thirteen studies found that patient morbidity and mortality are adversely affected by decreasing the total number of RNs on staff and decreasing the RN component in the skill mix (Aiken and Lake, 1992; Prescott, 1993).
- The higher the percentage of nurse staffing, the lower the mortality rate was in "magnet hospitals" (Aiken, Smith, and Lake, 1994; Aiken, Havens, and Sloane, 2000).
- The percentage of hours of care delivery by RNs in the RN skill mix is inversely related to a unit's rate of medication errors, decubiti, and patient complaints (Blegen, Goode, and Reed, 1998).
- There is an inverse relationship between RNs providing care and postsurgical complications of urinary tract infections, pneumonia, and thrombosis (Kovner and Gergen, 1998).
- In a study that looked at the effects of staffing in 80% of the nation's acute care hospitals, as the number of RNs per occupied bed increased, mortality rate decreased. It also found that as the number of licensed practical nurses and hospital administrators increased, the mortality rate increased (Bond, Raehl, Pitterie, and Ranke, 1999).
- Using the 10 American Nurses Association quality indicators in acute care institutions, the single most consistent and significant predictor was the percent of RNs in the nursing staff caring for patients. As the percentage of RNs increased, so did the patients' perceptions of satisfaction with care, pain management, education, and overall care. The higher nurse staffing per acuity-adjusted day was highly correlated with shorter lengths of stay. A statistically significant finding was that the lower the nurse staffing,

the higher the incidence of more preventable conditions—pressure sores, pneumonia, post-operative infections, and urinary tract infections (ANA, 1997; Moore, Lynn, McMillen, and Evans, 1999).

13. Why would using RNs instead of UAP make such a difference?

These findings are partially attributed to the fact that nursing is much more than objective tasks. Nurses constantly (often subconsciously) assess patients during all interactions, picking up subtle cues. They have the knowledge base and professionalism to make immediate, constant judgment calls and appropriately intervene, such as with a preventive measure.

Besides, compared to UAP, RNs have a higher productivity because they can do everything. One study found UAP have 40% downtime, compared to the RNs who only had 12%. UAP typically have a high turnover rate, and it consumes significant RN time to train and supervise them.

14. What factors should be considered for an ideal staffing mix in an acute care unit?

- Skill level of the nursing staff (e.g., all new graduates or experienced veterans)
- Knowledge level of the nursing staff (e.g., < 30% are technologically competent; and < 20% have been prepared to care for complex patients)
- Accessibility of ancillary service personnel (e.g., support available from central transportation, respiratory)
- Practice behaviors of physicians (e.g., typical frequency and complexity of orders)
- Patient acuity (e.g., rehabilitation or telemetry patients)
- Intensity and acuity of care (e.g., monitoring patients with Alzheimer's disease or central lines)
- The work environment (e.g., physical layout or proximity of ancillary services)

15. So tell me what average RN percentage I should have.

There is no absolute answer. The average current skill mix nationwide in acute care is 69%. Blegen, Good, and Reed (1998) found that the correlation of patient care benefits to the increasing RN component was true up to the level of 87.5% RNs. One expert recommends at least an 80% RN staff for critical care and a 70% RN staff for an acute care medical/surgical unit.

16. What are alternatives to using UAP for the assistive work?

Some managers are only hiring certified nursing assistants (CNAs), who are required to complete 75 hours of theory and practice and an examination. Other managers are hiring only other more highly trained persons, such as emergency medical technicians (EMTs) or paramedics.

Consultant Marie Manthey's studies found that auxiliary staff are used most effectively when the auxiliary partner can do 75% of what the RN can do. When that is the case, entire clumps of duties can be delegated rather than isolated tasks. She advocates an increased use of LPNs, especially in a partnering relationship.

Many hospitals are reporting success in recruiting student nurses ("interns") who have satisfactorily completed as least one semester of clinical work. These individuals already have some knowledge, experience, and sense of professionalism, and many choose to stay after graduation.

17. What types of staff arrangement are available to supplement my unit's full-time staff?

To cover vacancies in your schedule created by vacations, holidays, sick time, and educational absences, you need to select types of replacement staff. Choices include the following:

- Casual (PRN, per diem) staff
- Part-time staff
- Baylor Plan staff
- Float nurses

• Not replacing the absent staff member
• Substituting one classification for another (e.g., LPN for RN)
• Overtime
• Staggered or overlapping shifts
• Splitting the shift in half and extending previous and following shifts into 12-hour shifts (creating planned overtime)
• Staffing only part of the shift for the vacancy
• Travelers, such as a nurse contracted for a short-term employment (3–6 months)

18. How do I calculate my NCH?
The NCH is the average required hours of care per patient per day for all levels of nursing staff. This is the actual hours of direct patient care or production time. This includes regular time, overtime, and agency/temporary time but not orientation, education, or benefit (vacation, sick) time. Hospitals vary on whether a charge nurse position that does not take a patient assignment is included in this clinical patient care time.

$$\text{NCH} = \frac{\text{Nursing hours worked in 24 hours}}{\text{Patient census}}$$

19. What is total worked hours per day?
Total worked hours is a frequently used staffing assessment term that includes orientation time, vacation time, and other nonpatient care time. Worked hours includes all direct and indirect time on the unit (such as shift report), but excludes nonproductive time, such as vacation. One 2000 national survey found reported indirect time averaged about 17% on the medical-surgical units and was higher with telemetry because of the use of a monitor technician.

20. Explain the meaning of the letters HPPD.
Hours of nursing care provided per patient day (HPPD) by all the various levels of nursing personnel is a statistic used by some hospitals instead of NCH. It is determined by dividing nursing hours by the number of patients. However, clarify whether productive or total nursing hours figures are being used for the budgeting. Out-patient areas often use the term *hours provided per patient visit (HPPV)*.

21. Describe the difference between productive and total hours in the HPPD.
HPPD as productive hours includes all staff hours worked during a set time, divided by the number of patients treated during the same time to determine the average hours of care per patient. This is the same as NCH, actual time, or actual hours worked.
Total nursing hours are calculated by adding the hours worked and the hours not worked but paid for, such as vacation, sick, or workshop time, then dividing by the number of patients.

22. What are the current national averages for HHPD?
The Lawrenz 2000 national survey of actual staffing levels founds that the mid-range reported HPPD in hospitals by unit type was as follows:
• Medical-surgical units: 6.8 to 11.8
• Telemetry units: 7.8 to 11.7.
• Critical care departments: 14.6 to 25.5
• Emergency departments: 1.9 to 3.1; the average ED HHPD was 2.2 hours
• Labor and delivery departments: 17.9 to 24.0; post partum: 7.0 to 9.7; nursery: 6.5 to 8.7
• Pediatric units: 7.6 to 16.8
• Mental health units: 6.3 to 12.7

23. Talk about the criticisms of using the HPPD as a standard to measure productivity.
The bottom line is that the amount of time needed in direct patient care should be the driving factor for measuring productivity. When total HPPD hours are used, units with high se-

niority employees (e.g. more accrued benefit time) will be at a disadvantage—one that does not reflect direct care.

But even the use of productive HPPD often does not always accurately reflect the amount of nursing time required because it treats all hours of patient care the same. Patients are "sicker," requiring more nursing interventions, in the first hours of hospitalization compared to right before discharge. The increased throughput of patients results in more admissions, discharges, and transfers, which are the most workload intense periods in a patient's length of stay. Most hospitals report that the admitting process takes between 1 and 1.5 hours of nursing time. The midnight census as a staffing guide is criticized for similar reasons.

Measures that are more reflective of the required nursing time include patient turnover (admissions/discharges), patient activity (e.g., returns from surgery, post-procedural monitoring) and/or patient acuity levels.

24. I agree that not all patients are created equal. How do you account for patient acuity?

A common method is to have a patient acuity level based on the required nursing interventions rather than the medical diagnosis. A national staffing survey found that 37% of institutions were using some type of acuity system. Some institutions purchased a system; 23% developed their own. The problem is that only 28% of all institutions using any acuity system believed that it adequately met their needs.

25. Give an example of applying an acuity system.

PATIENT ACUITY LEVEL	MINUTES OF NURSING TIME	EXAMPLES OF NURSING INTERVENTIONS FOR THIS TYPE OF PATIENT
Level 1	20 min	Admission, discharge, one procedure
Level 2	60 min	Additional two to three procedures Administer one medication
Level 3	90 min	In-patient admission/transfer IV insertion, multiple medications
Level 4	180 min	Critical care admission Cardiac monitoring Multiple procedures/medications
Level 5	250 min	Cardiac arrest Major trauma victim

Multiply the number of each level of patients by the minutes for that level to obtain total nursing minutes in direct patient care.

For example, for an ED with 30,000 visits a year:

Level 1 $11,000 \times 20$ min   or 220,000 min
Level 2 $8,000 \times 60$ min   or 480,000 min
Level 3 $7,000 \times 90$ min   or 630,000 min
Level 4 $3,500 \times 180$ min   or 630,000 min
Level 5 500×250 min   or 125,000 min

A total of 2,085,000 minutes or 34,750 nursing hours or 16.71 FTEs.

This system typically does not include secretarial, housekeeping, administrative personnel, or supportive actions, such as ordering supplies, benefit time, and regulatory agency requirements. Most institutions have a different category for patients who are "maintained" or "held" in the ED after the acute interventions are completed because there is no available inpatient bed. See Jones's formula to deal with this in Chapter 10, Interacting within Management.

26. Are there other variations?

A variation for high procedural areas is to assign points to nursing tasks according to the amount of time they ordinarily consume. For instance, taking vital signs might be 1 point, administering an intravenous antibiotic is 3 points, and inserting a nasogastric tube with irrigation is 6 points. The cumulative patient point totals are then translated into nursing time,

This approach is a varying application of the Ambulatory Payment Classifications (APCs) systems used for capturing and justifying patient classifications and charges in outpatient settings. One criticism is that is does not capture many nonprocedural but time-consuming elements of nursing, such as answering families' questions.

27. What is an FTE?

The concept of FTE, or full-time equivalent, is often confused with position. A position is a single job for one person, regardless of the hours worked by the individual in that position. An FTE, however, is a standard of one employee working for 8 hour per day, 5 days per week, 52 weeks per year.

$$8 \times 5 \times 52 = 2080 \text{ hours budgeted for each } 1.0 \text{ FTE}$$

Examples: 1.0 FTE is budgeted to work 40 hours/week = 2080 hours /year budgeted
0.4 FTE is budgeted to work 16 hours/week = 832 hours/year budgeted

One FTE position may be split into two positions, such as one for 0.4 FTE (16 hours/week) and the other for 0 .6 FTE (24 hours/week). It takes more than 1 FTE to staff a position 7 days a week (1.4 FTEs [or 56 hours] for 8-hour shifts, 2.1 FTEs for 10-hour shifts).

28. How do I find out the number of FTEs I need if I know my ADC (average daily census) and NCH (nursing care hour)?

To find the number of FTEs needed when you have an ADC of 31 and NCH of 5.4:
Use 1.4 to equal 7 days a week with a FTE 1.0 working 5 days a week (7/5 = 1.4)
Use 1.14 to equal 0.14 FTE allotted for vacation, sick, and holiday coverage for each 1.0 FTE
Use 8 to equal 1 work day (excludes lunch hours)

$$\frac{\text{ADC} \times \text{NCH} \times 1.4 \times 1.14}{8} = \frac{31 \times 5.4 \times 1.4 \times 1.14}{8} = \frac{267}{8} = 33.4 \text{ FTEs/day}$$

29. Give me an example of how to determine a staffing pattern for my unit.

Your staffing pattern will be influenced by the type of care delivery system, the staffing mix, ancillary/support staff (unit secretaries, transportation), and the patient acuity.

Begin with your NCH. You have 33.4 FTE designated for your unit. If your NCH is 5.4 and your ADC is 31.1, you can develop a staffing pattern with some simple calculations using variations on the following formula.

First calculate the number of staff required for a 24-hour period using the formula:
NCH × ADC = hours needed per 24 hours
5.4 × 31.1 = 168 hours per 24 hours
Divide 168 by 8 hours per shift = 21 shifts/24 hours

This means you will need 21 nurses, each working an 8-hour shift, to cover the 168 hours of work.

30. How do you then find out the number of each type of staff?

Use the following formula:
Total FTEs needed × % staff classification × % per shift desired = number of individual classification needed to staff daylight shift

You want the daylight skill mix to be 75% RN, 20% LPN, and 5% NA.

You want the staffing distribution to be 50% of total staff on daylight, 30% on evenings, and 20% on nights.

You would calculate your RN staff pattern using the following formula:
Total staff × % RN × % per shift = RNs needed to staff each shift
21 staff × 75% × 50% = 7.87 RNs needed for daylight
21 staff × 75% × 30% = 4.72 RNs needed for evening shift
21 staff × 75% × 20% = 3.15 RNs needed for night shift
Total RNs needed for a 24 hours shift = 7.87 + 4.72 + 3.15 = 15.7 total RNs needed in 24 hours.

31. Can you put it all together for me?

Similarly, calculate your LPN staff and nursing assistant pattern using the following formula:

Total staff × % LPN (or NA) × % per shift = LPNs (or NAs) needed to staff each shift

% PER SHIFT/ % PER CLASSIFICATION	75% RNs	20% LPNs	5% NAs	TOTAL STAFF IN 24 HR
50% daylight staff	7.87	2.1	0.52	10.49
30% evening shift	4.7	1.3	0.315	6.32
20% night shift	3.2	0.8	0.21	4.2
Total staff required	15.77	4.2	1.1	21

32. Do I have flexibility to move positions around?

Yes. As you evaluate this pattern, you may decide the NA may not be needed on nights. You have the flexibility to move that position or make it a rotating position as long as the total remains 21 staff members per 24 hours.

33. How do I calculate vacation and holiday coverage?

Number of vacation hours × number of full-time people at that skill level = Total vacation hours per skill level (You would repeat this and then add the calculation if part-time staff is entitled to vacation hours.)

Total vacation hours by skill level ÷ 2080 hours = Number of FTEs at that skill level needed for vacation coverage. This calculation may need adjustment if you have employees with a large accrued benefit bank. Similarly, holiday coverage is calculated using the number of paid holidays (provided the position needs to be covered).

34. What percentage of staffing hours do other hospitals have for the nonworked nursing hours.

Deficit demands are events that result in a nurse not being able to work, such as leaves of absences, position vacancies, and sick time. In total, deficits due to these three reasons were reported at an average of 20.7%. Hospitals reported budgeting 10.8% of worked hours for nonproductive deficit time of sick time, holidays, and vacations. However, in units with a long-tenured staff, nonproductive time may be as high as 16%.

Sick time runs at an average of 5.0% in hospitals. The National Labor Bureau reports that sick time is 3% to 5% in most female-intensive organizations.

35. How do I factor in overtime?

Most finance departments will have a set acceptable standard of overtime that you will be permitted to budget. Overtime hours are likely to increase if you have many vacant positions or an unpredictable patient flow (e.g., recovery room, emergency department) In the Lawrenz 2000 survey, hospitals budgeted on average for overtime to be 4.4% of worked hours; but actual overtime use was 5.4% of worked hours. However, in some teaching and rural hospitals, overtime was as high as 30% of worked hours.

There should be a concern if overtime hours, either voluntary or mandatory, reach 13% to 15% of the budgeted hours or more than 300 to 350 overtime hours per person. Then staff burnout and turnover become an issue.

36. What about education hours?

Most hospitals have a standard allotment; 2.5% is the average amount budgeted nation-wide for staff education in acute care hospitals. This is considered low; most successful in-dustries usually allocate 5%.

37. What is productivity?

$$\frac{\text{Required staff hours}}{\text{Provided staff hours}} \times 100 = \text{Productivity}$$

38. What does it mean when I'm asked to justify variances in my FTE budget?

A variance is a discrepancy between the amount of dollars budgeted and the actual amount spent. Identify factors that·have positively or negatively affected your actual budget. You are then expected to devise a plan of action to control or eliminate those negative factors and capitalize on those positive factors.

39. What causes a budget variance?

The judicious manager tracks daily changes and seeks to vary staffing according to the needs. Possible causes of variances include the following:
- Improper initial budgeting of productive or nonproductive time
- Unanticipated increase in daily census
- Excessive use of sick time
- Excessive staff turnover, with or without replacement staff
- Extended orientation time
- Unexpected change in skill mix
- Unanticipated increase or addition of a service
- Unbudgeted education for mandatory staff inservices

40. Tell me what things to consider when I make the budget to minimize variances.
- New programs
- Community changes (new housing, another hospital closing)
- Change in the bed capacity of the unit
- Multiple anticipated staff vacancies
- Nursing shortage/average recruitment time for your region
- Local nursing shortage for experienced nurses in your specialty (requiring you to train your own)
- Number of employees with high accumulated benefit time banks
- Seasonal variances

41. Talk about the role of turnover as it relates to staffing.

Turnover is the rate at which employees leave their jobs for reasons other than death or retirement. It is calculated by dividing the number of employees leaving by the number of workers employed in the unit during the year and then multiplying by 100. Turnover is ex-pensive because of the recruitment and orientation costs of the new staff and the need to sometimes use more expensive staff (overtime hours, agency staffing) to fulfill the vacancy in the meantime.

Nationwide, the overall RN turnover rate is 20%; lower in teaching and rural hospital (10-11%) and higher (27%) in community hospitals. In addition, 20% of new RN graduates turn over in their first year of hospital employment. Anecdotally, new graduate turnover is as high as 50% in some institutions.

42. How does "station filled" staffing fit into all this?

Station-filled staffing means that an individual is placed "at that station (position)" regard-less of the current census or need. This is commonly used for smaller, independent depart-ments. For instance, a nurse has to be available in the out-patient gastrointestinal laboratory whether there are two patients or five patients scheduled. The position cannot always be cost-effective in terms of productivity but is essential as part of the hospital's larger mission.

43. What about the use of sitters?

Lawrenz Consulting's 2000 survey found that 0.8% of the budgeted nursing positions for sitters or companions (to avoid the use of restraints). Increasing use is predicted. The use of these personnel must be planned carefully because they can cost up to $18 an hour for agency personnel or staff overtime.

One way to account for the additional staffing needs for newer regulatory requirements is to multiply the nursing minutes by the frequency of occurrence and then convert the total minutes into FTEs. One emergency department was able to justify an additional FTE using this process for three of their new, time-consuming, mandatory department regulations.

44. Are there any other trends that affect my staffing budget?

Many nurses are reducing the number of hours they work, which creates staff hour vacancies even with the same number of people working. Nationwide, there is a 20% deficiency in available RN hours. Will agency nurses and traveling nurses be an answer?

Lawrenz found that the use of premium labor, overtime, agency, and travelers nationwide was 8.7%, which exceeded the budgeted amounts but is less than 3% of the total nursing budget. Interestingly, there is a decreasing trend from previous years in the use of agency and traveling nurses. Whether this represents hospitals deciding to work with a deficient number of staff or not enough of these premium labor nurses being available is not known.

45. Any tips for success?

- Maintain a budget tickler file with reminders you have gathered throughout the year.
- Get a good calculator; become comfortable working with spreadsheets.
- Set aside some time each week to review your budget, staffing patterns, and variances.
- Keep a list of the possible reasons for variances to help with the justifications.
- Work with someone who is budget savvy. Group efforts during the development phase can be helpful to the novice.
- Use financial terms when working with your chief financial officer (CFO). They speak a different language and aren't always "bilingual." For instance, don't say more staffing helps quality patient care; indicate that there is a good cost-benefit ratio. Stress the dollar amount when an improvement is needed to prevent a regulatory agency fine.
- Assume the role of an educator. Don't assume the person in the nonclinical CFO position understands the nature of clinical work. For instance, explain what is involved in obtaining an interpreter and why it is important. Then the CFO has a basis to consider your need if 25% of your patient population doesn't speak English.
- Have relevant data and statistics to demonstrate your needs. Even when it is true, it doesn't work to tell the CFO, "We're too busy." One manager came to the budget meeting with a small wagonload of supporting material.
- Negotiate. Everyone wants to feel they get something. One manager allowed a smaller nursing hour allotment per patient level in exchange for staffing that would be determined by acuity level rather than volume alone. The unit's high acuity actually resulted in an increase in FTEs allowed.
- Be able to quote standards or benchmarks from your specialty, professional organization, or the community or region's other facilities. It takes the need beyond personal opinion. It is a stronger point to be able to say "This figure is from the staffing formula presented at the annual meeting of the _____ association which is the official professional organization of xx,xxx nurses in the United States."

BIBLIOGRAPHY

1. Aiken LH, Havens DS, Sloane DM: The magnet nursing services recognition program. Am J Nurs 100(3):26–35, 2000
2. Blegen MA, Good CJ, Reed L: Nursing staffing and patient outcomes. Nurs Res 24(1):43–50, 1998.
3. Bond CA, Raehl CL, Pitterie ME, Franke T: Health care professional staffing, hospital characteristics, and hospital mortality rates. Pharmacotherapy 19(2):130–138, 1991.
4. Finkler SA, Kovner CT: Financial Management for Nurse Managers and Executives, 2nd ed. Philadelphia, W.B. Saunders, 1999.
5. Gilles DA: Nursing Management: A Systems Approach, 3rd ed. Philadelphia, W.B. Saunders, 1994.
6. Kovner C, Gergen PJ: Nurse staffing levels and adverse events following surgery in US hospitals. Image J Nurs Scholarship 30(4):315–321, 1998.
7. Lawrenz Consulting: Annual survey of hours: Perspectives on staffing and scheduling 19(3):1–6, 1999. www.lawrenzconsult.com
8. Moore K, Lynn MR, McMillen BJ, Evans, S: Implementation of the ANA report card. J Nurs Admin 29(6):48–54, 1999.
9. Tappan RM: Nursing Leadership and Management: Concepts and Practice, 3rd ed. Philadelphia, F.A. Davis, 1995.
10. Yoder-Wise PS: Leading and Managing in Nursing, 2nd ed. St. Louis, Mosby, 1999.
11. Zimmermann PG. Pierce B: Managers Forum: Staffing standards. J Emerg Nurs 25(3):216–223, 1999.
12. Zimmermann PG: Managers Forum: Staffing standards and benchmarks. J Emerg Nurs 27(2):179–181, 2001.

10. INTERACTING WITHIN MANAGEMENT

Camilla L. Jones, RN, BBA

The most important thing in an argument next to being right is to leave an escape hatch for your opponent so that he can swing over to your side gracefully without too much apparent loss of face.

Sydney J. Harris

1. What is organizational culture?

Organizational culture is the set of values that exist in an organization, which help people in that organization understand what behaviors or actions are acceptable or not acceptable. It contains one or more of the following concepts:

- A defined belief system
- Widely shared values
- Collective thinking
- Tradition
- Patterns of discoveries, developments, and adaptations

2. How has culture changed in nursing?

Our roots in nursing stem back to Florence Nightingale, when nursing was provided strictly as a humanitarian service to others. The business aspects of medicine have changed the way we provide care to our customers. These same aspects have changed the expectations of health care consumers. Even our customer base has changed. Patients used to dominate the concern of nurses. Now, the entire family has become a unit in the care that is provided. It is a rare hospital in this environment that does not consider patients, families, significant others, physicians, employees, vendors, and the media as a part of the customer base. A health care manager's challenge includes providing care and exceeding customer expectations globally while meeting a budget.

3. Why should understanding organizational culture be a priority to me?

Organizational culture is designed to enhance performance. If managers do not understand the organizational culture in which they are operating, they will not experience success in the work environment.

4. How can I determine what culture exists in my organization?

Mission statements reflect the organization's values and philosophy. To understand the organizational culture of an institution, look at key areas such as the following:

- Customer service
- Commitment to employees
- Concern for people
- Methods of control
- Empowerment
- Decision-making processes
- Career advancement
- Responsibility (collective versus individual)
- Delegation
- Evaluation processes
- Autonomy and entrepreneurial activities
- Management styles
- Ethics and compliance
- Procedural justice

5. How can I use my organization's cultural value system in day-to-day operations?

Organizational values should be emphasized in all areas of operation, from policy and procedure to socialization of employees.

6. Can you discuss employee compliance to organizational behavior expectations?

Even the interview process is not too early to discuss organizational values. All employees should be educated to understand organizational culture during orientation to ensure that the level of performance meets expectations. Some hospitals have required formal programs regarding ethics and compliance that are centered around the organization's values, mission statement, and philosophies. Managers must lead by example to ensure compliance and ethical behavior congruent with the organizational mission.

7. How can understanding the organizational culture affect my actions?

A manager can modify his or her own approach in communication to maximize effectiveness if he or she understands and embraces organizational values. For example, if a hospital has a "prestige" culture and seeks to present itself as the cutting-edge leader in new development or technology, citing recent research will probably be better received than a social emphasis, such as relief of suffering. As another example, a hospital's culture may encourage verbal communications. A memo or e-mail message may be discarded or overlooked, but a formal or informal conversation may produce immediate action. Modifying your communication style to match the culture will help you accomplish goals.

8. Do organizational cultures change?

Culture can be affected by the following:
• Strong networking relationships
• Technology developments
• Regulating agencies
• Industry advancements
• Reward systems
• Ownership changes

However, it is rare to have a major shift of any historical approach or attitude based on any one person's input or opinion. For example, it would be difficult to change a hospital's attitude toward nursing representation in meetings if the culture of the hospital embraced physician dominance in committee structure. The manager should expect to expend effort in negotiation and consensus building to effect change in well-developed cultural environments.

9. Discuss negotiation in organizational cultures.

Negotiation involves two or more parties who come together to discuss issues and compromise to meet synergistic goals and objectives. This is usually a "give and take" interaction and involves a win-win solution.

10. Describe networking.

Networking is the process of aligning oneself with others to obtain information, ideas, advice, power, and influence. It is *not* a short-term process and requires sincere effort on the part of the participants to establish honest relationships with others. The most effective networking includes socialization between the parties and creates personal bonds. There is usually a defined goal and even though the objective may be in the future, the relationship is being developed now. Networking helps the manager create motivation for compromise during negotiation. It can also provide a platform for information gathering and influence during decision-making.

11. Discuss consensus building.

Consensus building requires networking skills and is probably the most effective component of successful negotiation. It includes informal meetings, discussion, and subsequent agreement on issues or decisions on a personal level prior to formal decision-making processes. The key to quick consensus is productive information flow. The focus is on agreement, not method. If the consensus comes from the bottom up through interpersonal interaction, by the time it is presented to administrative levels, it can be presented with confidence, credibility, and agreement. The likelihood of approval improves dramatically when all parties agree in a positive "can-do" format.

12. What are the most effective methods or techniques in negotiating?
- Know what the other parties want.
- Include all stakeholders.
- Actively listen and clarify information.
- Avoid arguing or defensiveness.
- Collect and analyze data objectively.
- Clearly state objectives and be prepared to compromise.
- Give credit to those who do the work.
- Modify managerial style to facilitate communication.

13. Talk about managerial "style."
   The four predominant styles that emerge in communications and management are driving, emotional, analytical, and amiable. All styles have something valuable to contribute to a team effort or process. Each style has different motivational anchors but all styles are motivated by receiving feedback.

14. Describe the analytical style.
   Someone who is analytical wants factual data, such as graphs and statistics. It is important to collect enough data to make the "analytical" manager comfortable. A person with this type of style is helpful in identifying strategies that can benefit the process. But, realize that this type of person must feel that the decision is a sound one to experience "win-win."

15. Discuss the driving style.
   Someone who has a driving style feels most comfortable if he or she is in a leadership role in the process. These persons are motivated toward action and can get the job done. Allow this person to have control over an element of the process to facilitate buy-in. Be sure to give the "driver" credit to create a win-win situation.

16. Talk about the emotional style.
   A manager who has the emotional style must have an opportunity to vent concerns and frustrations. Managers with an emotional style are especially effective in helping identify how others in the organization will perceive the new process or negotiated decision. Give attention and reassurance when needed. Persons with an emotional style need to feel appreciated and involved to experience win-win.

17. What about an amiable style?
   Someone who is amiable should help with communications. Most "amiable" managers have many contacts, and this stakeholder can be a valuable asset in facilitating consensus building. Persons with amiable styles are usually motivated by being recognized as an integral part of the team.

18. How can I make sure my goals and objectives are met if others are unwilling to compromise?
   The most common causes of failed negotiation involve failed maneuvers to provide recognition or power. A good manager will freely give up recognition to meet objectives. Empowerment must be given without relinquishing power if it is needed to meet the desired goals and objectives. Consensus building is the most effective tool; those elements that cannot be compromised in a negotiation should be identified in an objective and nonterritorial

manner early on in the negotiating process. Compromise may be necessary. If no agreement can be reached, a higher authority may be necessary to create a "tie-breaker." The manager must be prepared that the decision might not swing in the desired direction.

19. What is the definition of power in management?
Power is usually defined as the ability to control, influence, or act individually or within groups to accomplish objectives despite resistance. Most experts agree that power can enhance or limit organizational effectiveness.

20. Is power "bad?"
Power itself is not bad; it is considered neutral. It is a mechanism to get things done. However, people who possess power may not use power in a way that benefits all parties. Unethical uses of power include the following:
- Using power strictly for personal gain
- Censorship
- Promotion of an autocratic environment
- Satisfaction of self-interests
- Closed communications

21. Is power the same as authority?
Authority is power that has been legitimized. It is usually manifested or vested in a position. Most managers are not able to sustain the influence of power if they depend solely on authority power. They must also have a balance of other types of power to maintain effectiveness in the workplace. The most powerful people may have been assigned initial power in an organization; however, they *earn* the power that makes them effective.

22. What are the different types of power?
There are five basic types of power:
1. Legitimate power (essentially authority) is assigned by the position
2. Reward power (control over the rewards an employee can receive)
3. Coercive power (ability to punish)
4. Expert power (control through information)
5. Referent power (influence through identification, charisma, and mentorship)

Expert and referent types are considered informal forms of power.

23. What is the difference between personal, organizational, and executive power?
Personal power is usually identified as a characteristic of "influence ability." It exists within the person, regardless of their assigned authority. Personal power requires expert and referent power qualities.

Organizational power is usually identified as the ability to accomplish organizational goals through others. Organizational power includes elements of position power and executive power. This can include the ability to accomplish career goals or climb the organizational ladder.

Executive power is the use of influence to motivate employees in a positive manner to accomplish both organizational and personal goals. Executive power is the most valuable type of power to possess.

24. What are the goals of power?
Key Business Skills for Nurse Managers by Leann Strasen effectively defines the goals of power for nurse managers as the ability to be able to do the following:
- Get things done
- Implement one's ideas or visions
- Obtain physician support
- Provide appropriate human and capital resources
- Provide adequate salary
- Make a significant contribution to the organization or profession
- Survive in a difficult world

- Advance in career, economic, and professional status
- Obtain respect from colleagues
- Avoid frustrations of ambiguity in a competitive environment
- Be accountable for significant issues

25. How does style influence the effectiveness of power?

Some models suggest that growth of power style develops much like Maslow's Hierarchy of Needs. The least developmentally mature managers rely on assigned or legitimate power. As a manager matures, the model suggests that mangers move through developmental stages, using manipulation and influence, until they can rely on elements of personal power, applied as executive power.

26. Can power style be changed?

Personal power style is largely influenced by experiences, even those early experiences within a family structure. Style can be changed if the individual is motivated to change. Experiencing an effective mentor is probably one of the most common denominators that cause managers to change styles. However, managers should never expect to change the styles of others.

27. Talk about politics in the work environment.

Some form of politics exist in every work environment. Self-interest is usually acknowledged as a primary goal. Politics usually increase when resources are limited. Persons with political savvy can increase their personal and organizational power. In essence, politics is like a game. There are players in positions and a strategy. Strategies often involve defensive posturing, offensive posturing, collaboration, and, sometimes, bowing out of the game. Observant behavior and knowing who is in the game are required to determine which strategy to engage. It is easy to see the value in networking as a resource in playing the political game as it provides a mechanism to identify weaknesses and strengths that exist within the organizational or political culture. One of the most important rules for successful play in the "game" is to pick and choose your battles. If you are involved in a tug-of -war, no winner can emerge. Always try for a win-win scenario if at all possible.

28. How can I exist in a political environment without becoming "political"?

The political process depends on effective consensus building. Seek to discover and understand other players' needs and wants. One element of consensus building is the concept of future obligations. This very political situation stems from the old adage "I'll scratch your back if you scratch mine." It is different from a coalition in that goals are individualized and there is a predetermined expectation attached. The future obligation pops up when the player calls in a favor, for example, workers exchanging shifts. As long as collaboration occurs with predefined rules and expectations, and it is done honestly, this practice can strengthen relationships rather than create political "gamesmanship."

29. How important is it for me to play politics up the ladder?

Even if it is not your ambition to "move up the ladder," it is very important to understand and engage in organizational politics to "remain on the ladder" or to persevere in a complex work environment. The alternative is to be uninvolved. Politics are normal processes that exist in organizations. Each boss has his or her objectives, which are tied to political processes in one way or another.

30. How important is it for me to play politics with my employees?

Some mangers believe that the best political tactic is to come in strong and strict, then relax later as employees come into compliance. Some managers believe that it is most effective to come into a department in a nonthreatening, "I'm going to be your good friend" mode to gain cooperation. I believe that neither of these methods is as effective as setting down clear, honest expectations.

31. What do I need to know about politics and inherited employees?

It is critical that the manager assume a supervisor's role upon assuming the position, even when brought in from the ranks. Give expectations in a direct but respectful manner soon after assuming a new management role or a major change. The manager should encourage each employee to evaluate whether he or she can support the expectations. If the workers cannot, they must decide whether they want to continue working in that environment. Two common dialogues used to communicate this concept are "willing and able" or "on the ship or off the ship."

32. Give me the "willing and able" dialogue.

"Most employees are able to perform a job with adequate resources and training. Employees must ultimately decide whether they are willing to perform the job. If you are not willing to perform the job, then this job is not right for you and you must decide whether you want to stay here with little chance to succeed."

33. Provide the "on the ship or off the ship" dialogue.

"These are my expectations and this vision is where the department is going. You have to be on the ship to get to that destination. Every employee gets to choose to be on the ship or off the ship. You can't swim alongside; you can't row in the opposite direction; you have to be on or off. If you want to go to that destination on this ship, we need you. But if you are not going in same direction I am taking this department, you must choose to get off the ship."

34. Talk about the use of the "grapevine."

The grapevine is the informal communication system that exists within an organization and it is one of the most useful tools for getting positive information out. However, it is important for the manager to separate the rumor mill from the grapevine and identify acceptable entry links through credible employees. The information that is spread through the grapevine must be trustworthy or the manager will lose credibility. The grapevine is never quiescent and it will spawn its own news if legitimate news is not available. The manager can "feed" the grapevine at advantageous moments to boost morale, set expectations, or prepare employees for change. In addition, the grapevine can send information back to the manager, which may provide an accurate barometer of employee morale, satisfaction, or concerns. In some ways, the grapevine is one of the primary sources of feedback to the manager.

35. What are some key strategies if I decide to climb the ladder?
- Increase personal power
- Look for the right boss
- Make your bosses' objectives your objectives
- Support your boss
- Look for an effective management mentor
- Develop good interpersonal relationships
- Help others achieve their goals
- Be friendly
- Get to know everyone's secretary
- Learn to negotiate
- Analyze the adversary
- Be visible
- Dress the part

36. What is collaboration?

Collaboration is an interdisciplinary interaction in which interaction is necessary to achieve compatible goals. The goals between the parties may not be identical; however, the process must be agreed upon and compromise is usually involved.

37. Is a collaborative the same as a coalition?

A coalition is a form of a collaborative. It operates on a concept of synergy in which the sum of two goals exceeds what either individual could accomplish on his or her own mastery. Coalitions form when parties join forces, usually to accomplish common goals.

38. What value does a collaborative serve?

A collaborative effort promotes innovation and can resolve differences between parties. It promotes productivity by creating new goals and objectives that supersede the original ones through finding common ground. It is the ultimate win-win situation.

39. Can conflict cause problems in the process?

Conflict is frequently present. If conflict escalates or remains unresolved, it can cause major disruptions in an organization. Nurses and physicians who "duke it out" on a nursing unit can leave the staff shaken, the unit operations fractured, the physician agitated, and the patient afraid that no one is looking out after his or her best interests.

Although conflict is generally thought of as unproductive, focused conflict can generate opportunity and stimulate healthy competition. The reaction to conflict is dependent on goal compatibility and finding common ground so that a compromise is desired by both parties. In the hospital, patient care is frequently that common ground.

40. How important is relationship to the process?

Previous networking establishes relationships that provide motivation for both sides to compromise and avoid power struggles. This is an important reason to always seek networking opportunities early in a business situation, before conflict is an obstacle.

41. Discuss tips for communication during conflict.
- Let the other person/side speak first.
- Listen and verify that you have understood the point of view.
- Withhold judgment until all facts are out and all sides have spoken.
- Work toward a solution that allows everyone to "save face," particularly a senior administrator or physician.
- Avoid offending or using challenging language. It makes the other party retreat and defend rather than work toward an acceptable compromise.

For more discussion on this topic, see the chapter on negotiation.

42. How do I make sure the message I intended to send is received well?
- Communicate in a manner that the other party will relate to and understand.
- Maintain a global view. If too much time is spent stating "my people need this or that," the manager will be perceived as narrowly focused, and credibility will be lost.
- Allow other parties to speak first, taking notes.
- Seek common ground to tie in goals during your presentation.
- Avoid defensiveness at all costs.

43. What if a volatile issue arises or a decision seems imminent that will not work?

You may want to "hold your cards to the vest" at this time. Most decisions in collaborative efforts are not made in the first meeting. Ask for time to collect information and then use the time to do some informal consensus building.

44. What are some specific things to keep in mind when collaborating with physicians?
- Work with the clinical experts with whom they have pre-established relationship.
- Schedule meetings at the most convenient time for everyone involved
- Allow the physician to present his/her information first.
- Connect your goals and objectives to the physician's goals

• Avoid defensiveness or confrontation.
• Try for a compromise, but be willing to lose the battle to win the war.

45. What are some specific things to keep in mind when collaborating with administrators?
• Administrators need factual, not anecdotal, information. As they say, "In God we trust, all others bring data."
• Use bullet-style presentations that summarize.
• Do not "sweat the small stuff." Focus on outcomes rather than how to get there.
• Consensus build before you get to the negotiating table.

46. Can you give an example?
In our emergency department, we sometimes "hold" admitted patients until an in-patient bed is ready. This requires additional staff, but it isn't effective to simply tell the chief operating officer (COO) or chief nursing officer (CNO) that "we are really busy" and we need more resources. I developed the following formula to justify our increased staff numbers.
Standard, benchmark, or fixed information:
Average length of stay (LOS) = 140 minutes
Variables:
X = census
Z = adjusted census
Y = number of patients in ED longer than 6 hours
T = average LOS in minutes of Y
The formula uses the referenced fixed and variable data to demonstrate increased volume represented:

$$Z = \frac{(TY - 140Y) + X}{140}$$

The average LOS in this ED is 140 minutes. If 83 patients came to the ED in 24 hours and 10 stayed more than 6 hours at an average of 513 minutes, the following adjusted census formula is true:

$$Z = \frac{(513 \times 10) - (140 \times 10)}{140} + 83$$

$$= \frac{5130 - 1400 + 83}{140} + 83$$

$$= 26.64 + 83 = 109.64 \text{ patients (adjusted census)}$$

The adjusted labor-hour per patient ratio (109 patients instead of 83) helps the COO and CNO understand why more labor-hours were needed to care for patients, even though the overall department census did not increase on this day.

47. What are things to keep in mind when collaborating with peers?
• Communicate in a manner the other party can understand.
• Remember that managerial peers possess the same passions about their own units as you possess for your unit. If limited resources exist, there will definitely be competition.
• Avoid focusing on individual needs. Look for connected goals.
• Avoid making comments that suggest how other departments should change operations. Instead, ask questions that allow the other manager to come to a conclusion on their own.
• Discuss what you, not they, can give and take.
• Avoid aggressive confrontation. Think "save face."
• Give credit away whenever possible. Keep focused on the outcome rather than who did what to get there.
• Take breaks if conflict is becoming too disruptive.
• Be sincere. Demonstrate good faith.
• Don't be afraid to apologize.

BIBLIOGRAPHY

1. Brooks E, Odiorne GS: Managing by Negotiations. Malabar, FL, Krieger Publishing, 1990.
2. Edler R: If I Knew Then What I Know Now: CEOs and Other Smart Executives Share Wisdom They Wish They'd Been Told 25 Years Ago. New York, Berkley Books, 1997.
3. Jurrens WG: Junior Executive NEC: Interview. Austin, TX, 2001
4. Marett BE: President's message: Emergency nursing in perspective: Mentoring, sharing, supporting. J Emerg Nurs 26:401–402, 2000.
5. Meinecke J: No nurse is an island. Nurs Manage 31:35–36, 2000.
6. Moorehead G, Griffin RW: Organizational Behavior. Boston, Houghton Mifflin, 1995.
7. Strasen L: Key Business Skills for Nurse Managers. Philadelphia. J.B. Lippincott, 1987.

11. MANAGED CARE CONCERNS

Robert D. Herr, MD, MBA, CMCE

Then, as now, however, the experts did not always see eye to eye. Although everyone agreed that phlebotomy and the administration of purges could be positively beneficial, even for the hale and hearty, there was some difference of opinion over the most effective dates for ridding the body of unwanted humours. According to one English vernacular source, dropsy could be prevented by letting blood on 17 September, migraine by a similar exercise on 3 April and blindness by a repeat performance eight days later. But in 1437 a lively controversy erupted at the University of Paris over the best time for taking laxatives in January.

Carole Rawcliffe, 1995

1. What is managed care?

The term *managed care* is a pejorative for any involvement of a "third party" in medical care for the purposes of supervising the cost of care. Usually the third party is a payer of all or a portion of the cost. However, the payer can hire a firm to oversee the costs of care on their behalf, paying the firm a fee for doing so. This firm then manages the care costs by seeking discounted fees from practitioners and facilities, limiting payment only to certain areas "covered" under the health insurance, and denying payment for procedures and treatments that are not "medically necessary."

The spectrum of managed care plans is wide. It ranges from Veterans' Hospital, which salaries practitioners and owns facilities, to discounted fee-for-service Medicare or Workers Compensation. In those arrangements, you can go to any practitioner who participates in the plan; that is, who signs a contract agreeing to the fee schedule and certain regulations of the plan.

2. What are the key terms and characteristics in understanding managed care?

- *Enrolled member*, meaning an individual whose premium has been paid for that month
- *Participating provider*, namely a doctor, midlevel practitioner, hospital, or clinic that sees an individual member
- *Claim*, or bill submitted by a participating provider to the managed care company
- *Fee schedule*, or agreed upon rate of reimbursement to the provider
- *Capitation*, or monthly fee that covers all enrolled members for a particular service
- *Disenrollment*, or removal of individual from group of those care costs are covered by the managed care plan, usually because of failure to pay the premium
- *Authorization*, or commitment of the plan to pay for care
- *Denial*, or refusal of the plan to pay for care
- *Medical necessity*, or premise for determining whether a service is covered under the plan
- *Noncovered*, or outside of coverage, or a benefit such as prescription drugs that is not a purchased benefit by the member or the member's employer
- *Utilization review*, sometimes called *care management*, or the process for tracking the care and determining if the care is medically necessary.
- *Restricted access plans*, requires contact with a primary care physician prior to payment for specialty care
- *Point of service* plan gives a discount for contact with the primary physician before a specialist is seen but allows direct access to the specialist for a higher copay, coinsurance, or deductible

3. Let's be honest. Isn't managed care really about shareholders making money?

Managed care conjures images of unhappy patients, frustrated practitioners, and faceless bureaucrats who, according to stereotype, deny vulnerable people expensive medical care in order to line their own pockets.

To be fair, many firms do earn the pejorative by only managing costs instead of improving care. Real managed care derives from improving the coordination of medical care by encouraging preventive care (e.g., immunization, mammography), systematic record keeping, or directing members to a primary care practitioners' office where care can be coordinated. Coordinating care improves information given to consultants, reduces redundant testing, directs referrals to the right consultant at the right time, and helps prevent errors from incompatible medications and conflicting treatment regimens. Coordinating care can reduce costs not through denying care, but through satisfying individuals with the appropriate level of care that optimizes their outcome of treatment, satisfaction, and feelings of support and trust not just in their practitioner, but in the company they work for.

4. What are some opportunities and benefits from the decision to work more closely with a managed care plan?

"Managed care groups could conceivably help practitioners forge a new doctor-patient relationship free of burdens such as cost, access, time, and administrative hassles."—David Nash, MD, MBA (1994)

David Nash's vision of managed care reducing hassles to practitioners is nearly a reality, with certain offices that demonstrate cost-effective care of high quality. I have seen both hospital-based and clinic-based nurse managers who have worked closely with one or more health plans to earn exemption from preauthorization requirements for surgery and referrals.

Even if you need to call for authorization, using the right form and knowing when and when not to call for authorization will help. A well-working system will reduce the hassle to patients, paperwork, and rework, while it increases payment and increases office staff and practitioner satisfaction.

5. What is in it for hospital nursing?

Hospital-based nursing bears the burden as a high-cost area of care from health plans' focus on hospital in-patient days. Most hospitals are already using some form of pathway for in-patient care to make care more efficient and consistent and to build teams (Renvoize et al., 1997). This benefits clinical quality. The overwhelming number of decisions in inpatient general medicine rests on evidence from sound clinical trials. However, there is room for improvement. One study found that 10 of 150 charts of medical in-patients had decisions that could have been improved significantly through adherence to a guideline (Michaud et al., 1998). The managed care plan is likely also to be interested in efficiency. Working with the plan could help the hospital staff adopt a wider use of guidelines, while tracking the use through its utilization management (UM) personnel.

Working with the managed care plan exposes the staff to the resources of the entire chain of care from the out-patient setting to the emergency department (ED) to in-patient care to rehabilitation to home or long-term care. The health care system works best when high-risk, high-cost, acute in-patient care is used appropriately and efficiently. The end result is quality, cost-effective care.

The plan can also benefit the hospital's bottom line. Hospitals are reimbursed through Medicare on a diagnosis-related group (DRG) basis. The hospital gets a sum based on the DRG diagnosis rather than the billed charges or length of stay. The hospital wants Medicare patients evaluated and discharged in a timely, though safe, manner. Working with the plan's utilization review (UR) nurses will help accomplish that.

As the hospital proves its cost-effective operation to the plan, it will begin to transfer out-of-network patients to be admitted to your hospital. This can improve the hospital's payer mix and volume.

Working with the plan's UM can support getting more staffing and services. The managed care plan's UM staff is frequently on site at the hospital, sparing the hospital budget's for that type of position. The managed care plan's UM nurses typically identify potential avoidable days or payment denials based on delay of care, such as not having diagnostic tests available on weekends or holidays. The hospital administration will have to view the cost of this lost revenue against the cost of providing the service or staff. The benefits of additional services become apparent. Your role can be to raise the appropriate questions with the hospital administration.

6. What's in it for clinical nursing?

Clinic-based nurse managers benefit from maintaining status as a preferred provider in the managed cared plan. Demonstrating efficient use of the hospital, ED, and ancillary testing can earn exemption to UR/preauthorization requirements. This improves your throughput of patients. This in turn increases your clinic's value to the managed care plan, and they will direct more referrals to the clinic.

7. What's in it for practitioners and their practices?

All practitioners can favorably influence managed care plan coverage and policies specific to their practice. Managed care plans usually welcome participation in committee work in quality assurance (QA), UR, pharmacy and therapeutics (P&T), or medical technology review.

When I served as medical director of a statewide HMO, I was surprised by how much a practitioner could influence coverage through reviewing appeals. The practitioner would be sent cases in his specialty that were denied coverage by the medical director. The member would then appeal the decision. The practitioner would review the case in light of the literature and managed care plan guidelines and comment on appropriateness of paying for the care.

I have seen practitioners gain an audience within the managed care plan for articles that influence coverage decisions, especially in controversial areas such as plastic surgery, dermatology, allergy, and family practice.

Any clinic practitioner can help get claims paid promptly by establishing relationships with claims staff that promotes payment of "gray" area claims. The claims staff then will call you for clarification before paying, rather than just denying the claim and requiring you to appeal the denial.

Another benefit of working with the managed care plan is discovering more options for care that may be offered by the plan. For example, terminally ill patients may be completely covered for hospice care. Chronically ill patients may qualify for case management that gives them added attention and helps your office implement a care plan.

8. Is it best to join many plans to maximize the managed care opportunities?

Each of the mentioned benefits depends on establishing an ongoing working relationship with one to three managed care plans. Many providers have six or more plans, and then this is impossible.

Efficient use of scarce time suggests that it is best to concentrate on major plans with greatest revenues to your practice. Some benefits hinge on relationships with managed care plan employees in claims and provider relations. Therefore, focus on stable plan with employees who will remain with the company.

9. I get so frustrated dealing with a managed care plan bureaucracy. I don't see where it is worth it.

Actually, tolerating the managed care plan bureaucracy will distinguish you as a quality practitioner. Establishing an effective working partnership requires putting up with frustrations, such as periodic long telephone queues, multiple call transfers, misplaced and mispaid claims, and communication breakdown. It is no secret that few practitioners or their staff will tolerate this. Most give up.

Your ability to work with the company representatives will distinguish you and can result in considerable influence and power at the managed care plan. You can be a big fish if you want to be. A few perks will come your way, such as a "backline" to get around the telephone queue. Always ask for the same person in claims, utilization, or other department.

If possible, choose the managed care plan to enroll you and your employees for coverage. Paying revenue to the managed care plan puts you in the position of customer as well as provider. You then have a great opportunity of getting to know the plan from multiple perspectives.

10. What are the steps in joining a managed care plan as a provider?

1. First understand what the plan wants in the spectrum of its managed care. Each of these distinguishes the company:
   • Along axes of management oversight for members
   • Of local versus national company
   • Of population insured
   • Of who has financial risk for cost of care

2. Take stock of your perceived importance to the plan in terms of its members and dollars. Are you a big fish or a small fry? Is this the plan for you?

3. Discuss joining this plan with the managed care office at your hospital or physician group practice.

4. Arrange one or more meetings with managed care plan representatives discussing what the areas of difficulty will be.

5. Try it out. Encourage meetings of people you depend on such as billing, front office, and so on with managed care plan representatives to air issues.

6. Work with the managed care plan to resolve problems. After you have seen enough patients, you will understand what difficulties have emerged. Collect specific cases (patient name and managed care plan number with date of service) and forward them to the managed care plan in advance of the meeting so that their history can be researched.

11. What do you do if you are told your organization (or physician) has just become a participating providing in a managed care plan?

Contact the Office of Managed Care at your organization to determine what is expected of you and what you can expect of the managed care plan. Ask specifically about facility fees and professional fees since contracts will address them separately. However, your decisions will likely have an impact on both areas. Also, seek a direct communication to the provider representative at the managed care plan. Direct remaining questions to that individual and arrange regular meetings to discuss concerns.

12. How do you recognize managed care plan patients?

My experience shows that few people, including me, truly understand all of their insurance coverage, even when they need it. Health insurance is no exception. Policy language has been simplified compared to 10 years ago, but there is still a gap between the enrollee's hope for universal coverage and the reality of the low-cost plan they purchased.

An individual may not recall that they changed managed care plans since their last visit. In fact, the individual can stay with the same managed care plan and change coverage, deductibles, provider networks, and need for preauthorization. Managed care plans themselves complicate things when they change the appearance of membership cards and send them to members who have had no change in any coverage.

Few individuals understand how a small change in health insurance can totally change the way their care is delivered. I recall one example of trying to arrange an air evacuation from a remote clinic in a national park. I contacted a managed care plan listed on a patient's card. We arranged a receiving physician, booked a fixed wing aircraft, gave report to both the physician and the receiving ED physician, and loaded the patient into the ambulance. As the ambulance doors were about to shut, the patient's wife produced another membership card to a different health plan. He had dual coverage, but the new plan rated primary coverage. Each of the previous arrangements for transfer had to be changed. It was exasperating.

The point is to routinely ask about change in health insurance whenever a patient presents, especially established patients. Many companies offer benefits to domestic partners of employees, and the patient may have a card with a same-sex partner as primary policy-holder. In addition, place signage that alerts potential patients to your new participation when your organization joins a managed care plan as a listed provider.

13. How do you handle it when a specialist to whom you just referred a patient cannot see the patient without a referral approved by the managed care plan?

Some plans are moving away from the primary physician as a "gatekeeper," but most of those plans allow direct access to the specialist only for a price. The patient pays either a higher deductible or higher coinsurance or co-pay.

If the managed care plan policy requires this, it likely wants to make sure the patient goes to a network provider. Ask the plan why they require preauthorization of referrals. The need could be addressed over the phone with a plan representative if it is due to "medical necessity" or "direction to a network provider." The payoff is that once you understand the rules, you can spend less time on the phone and less re-work from retracting or modifying referrals already given to patients.

This advice also applies to the case in which the specialist will not schedule the patient without preauthorization. This UM strategy may be intended to keep the member in the preferred provider network. The plan provider relations (PR) representative checks whether the specialist is on the list and, if not, gives a choice of those who are.

14. Information was sent to the office showing excessive referrals to some specialties. You are asked to begin notifying the managed care plan prior to making these referrals. Now what?

It sounds like you are being subjected to scrutiny for unconventional referrals. Ask questions.

- *How large a "net" did they throw that caught your practice?* Because a generalist typically can refer to 20 different specialties, odds alone will cause some categories to be significantly high and others significant low without truly inappropriate referrals.
- *What was the size of the sample?* A low sample size of members can cause a few referrals to distort things, again without indicating the need to change.
- *Which practitioners are being compared?* Internists, family practitioners, pediatricians, and general practitioners will all have different referral characteristics; comparing among them is not too helpful. Comparison within a specialty can be useful.
- *Is the information adjusted for Medicare-aged patients?* This group of patients typically has a higher rate of referrals.
- *Do the specialists to whom you refer have expanded robust practices?* For instance, neurologists performing their own electroencephalography or electromyography, or dermatologists doing surgery? This means that high referrals to one specialty are associated with lower referrals to another specialty. If so, the managed care plan should cluster their referral rates together in these specialties before attempting to compare your practice with their information.

15. What if none of these distinctions apply?

Then the information may be helpful. Each practitioner or team practices differently, and referral patterns can speak to their comfort with handling certain conditions themselves. This not only can cost the managed care plan more but also can cause inconvenience to patients who must undergo the referral.

Practitioners may need to enhance their skills in weaker areas, perhaps with the help of the managed care plan or its network specialists giving inservices. I have seen orthopedists give successful half-day seminars in "office orthopedics" to internists to reduce the number of "unnecessary referrals" to them. In my experience, this proactive approach works better than having to call the managed care plan for preauthorization and of course is less "hassle" to the plan's preauthorization department as well.

16. A managed care plan representative has presented data showing that the length of stay and number of hospital admissions is higher for my organization than for other organizations. Now what?

First, you want to determine the intent of the communication. Most likely, the managed care plan would like your organization to reduce its hospital admissions or length of stay.

Second, determine whether the data are truly comparable:

• Have the admissions been adjusted for your group's number of members or member-months?

• Is their adjustment for number of Medicare beneficiaries (who typically get hospitalized at five times the rate of those not getting Medicare)?

• Are there outliers whose long stay or frequent re-admits slanted the overall data?

If the answers show that your group is comparable to others, and your hospital admits or lengths of stay are higher than others, it's time to take stock of your practice and its overall higher expense to the managed care plan.

17. How do you resolve issues in preauthorization for surgery? We do not have the staff to spend time on the telephone to get preauthorization.

There are two common problems. The operating room (OR) scheduling won't schedule the managed care patient for surgery until it is cleared with a managed care plan, or the managed care plan has added a frequently-performed procedure (e.g., hysterectomy) to its list of surgeries requiring preauthorization. Both situations speak to the managed care plan fearing it will have to pay for unneeded surgery. It is best to find out specifically how you can exempt your practice from these requirements. Contact the MC Plan provider relations representative to determine its preauthorization policy. You may be able to exempt your office from it if the utilization is in line with what is expected.

If you can look at your own practice data by payer class, this may persuade the managed care plan to exempt you. Otherwise, you have to rely on their data. You should review it carefully, asking the same questions you would about referral patterns (see question 16). No managed care plan likes to give preauthorization, and hysterectomy is one of the toughest procedures to preauthorize.

Of course, the preauthorization is not needed and will not be obtained if the surgery is not covered under the plan, such as cosmetic surgery. Patients will have to decide whether they are willing to pay for it.

18. The patient wants an excision of a lipoma. He says it is irritating him and is not "cosmetic surgery," but his managed care plan is very strict. What do you recommend?

You owe it to the patient to accurately document the extent of his discomfort and any supporting evidence that the condition is a threat to health or life. You owe it to the managed care plan to likewise adequately document the condition and diagnosis. Just keep a professional distance from the patient's concern about payment. Ultimately, the issue is between the patient and his insurance carrier.

You are the medical expert, but do not lose sleep or intentionally misrepresent a condition solely to justify coverage. Doing so can lead down a slippery slope of deceit. I have seen more than one patient threaten to expose a practitioner who previously had gone out on a limb to justify insurance payment for a cosmetic condition. Such patients tend to ask for other favors. A few will seek to manipulate you into clearly illegal activity, and you are vulnerable because you have more at risk than they do, such as medical licensure, narcotic prescribing privileges, and good will of the public. Lastly, patients enjoy legal rights to confidentiality that you as a physician or nurse do not. Imagine how you will explain things to a reporter when you cannot mention the patient's condition, diagnosis, medications, or medical history.

19. How do you respond in the emergency department to the managed care patient?

Federal laws under COBRA and EMTALA have repeatedly said that patients must be seen and stabilized without regard to their method of payment (Herr, 1998). While this law originally guaranteed the rights of the uninsured to emergency care and treatment of active labor, its interpretation extends to any barrier between the patient and initial assessment and treatment. This initial care is called the "emergency screening examination." Although the law does not specify what a screening examination actually entails, the overriding rationale is a common sense approach to giving the patient the essential treatment until his or her life or limb is no longer threatened. Once the patient is stabilized, the screening examination has ended, and form of payment can be considered.

The managed care plan cannot delay care for preauthorization as long as there is an emergency. What defines an emergency? Most states and the federal government through Medicare and Medicaid have adopted the so-called prudent layperson definition (Herr, 1998). Any condition of sudden onset, including severe pain, that a prudent layperson possessing average education would consider an emergency should be considered an emergency under the law.

20. How long do you wait to have the managed care plan physician call back if the patient needs a hospital admission?

The most recent EMTALA law specifically cites the obligation of the emergency physician to contact the managed care plan for post-stabilization treatment. However, if the managed care plan does not respond within 30 minutes, there should be no obligation to the managed care plan. You should go ahead and admit the patient just as you would if the patient were not covered under the managed care plan.

21. How do you handle it if the managed care plan calls back and wants the patient transferred to a designated hospital for admission?

Federal law protects patients from involuntary transfer and requires their written consent prior to transfer. However, the managed care plan does not have to pay for the post-stabilization care at the out-of-network facility. Therefore, you need to tell the patient that the plan will pay for the admission only if he or she agrees to the transfer. Offer to admit the patient to your facility and leave the decision to them. Most will agree to the transfer.

Your professional obligation is to be relatively certain that the risks of transfer are minimal. If you foresee that the patient's life is at risk, or that the receiving facility does not have the resources to care for the patient, then you should use your professional judgement. You should inform the managed care plan of this, state your opposition to the transfer, and give the patient the benefit of your opinion about the risks. Then, you can encourage the patient to stay for admission and appeal the coverage decision.

If the managed care plan still desires the transfer, you have the right to demand that care be transferred to a managed care plan physician *after* that physician has physically appeared and examined the patient. I work at a Kaiser-affiliated managed care plan and we have on-call physicians who will appear in an ED, accept responsibility for the care, and ride in the ambulance with the patient. This arrangement has worked out very well for the transferring ED and the patient.

22. Our problem is that managed care plan UR staff will call the hospital and indicate we should discharge a patient, as he no longer needs to be there. What is the best way to handle that?

This kind of call is always provocative. Ask for the basis of "decertifying" coverage of the hospital day. The managed care plan will quickly tell you what basis it has for deciding to stop coverage. If you disagree, the decision should be appealed by either the hospital or the patient. Such "urgent" appeals require review by the managed care plan medical director or a designee. Appeals under Medicare must be completed within 72 hours.

Of course, if you feel that the patient's continued stay is discretionary, or due to social circumstances, you can either discharge the patient as suggested or enlist the managed care plan's support to provide adequate alternative to hospitalization.

23. What do you recommend if a patient or pharmacist says the medication prescribed is not covered by his managed care plan?

After double-checking to make sure the prescription accurately reflects what was ordered (prescribing errors happen!), ask the physician to change it to some comparable drug (if it exists). You can get a lists of covered medications in the same class from the pharmacists, the Plan's provider representative, or a published formulary (if you can find it in the office).

24. How about if the patient requests a change in the diagnosis to a condition covered by the managed care plan?

Although it is insurance fraud to blatantly misrepresent a diagnosis to get payment, my experience is that the patient is often right. The diagnosis was accurate, but another related diagnosis would also be accurate and be reimbursable under insurance.

25. How do you handle it when a patient has a change that means he or she is now out of the managed care plan?

The managed care plan UR staff or patients themselves can inform you that due to an employer-initiated change you are a not a participating provider in the new plan. No one can tell a patient whom to see or not to see. However, a managed care plan can decline to pay for the care under the plan's terms, with certain provisions of coverage mandated by the State Insurance Commission.

One provision is the right of an individual to "continuity of care." State laws differ on the definition of this, but in general it means that the managed care plan must pay for care if the patient suffers from an acute medical condition, including illness or injury. I have seen practitioners try to overinterpret this to apply to any member who has a chronic illness. However, it is more fairly applied to individuals undergoing intensive care or any care during which a change in attending physician or facility could threaten their recovery.

26. How do you resolve issues in a patient whose insurance has expired?

For whatever reason, some people collect expired membership cards instead of destroying them. How do you know for sure if he is still a member? The best way is to call the managed care plan to verify coverage. It is a good idea to do this if the member is about to run up a big bill for treatments that could be deferred until later or you need to make a pivotal decision about referral, testing, or hospitalization.

There is still a loophole. The managed care plan may not cover the patient if the employer did not let the managed care plan know the member was no longer covered (see your contract language) In this case, you could still be left "holding the bag" and not get paid.

27. At the end of the patient's evaluation, you find that the patient is a member of a managed care plan that your organization does not participate in as a provider.

You want to encourage the patient to check with their managed care plan for follow-up care or prior to referring for testing or consultation. Your office will likely get paid in full if the visit fits into one or more of several categories. These include (1) an emergency medical condition in the member's perception, (2) you are continuing care from previously when you were a provider in the member's health plan, or (3) the member needs care but is not close to a contracted facility or provider. You could even get your full fee from the plan. If the plan decides not to cover the payment, you are usually able to bill the member for payment.

28. When can you balance-bill the patient?

Most managed care plan contracts allow you to balance-bill the patient only if the patient and managed care plan agree that this is not a covered service, or the member's coverage has expired. Most provider contracts stipulate that you cannot balance-bill the member if you provide a service that is not "medically necessary." This means if the coverage is denied, you will not be paid and the patient does not need to pay. Keep in mind that if the hospital day is denied, so too may be professional charges for consulting or attending practitioners on that day.

29. What other payors should I concede?

There are some rules of thumb for suspecting there is another insurance that may pay. The following are generalizations that you can use to ask about other coverage:

- Occurred at work—Workers Compensation ("Labor and Industry" in some states)
- Age over 65 years—Medicare
- Children—Medicaid or CHIP
- Disabled—often Social Security Disability (SSI)
- Nursing home patient—often Medicaid

30. How should we handle a patient's request for release of their medical information to a new provider?

There are new considerations related to the Health Insurance Portability and Accountability Act (HIPAA). These new privacy regulations were signed in by President Clinton, published December 28, 2000, and must be implemented for employer-sponsored group health plans by April 14, 2003.

HIPAA tightens patient confidentiality and the release of medical information (related to past, present, or future conditions) in nonemergencies. Violators are subject to civil penalties and prosecution, with the determining factor not based on the actual harm done but "on the willingness of the covered entity to achieve voluntary compliance."

According to HIPAA, no information can be released without a signed statement from the patient giving permission and specifying the intended recipient and the scope of information to be released. The only exception is when the life of the patient is in jeopardy.

31. We received a form requesting a managed care patient's record be copied—at our expense—and forwarded to managed care plan on a patient who is appealing his coverage for the visit. Are we required to do that?

This form refers to the contract with the managed care plan. Many contracts refer to the right of the managed care plan to review all medical records on its members. Many contracts also require that the copies be made at the expense of the provider, be it hospital or medical practitioner. In contrast, most attorney's offices will offer reimbursement for copying records. Then again, the attorney may be suing you; the managed care plan usually is not.

BIBLIOGRAPHY

1. Congress adopts prudent layperson standard for Medicare/Medicaid enrollees. Managed Care Emerg Depart 1:90, 1997.
2. Herr RD: COBRA and the required screening examination. J Emerg Nursing 24(2):180, 1998.
3. Herr RD: Managed care and the emergency department: Nursing issues. J Emerg Nurs 24(5):406–411, 1998.
4. Michaud G, McGowan JL, van der Jagt R, et al: Are therapeutic decisions supported by evidence from health care research? Arch Intern Med 158(15):1665–1668, 1998.
5. Nash DB: Overview. In The Physician's Guide to Managed Care. Gaithersburg, MD, Aspen Publications, 1994, pp 1–11.
6. Rawcliffe C: Astrology and the occult. In Medicine and Society in Later Medieval England. London, Sandpiper Books Ltd, 1995, pp 82–104.
7. Renvoize EB, Hampshaw SM, Pinder JM, Ayres P: What are hospitals doing about clinical guidelines? Qual Health Care 6(4):187–191, 1997.

12. BUSINESS STRATEGY

Polly Gerber Zimmermann, RN, MS, MBA, CEN

Without a strategy the organization is like a ship without a rudder, going around in circles. It's like a tramp; it has no place to go.

Joel Ross and Michael Kami

1. What is strategic planning?
A strategy is action planning in response to a comprehensive analysis of a business in relation to its industry, its competitors, and the business environment for both the short- and the long-term. It is the total business plan on how the organization will achieve its goals. This usually involves an external assessment to look at opportunities and potential threats and an internal assessment to identify its strengths and weaknesses. It can be done on a network, an institution, or a unit basis.

2. Is strategy the exclusive element?
Strategy is just one of the elements typical of the best-managed companies. The strategy must fit the organization and be interwoven within its fabric. The other six are
- *Structure:* organization; policies, procedures, and processes for making decisions and interacting with the outside environment
- *Style:* culture (aggregate of behaviors, thoughts, beliefs, and symbols); the common way of behaving and thinking among employees
- *Staff:* human resource systems, including training, wages, motivation
- *Skills:* distinctive abilities (newest technology, bilingual staff); employees will know how to do their jobs and keep current with innovations
- *Systems:* procedures, formal and informal, by which an organization operates
- *Shared values:* guiding concepts

3. How does this relate to a mission statement?
All of these strategical elements are combined into a mission statement, which is a statement of goals and priorities. The mission statement should be clear, concise, and inspiring. A good mission statement should be market oriented, realistic, specific, and motivating; illustrate distinctive competencies; and provide a vision.

4. Give an example.
Many health care organizations tend to have similar statements that are long, bland, and tedious. After hearing a mission statement such as "We will give the best health care possible." I personally am tempted to ask, "Is there any healthcare organization in American whose goal is to give mediocre or inferior care?"

Look at the business world to understand the distinctions that are possible. For instance, Federal Express's mission had used a simple direct guarantee: to deliver the package overnight. Regardless. Compare that to Chrysler's mission, which emphasizes key aspects of implementation: Our primary goal is to achieve consumer satisfaction. We do it through engineering excellence, innovative products, high quality, and superior service.

5. I'm still not convinced strategy is needed. Our goal as nurses is to provide health care for people.
You need direction. A famous passsage from *Alice in Wonderland* sums it up:
Alice: "Would you tell me, please, which way ought I to go from here?'

Cheshire Cat: "That depends a good deal on where you want to get to."
Alice: "I don't much care where..."
Cheshire Cat: "Then it doesn't matter which way you go."

6. What are the five forms that strategy can take?
Plan, ploy, pattern, process, and perspective.

7. Talk about the levels of strategy.
Strategy takes place on three different levels:
1. Functional: value activities you engage in (e.g., an out-patient clinic adds a new service)
2. Business: fighting competition (e.g., your hospital tries to be the provider of choice for childbirth)
3. Corporate strategy: "What business should I be in?" (e.g., is it prevention or cure or hospice? pediatrics or maternity or elder care?)

8. What generic business strategies can hospitals implement?
- *Cost leadership:* Offering the lowest cost to the patient (even if you are a loss leader) or doing so many procedures that you have economies of scale (e.g., costs you less).
- *Differentiation:* Make your service different in the mind of the consumer (often through advertising), using slogans such as "we care more" or "we're the experts" or by emphasizing location. One emergency department (ED) markets only a 60-minute wait to see the doctor in the ambulatory emergicenter, or the visit is free. This strategy creates a competitive advantage by offering unique customer benefits, which often helps compete against lower-cost rivals.
- *Focus:* Concentrate on one market segment and know it very well. This narrow segment emphasis is often on quality or benefits. Examples include the pediatric hospital or Alzheimer unit.
- *Middle-of-the-road:* Institutions that do not pursue one of the above general strategies often lack a focus. They may survive, but they are vulnerable to more focused competitors and will have difficulty reacting to environmental change, such as an economic downturn.

9. Discuss integration.
Integration means that you are participating at various spots in the value chain. For instance, the hospital providing a visiting nurse or health screening service, in addition to acute care, meets the patients at various places on their continuum of health.

10. How often should the business strategy be reviewed?
Five years used to be the conventional wisdom. In today's fast-paced, changing society, most say a 3-year (or sooner!) plan is best.

11. What are business units?
All hospitals have multiple "products" or units (e.g., each type of nursing unit) that make up its business portfolio. The famous Boston Consulting Group (BCG) studies showed that high market share was significantly correlated with higher return on investment and lower costs because of the learning curve effect. Therefore, it is best to have a stable, high market share in some businesses to fund the cost needs of other businesses. Some common terms heard to describe them, taken from the BCG Growth-Share Matrix, include *question marks, stars, cash cows,* and *dogs*.

12. Tell me what these terms mean.
Question marks: high growth, low share. This will take a lot of resources to grow it or it must be phased out.
Stars: high growth, high share. This will require continued investment to maintain its share.

Cash cows: low growth, high share. These areas generate the profits for other areas.

Dogs: low growth, low share. These are often either eliminated or kept because they contribute to other organizational goals.

For instance, an out-patient department may have a "star" in the flu vaccination program, a "cash cow" in the pediatric immunization program, a "question mark" in the weight loss clinic, and a "dog" in the organ transplant clinic.

13. Tell me about the Porter Five Forces Theory.

Any business entity has at least five major forces to deal with from competitors in the market place:

1. Threat of substitutes
2. Threat of new entrants
3. Bargaining power of suppliers
4. Bargaining power of buyers
5. Intensity of rivalry among competitors

14. Our hospital wants to grow. What are the ways to expand the market? Isn't there just a limited amount of healthcare needed?

The Ansoff Grid is a common reference to identify four growth strategies for product or market expansion.

	Existing Products ↓	New Products ↓
Existing Markets →	Market Penetration	Product Development
New Markets →	Market Development	Diversification

Using the grid will help direct the types of activities that can result in a larger share of the health care market. For instance, they may seek to do more penetration or capture of the local area through contracting with various HMOs as a preferred provider. On the other hand, they may tack diversification by attempting to expand into a new market, such as occupational health, or a new product such as widespread marketing about the importance and availability of bone density screening.

15. What are the 4 P's of marketing?

Product, Place, Price, Promotion. Which one any institution will choose to use will depend on marking analysis, planning, control, and implementation. Considerations include microenvironmental forces (such as suppliers, competitors, and human resources) as well as macroenvironmental forces (demographics, technology, cultural, economic, and political).

Marketing often involves whether that institution is the leader, challenger to the leader, or a "follower." Often larger, well-known, affiliated hospitals will promote themselves as the leader while a community hospital might emphasize that your care is just as good (or even better because it is more personable) as at a leading hospital.

16. Can you given an example?

A hospital could emphasize its unique or best product (which is often service, technology, or staff for hospitals), its convenient location ("your neighborhood health care provider"), the reasonable health care prices among today's rising costs (and the cost effectiveness of using its prevention services), or promoting awareness of its availability and (superior) services.

Promotion will often team up with other organizations for co-marketing, such as offering reduced-price mammograms during October's Breast Health Awareness Month or free screening for diabetes during National Diabetes Month in November. Findings are given to the patient, usually along with a referral to a hospital-affiliated health care provider in that area.

One general medical clinic specifically had the nurses speak to patients about all of the prevention services available for them and their family at the hospital. As a result, there was a significant increase in utilization of the hospital's services from the established patients and their families.

17. What is market segmentation?

It is not possible to be all things to all people. The term simply means deciding where the institution's resources will be directed. Deciding that usually involves demand forecasting, market positioning, and market targeting.

For instance, a new clinic might be developed because of the predicted epidemic of diabetes type 2 patients or a new emphasis on language interpretation and ethnic advertising might be pursued as a result of a different ethnic group moving into the neighborhood. Some hospitals even actively recruit and reward bilingual staff, advertising that "We speak your language."

18. I find this talk about marketing so shallow. I went into nursing to help people, not "sell a product."

Studies show that approximately 80% of nurses are motivated by altruistic goals. But today health care is also a business. Understanding and working with the hospital's marketing of its mission and strategy will help your effectiveness, especially if you desire to grow a new program.

I liken marketing to the wrapping we put on a gift. Wouldn't your perception and reaction to a gift of a priceless antique book be different if you received it in a rumpled, torn paper bag rather than a nice box with foil wrapping and a bow? Marketing doesn't change what health care providers do so much as change the patient's perception. It enhances the patients' awareness and appreciation of the available quality care we are providing.

19. Explain synergy.

Synergy is used for the benefit of two or more businesses combining resources in the belief that together they can perform better. Commonalities that they might share include the same buyers, the same database, same products, or sharing managerial know-how. Examples in health care could include long-term and acute-care networking, or two hospitals merging and having either only one pediatric unit or one unit for stable children and one for the critically ill.

Network failures are often attributed to inadequate commonalities. For instance, a for-profit, unionized, small, rural hospital united with a religious-owned, nonunion, large inner-city hospital. A year later, they "divorced."

20. Any tips on how to work with my hospital's mission and strategy?

- *Know the basics of strategy.* Be able to use the appropriate terms so that you can present your needs in a perspective that is meaningful to the "financial types." You'll be in a better position to lobby effectively for resources if you can talk about how targeting this segment will allow for diversification of the market rather than just emphasizing that you believe it meets a need.
- *Work to enhance the synergy between your department and the hospital's mission and strategy.* What you may choose to emphasize in your rehabilitation unit (or to even justify its existence) may depend on whether the hospital is striving to be the number one provider for trauma victims or hip replacements.
- *Dovetail promotions with established health observance and recognition days.* That way you can often obtain advertising in the local paper through an article. Offer knowledgeable staff speakers on special topics (such as the hospital's eye clinic or same-day eye surgery during May's National Sight-Saving Month) to local community groups. A calendar listing these observance days can be purchased from the American Hospital Association.

• *Consider writing about a program in a professional journal.* Even if your program isn't the first of its kind, write about an aspect of your experience. This could be anything from lessons learned to marketing. Provide pictures; it draws in readers.

Then call the local paper to notify them that your hospital's new program was featured in that professional journal. This often results in free publicity while promoting the image in the community that you are on the cutting edge.

BIBLIOGRAPHY

1. Byrne J: Strategic planning. Business Week, August 26, 1996.
2. Peters TJ, Waterman, RH: In Search of Excellence: Lessons from America's Best Run Companies. New York, Harper & Row, 1982.
3. Silbiger S: The Ten-Day MBA. New York, William Morrow, 1993.
4. Thompson AA, Strickland AJ: Strategic Management, 7th ed. Homewood, IL, Irwin, 1993.

III. Staffing

13. RECRUITMENT AND RETENTION

Camilla L. Jones, RN, BBA

The five most important words in the English language are "I am proud of you."
The four most important words are "What is your opinion?"
The three most important words are "If you please."
The two most important words: "Thank you."
The least important word: "I."

Robert W. Woodruff

1. Talk about the current nursing shortage.

The current international registered nurse (RN) shortage is predicted to be worse than any previous one. The Bureau of Labor Statistics projects the need for RNs will rise 25% by 2005, and 36% by 2020. One 2000 survey found that 11.4% of the budgeted nursing positions nationwide were vacant. The reasons include the following:

- *An aging nursing workforce.* The average age of nurses is 44 to 46 years. Baby Boomers (those born between 1946 and 1964) will start to retire in or before 2011. California predicts that 50% of its nurses will no longer be practicing by 2012.
- *Declining nursing school enrollment for new nurses, with an older nursing student.* The average age of the new graduate nurse is 31 years. Baccalaureate nursing program enrollments have decreased for the fifth consecutive year.
- *Increased opportunities within and outside of nursing.*
- *Growing demand.* The Bureau of Labor Statistics predicts that the RN job market will grow 23% by 2006. By 2020, the prediction is that the need for RNs will rise by 36%.
- *Changing post-Baby-Boomer Demographics.* A smaller pool for future workers is coupled with increased volume and acuity in health care. The population of those 82 years of age and older is growing at a rate that is six times faster than the growth of the rest of the population. The U.S. Census Bureau estimates that by 2020, the number of people 85 years or older will have doubled.
- *Increasing preference of "graying nurses" to work part-time.* This trend creates vacant staff RN hours, even with the same number of working nurses.
- *Resulting ramifications of health care re-engineering.* Job redesign has excessively burdened the RN. As early as 1996, American Hospital Association President Dick Davidson warned about the "thinning" of nursing staff. As a result, there has been an exit of many experienced, but overwhelmed, nurses from the profession.

2. Discuss staffing solutions hospitals are seeking. What are the concerns regarding these solutions.

One recent survey found that most hospitals have resorted to the usual means of overtime, in-house staffing pools, temporary agencies (83%), travelers (74%), and on-call staff (73%). Financial incentives, including sign-on bonuses (84%) and bonuses for voluntarily increasing hours for a period of time (e.g., summer vacations) are increasing. Referral bonuses, retention bonuses, and relocation assistance are infrequently used. Many believe, however, that most of these are band-aid solutions that do not build loyalty.

Hospitals report focusing on scheduling flexibility. This includes returning to using weekend-only positions and enhanced central resource pools. In addition, they are "growing" their own nurses through new graduate nurse programs and student scholarship programs.

Some experts point out that the problem is not a shortage of nurses per se but a shortage of nurses willing to work in the current conditions. Of the top 11 JCAHO sentinel events, 5 have a proven relationship to staffing and 3 have an anecdotal relationship to staffing. It is predicted that if conditions improve, with a focus on helping rather than business, many nurses will be willing to return to the bedside.

3. What time spans can I expect to hire a nurse to fill a vacancy?

Lawrenz Consulting's 2000 nationwide actual staffing survey found hospitals reporting increasingly longer spans of time needed to hire a nurse. On the average, it took 13.3 weeks to hire a medical-surgical nurse and 16.6 weeks to hire a specialty nurse.

4. How can I entice nurses into my region?

Learning to compete in the nursing market is a crucial managerial behavior. Stress opportunities for growth in the employment environment. Promote the local community and its positive qualities. Today's worker is looking for a balance between work and leisure. Evaluate every asset that the work and community environment possess and sell, sell, sell! An applicant will move some distance to an area that can offer the right amenities.

Consider these marketable assets:
• Natural resources like skiing, hiking, or boating
• Cultural resources
• Low crime rate
• Excellent local school systems
• Nearby universities

5. OK, they like the region. What is the next step?

Once the manager has attracted the applicant, the work environment must be marketed. Most nursing applicants are looking for a work environment that has a consistent structure, elements of autonomy, and a cohesive atmosphere that can support the applicant's goals and objectives. A note of caution: the manager must be honest and offer only what the work environment can actually deliver.

6. Where should I look for new recruits?
• Local, regional, and out-of-state nursing programs
• National and local seminars
• Localities that are closing hospitals or downsizing
• Association newsletters
• Local and regional association meetings
• Countries outside of the United States, especially Canada

7. Talk about recruiting nurses from Canada.

One study found that nearly 1 in 10 Canadian nursing graduates from 1995 to 1997 migrated to the United States. There are 15 nurses leaving Canada for the United States for every U.S. RN who migrates to Canada. Canadian nurses are interested in coming to the United States because of limited work opportunities stemming from their own country's health care budget cutbacks since 1995. Approximately 50% are employed in Canada on a part-time or casual basis, and two-thirds of these nurses claim that it is not by choice. Increased resources in technology, the ease of transfer into specialty areas, and a good exchange rate make U.S. opportunities very appealing.

Employers relate that the Canadian nurses are well trained and have excellent skills. Canadian associate degree nursing programs continue during the summer and include about 2000 clinical hours. An added benefit: language is never a problem!

8. Describe the visa requirements.

Any Canadian citizen who has completed the necessary education and has a nursing job offer can obtain a TN (Trade NAFTA) Visa under the 1994 North American Free Trade Agreement. It is a nonimmigrant (temporary) visa that allows certain professionals to come to the United States to provide services to a specific employer for a specific position. It is issued initially for up to 1 year but can be renewed annually for an indefinite number of times in 1-year increments. The nurse may change employers or work for two employers at the same time, as long as permission is obtained from the Immigration and Naturalization Service. A spouse and unmarried children under the age of 21 can travel with the TN visa holder under a category called TD (trade dependent).

Many U.S. hospitals use Canadian job fairs to meet interested applicants not only for nurses but also for pharmacists, radiology technicians, physical therapists, or occupational therapists. There is usually a 3-month wait for the nurses to obtain the license reciprocity.

9. I haven't heard of international recruiting before. Is the United States the only country doing this?

The nursing shortage is a global problem, and many countries are attempting to attract nurses. New Zealand has recruited from Britain, Canada, and South Africa; Northern Ireland has looked toward Spain, Germany, and Denmark; England was advertising in Trinidad and Tobago; and Canada sought to recruit U.S. nurses.

10. What specific elements do applicants look for in a work environment?

It really is true that money is not the only draw. Many an applicant has left a well-paying position for a change of pace or a healthier environment. The following is a short list of desirable workplace amenities applicants seek that can be demonstrated during the interview process:
- Respect of the applicant's time
- Assertive friendliness
- A manager with comprehensive listening skills
- Consistency in human resources practices
- Competitive wages and differentials
- Relocation packages
- Flexible scheduling
- Travel time reimbursement
- Tuition assistance/college collaborations
- Specialty training opportunities
- Goal-based bonus programs
- Incentive programs
    - Attendance
    - Flexible coverage
    - Competitive on-call rates
    - Incentives for extra work
- Structured and/or extended orientation processes
- Mentorship programs
- Administrative visibility
- Cohesive teamwork (clinical and managerial)

11. What are the most important benefits nurses look for?

In a recent survey, respondents rated the following benefits:
- Medical coverage, 95%
- Dental coverage, 85%
- 401k or other saving plan, 85%
- Tuition reimbursement, 80%

- Pension plan, 80%
- Some freedom to choose work schedule, 80%
- Life insurance, 60%
- Eye care coverage, 55%
- Maternal/paternal leave, 35%
- Profit-sharing plan, 27%
- Annual or semiannual bonus, 20%
- Childcare, 15%
- Eldercare, 10%

12. I've spent lots of time and effort getting the applicant here and we are short-staffed. I'm afraid I'll lose the applicant.

Matching the applicant's goals, objectives, and expectations to the facility's mission and philosophy is crucial in not only recruiting but in retaining the applicant. The department and the job should have been realistically presented to the applicant no matter what understaffing issues exist. Recruited employees who become disenchanted or feel misled by the recruiter leave their new work environments discouraged and bitter toward the institution. Many times, the ex-employee will remain in the area, employed at a competing hospital. This is not only expensive, but the inevitable "grapevine" can be detrimental to local recruitment efforts.

13. What can I do during the interview to make sure I get enough information to make a good decision?

Never schedule less $1\frac{1}{2}$ hours for the interview. The interview process should be bidirectional. In this day and age, the manager is also being interviewed.

It is most effective to gather information first. Initiate the interview by collecting information regarding clinical competence. Make questions open-ended. Asking the candidate to discuss their strongest and weakest clinical skills will give insight into clinical competency and orientation needs. Do not rule out a candidate if he or she doesn't have a particular skill set but does appear motivated to learn. Skills can be taught; work ethic is much more difficult to change. Spend the most time assessing the candidate's motivation, work behavior, and expectations.

14. List some questions to help assess a candidate's work ethic and potential "fit" in the work environment.

1. What is important to you in a job?
2. What motivates you the most (keeps you in a job when the going gets tough)?
3. What types of work environments do you enjoy?
4. What types of people would you rather not work with?
5. Would you rather do a job, design it, evaluate it, or manage others doing it?
6. Which of your previous jobs was the most satisfying and why?
7. Which of your previous jobs was the most frustrating and why?
8. Tell me about a conflict with a coworker and how you resolved it.
9. Describe a situation when you had to deal with a difficult customer and how did you handle it?
10. Tell me about a problem you solved with others and what your contribution to the process was.
11. What accomplishment from your previous jobs did you take most pride in?
12. Tell me about the best supervisor you ever had.
13. Tell me about your worst supervisor. What made it hard to work for them?
14. What do you consider your greatest personal strength?
15. What do you consider your greatest personal weakness?
16. Where do you see yourself 5 years from now?
17. Describe your ideal job.
18. What special skills do you have that qualify you for this job. Why should we hire you?

The new manager might be surprised how much this interview style can impact management style. It's hard to hold onto a management behavior that candidate after candidate identifies as one the "worst supervisor" utilized.

15. How can I learn whether the applicant values what I value?

Select four or five hot spots or work behaviors that are important to you and have candidates place themselves on a 10-point scale regarding those points. For example, on a 10-point scale (1 being the lowest, 10 being the highest) rate yourself on:
- Punctual attendance and reliability
- Customer service
- Teamwork
- Organization
- Loyalty

16. How much information should I share about my department and management style during the interview?

Give the candidate information about the department and facility mission. The candidate should walk out of the interview with a clear picture of goals and objectives that are important to the manager and hospital. Some managers will give a history about how far the department has come in the past 3 years to emphasize the unit's future potential.

17. How do I compete if another hospital is also recruiting the applicant?

This is a tough scenario. A manager can practically get into a bidding war with another facility if the candidate is experienced, qualified, and has flexible attributes. It is important to remember that under every circumstance, new applicants are looking for managers who are fair and attentive,and who seem interested in the applicant's goals. These workplace qualities consistently rank higher than money. Gain an edge by
- Keeping the applicant informed.
- Presenting a pay structure that is fair and consistent.
- Facilitating the hiring process.
- Offering any flexibility in regard to scheduling.
- Reviewing the interview and conveying again all elements of your workplace that meet or exceed the candidate's expectations.

18. My hospital delays the hiring process to get a drug screen and a background check. How do I deal with this if I'm anxious to hire the candidate?

The applicant should be informed at the first interview about the hospital processes. Complete the drug screen after the first interview if the candidate is being considered. If a background check is required, the process should be explained with an estimated date of completion. Some hospitals will hire the candidate prior to the background check on the condition that continued employment will depend on the satisfactory background check results. It is always helpful to alert the candidate to bring their driver's license, nursing license, certifications, and any health records or immunizations with them on the first interview.

19. Should I let the applicant know right away that I want to hire him or her?

The manager should clearly and supportively communicate that the hiring process is not completed until all hiring requirements have been met, including a physical if applicable. The manager should certainly indicate whether the candidate is being strongly considered and has met all other qualifications for the position.

20. Should I commit to a base rate of pay on the first interview?

It may be desirable to quote a base rate or range at the time of interview, especially if the manager is confident that the institution is highly competitive. Most full-time candidates expect a review of their application and experience prior to a base rate quote. Applicable differentials, tuition reimbursement, benefits, and bonuses are usually of interest to the candidate and generally are more concrete. Keeping a benefit summary sheet handy for the first interview is effective.

21. How do I attract nurses to my specialty unit? There aren't enough experienced nurses out there.

- Hold open houses where hospital and community nurses can see the environment.
- Offer the opportunity to just buddy with a nurse for a day, without giving care. This often helps overcome initial hesitancy.
- Have flexible "PRN" pool options. Managers can often entice nurses to sign on for regular employment after having positive PRN experiences.
- Use employee referral. Word-of-mouth is powerful in bringing other nurses to explore the opportunity.

22. How long does it take for a newly hired nurse to become productive? How much does it cost?

It will depend on the individual's experience (years and previous work environment), base pay rate, and personal flexibility. "Seasoned" nurses can reach maximum productivity in 3 weeks; nurses new to a specialty usually take at least 6 weeks; and new graduates can easily require 6 months or longer. Experienced staff adapt more quickly but are paid at a higher rate.

Some costs are universal, such as the hospital-wide orientation time, benefits, and any incentive payments. Otherwise, depending on all of these factors, the orientation cost can be anywhere from $1800 to $17,000. That is why it is so important to work toward retaining good staff.

23. Besides the orientees' time and wages, are there any other aspects I should consider?

Preceptors' own patient care productivity typically decreases during the time they spend orientating new staff, particularly at the beginning of that period. Some educators even recommend that the extra time needed for explaining and showing should be built into the staffing pattern. They suggest that the preceptor with a new graduate should only have a half-assignment the first week.

24. How can I make sure I keep the recruited employees I have attracted?

A recent survey of 300 candidates listed the top 10 reasons nurses left positions.

1. Lack of growth
2. Lack of leadership
3. Staffing levels
4. Hours
5. Desire to work for and with people who care
6. Desire for a team atmosphere
7. Lack of organizational stability
8. Pursuit of more money
9. Lack of communication
10. Desire to be respected

Look where "money" is on the list. Although money is an effective recruiting tool, the work environment and meeting employee goals and objectives are most important in workforce retention. These work environment qualities are a result of "top-down" influence.

25. I know some of the flexible pool nurses have left for agencies where they could earn more money. How can I compete?

One hospital created its own agency with unique requirements. Nurses commit to work for 32 hours per week for 12 consecutive weeks, with a weekend requirement. In exchange for this commitment, the nurse receives a pay rate that is higher than the outside agency (but no benefits). The hospital offers a limited number of these positions to experienced nurses with the appropriate certifications. Initially done as a retention effort, it became a powerful recruitment tool with three times more applicants than positions.

26. Besides money and benefits, what programs keep good nurses?
- Adequate orientation and mentorship
- Career ladders
- Educational opportunities (seminars, inservices, certification programs)
- Flexible scheduling
- Empowerment (practice committee, operational PI teams—troubleshooters)
- Leadership programs
- Positive feedback (public commendation board)

27. Any other factors?
Often nurses entering a new specialty will hit a "hump" period between 3 and 6 months. They become frustrated with all the knowledge, processes, and changes of the new environment. Without having many established friendships among the staff, or in the face of no support, they want to quit.

This may occur because orienting nurses have preconceived self-imposed expectations regarding how long it will take to feel comfortable. When that doesn't happen, they feel inadequate, which can cause them to become dissatisfied.

This phenomenon is so common that this author has incorporated a routine discussion of the subject during all new employee orientations. It has helped to make new staff aware of this so that it can be recognized and dealt with. Try to spend some extra time with new nurses if any signs of discouragemen crop up. Otherwise, the staff member can feel alone and regard quitting as the only option.

Helping staff set realistic expectations in the first place helps. And, usually if they just persevere, they can go "over the top" within another month or so.

28. Discuss exchange programs.
Usually an observational or shadowing experience, exchange programs allow nurses to experience a specialty environment related to their usual clinical work. For instance, a staff nurse on a postoperative floor watches surgical cases or an emergency department (ED) nurse watches cardiac catheterizations. Unless the program is strictly voluntary, the employee is paid for his or her time as an educational experience.

29. Describe the benefits of an exchange program.
An exchange program promotes staff understanding of the interdependence of patient care and operations between the different areas. Nurses who witness internal organs being manipulated during a procedure can understand why a postoperative patient needs the analgesics. Staff often return stimulated, with some suggestions for improvement. In addition, meeting other nurses establishes relationships and enhances cohesive teamwork.

30. Is this cross-training?
No. Institutions/networks that want to train staff to work in more than one similar unit within the hospital or between hospitals within the network must provide a formal (though usually abbreviated) orientation to the new unit. Some of the advantages of this type program are personal growth for the employee and increased flexibility for the hospital.

BIBLIOGRAPHY

1. American Health Consultants: ED nursing salary survey. ED Nurs 4:22, 2000
2. Bozell J: Breaking the vicious cycle. Nurs Manage 32:26, 28, 2001.
3. Cavouras CA: Nurse staffing levels in American hospitals: A 2001 report. J Emergency Nurs 28:40–43, 2002.
4. Edler R: If I Knew Then What I Know Now: CEOs and Other Smart Executives Share Wisdom They Wish They'd Been Told 25 Years Ago. New York, Berkley Books, 1997.
5. Zimmermann PG: The nursing shortage: What can we do? J Emerg Nurs 26(6):579–582, 2000.

14. STUDENT NURSE EXTERN PROGRAMS

Camilla L. Jones, RN, BBA

In order that people may be happy in their work, these three things are needed:
They must be fit for it
They must not do too much of it;
And they must have a sense of success in it.

John Ruskin

1. Can a student nurse extern program help my recruitment efforts?
The catch phrase of the day is "grow your own." It is a very effective way to develop healthy expectations in a future workforce. Student nurse extern candidates should have completed at least one clinical rotation. They work as assistive personnel and should have their own unique job description. The position allows the extern to use skills (e.g., catheterization) or work in areas (e.g., obstetrics, pediatrics) that they have successfully completed in the nursing program. Many then choose to stay on at the unit or hospital after graduation.

2. This sounds great! Is there a downside to a student nurse extern program?
The downside is that the student nurse extern is usually counted as a staff assistant position and uses budgeted labor hours. The extern's ability to truly "extend" a nurse is limited, and many student nurses are not as satisfied if they simply do "aide" work. They must be provided appropriate orientation as described in the job description, even though they are familiar with many of the basics, from vital signs to asepsis. In addition, it is a given that within 1 to 2 years, this worker will either leave or need additional orientation upon graduation. An extern program is not a substitution for new graduate or nursing orientation.

3. How do I communicate with administration to gain support of a student nurse extern program?
Communicate the pros (and cons). Emphasize that this type of program demonstrates vision. Key elements include the following:
1. Nursing shortage strategy
   • Current supply deficit
   • Graying workforce
2. Future workforce opportunity
3. Future relief strategy for eliminating costly agency coverage
4. Future relief of closed, unstaffed beds

4. How do I find acceptable student nurse recruits?
Current nursing students who function as aides are usually eager to become a student nurse extern and capitalize on additional opportunities. Many programs offer some tuition reimbursement in exchange for a commitment to work at the institution after graduation. It becomes a win-win situation.

5. What about extern candidates outside my hospital environment?
- *Build relationships with area colleges and technical schools.* Offer to speak at student nursing association functions or in the leadership class.
- *Request an opportunity to talk to the students about the program with any school of nursing that uses your hospital for clinical experiences.* Offer to provide leadership shadowing.

• *Offer involvement in local college or technical school advisory boards.* It will give you opportunities to network about programs and market trends.
• *Interact with the students on your unit.* Invite them to your professional meetings.
• *Address grade schools, high schools, and volunteer programs.* These are ground-level entry points for future workers. Think like an investor: results are not instantaneous.

6. How can I make sure my student extern program doesn't backfire?
Selection is important. Screen and interview these candidates in the same manner you would any other applicant to determine expectations and fit. In addition, request a letter of reference from clinical instructors about clinical competence, initiative, and work ethic.

7. How is a nurse internship/residency program different?
These types of programs usually offer didactic classes, in addition to traditional clinical orientation, to prepare nurses for a specialty unit. An employment commitment or relationship is usually required. In one residency example, 11 area hospitals went together to create an emergency nursing course. Participating hospitals sent either new hires or cross-training nurses free of charge. The hospitals provided instructors for the didactic portion of training and identified preceptors for the clinical experiences. Additional support was obtained from suppliers and community agencies (e.g., organ procurement, intraosseous needle insertion).

Many facilities report that in addition to "growing their own" specialty nurses, classes and training opportunities often work as a recruitment tool. Some community nurses may also take the course for a fee to "try out" the specialty, exposing them to the hospital and its positive qualities.

8. Some of the staff are not really supportive of the students who are working in an extern position. How can a manager enhance staff support for nursing students?
It is key to have a professional environment that supports beginning nurses. Make this expectation a normal part of your unit's culture and work experience. This includes the following:
• Selecting, training, and rewarding the most positive preceptors you can obtain.
• Have a structured curriculum or matrix in place. Make sure all staff understand the content and limits of the student nurse extern experience.
• Augment the importance of this experience by discussing mentoring during new hire orientation, making it a part of the staff's annual evaluations, and providing rewards or recognition for preceptors.
• Include the topic on a regular basis in staff meeting agendas.

If someone continually behaves in an inappropriate, nonsupportive manner toward student externs, then the individual should be counseled as he or she would for any other unsatisfactory aspect of the job performance. For additional discussion on this issue, see Chapter 21, Ongoing Staff Education and Professional Development.

BIBLIOGRAPHY

1. American Health Consultants: ED nursing salary survey. ED Nurs 4:22, 2000.
2. Bozell J: Breaking the vicious cycle. Nurs Manage 32:26, 28, 2001.
3. Edler R: If I Knew Then What I Know Now: CEOs and Other Smart Executives Share Wisdom They Wish They'd Been Told 25 Years Ago. New York, Berkley Books, 1997.

15. NEW GRADUATE NURSES

Camilla L. Jones, RN, BBA

Who dares to teach must never cease to learn.

John Cotton Dana

1. Why would I want to hire a new graduate?

We are on the edge of a severe labor shortage. Hiring new graduates is a manager's opportunity to have an impact on the workforce of the future. In addition, new graduates bring energy, enthusiasm, idealism, flexibility, and creativity to a department today. These qualities are critical to help our profession begin to solve tomorrow's problems, some of which we have already begun to experience.

2. What is the best method to attract new graduates?

It's definitely a job-hunter's market out there. New graduates have more opportunities than ever, not only to land a job *and* a hire-on bonus, but also to take advantage of opportunities to train in desirable fields of nursing. New graduates today are interested in building their marketability and building relationships. A manager will have the best opportunity to build relationships with future workers if the hospital or department is actively involved in clinical outreach to area nursing programs. Student extern programs, particularly in critical care settings, provide a synergistic solution. They can be effective in nurse extender positions, and, by the time the student graduates, the new graduate has a realistic impression of departmental operations, expectations, culture, and workload.

3. What are the most important things to know prior to hiring a new graduate?

Gaps will exist in the new graduate's clinical skills, critical thinking, and decision-making processes. These variables require an organizational commitment to extended orientation. However, it is less expensive to put up-front dollars into mentorship programming than it is to pay the recruitment costs for the inevitable turnover that will occur if new graduates are hired without adequate training.

Dollars are not the only resource you will have to prepare to deploy with new graduates. Many new graduates emanate from the Generation X culture and require your involvement. They want the following:
- Good jobs that are stimulating
- Conversation that gets to the point and then moves to action
- Meaningful feedback, frequently
- Diversification and keeping options open
- To advance their own goals and objectives

For further discussion on this topic, see Chapter 28, Managing Generation X Employees.

4. How can I prepare my unit and existing employees for new graduate employees?

New graduates are not unlike any other new employee in that they seek to be accepted when they start a new job. The nursing field has always granted acceptance for a demonstrated skill level. These less-experienced nurses depend on the goodwill and clinical maturity of the existing staff to survive the initial employment period. Unfortunately, sometimes they find themselves in hostile territory.

There must be a bidirectional effort by all parties to recognize the value and potential of each individual. This can only happen from the top down. The manager must instill a commitment in staff members to coach and develop new graduates into experienced team members.

This process is self-perpetuating. The new graduate who is offered the unit's best in preceptorship will become a loyal, skilled employee who can forward his or her training experiences to other new graduating employment candidates.

5. How is orientation different for the new graduate today than it was 20 years ago?
Experts cite three factors that make assimilation more difficult today:
1. Re-engineering and loss of the clinical nurse specialist role, as well as experienced staff, on an established unit
2. Higher patient acuity and turnover consuming the time in which educational needs were traditionally met
3. Health care's high-tech environment and increasingly rapid turnover of knowledge

6. How can I best integrate the new grad into my department and ensure that standards of care for the patients are met?
Mentoring, training, and a lengthy orientation are the answers.

7. Describe what to include in a new graduate orientation.
Student nurses are rarely assigned more than two patients at one time, nor are they trained for the department-specific clinical nuances (doctor preferences, politics). Specific classroom and clinical instruction should include a multiple patient environment, time management, prioritization, and clinical skills (for review and competency verification).

8. Give an example of one successful new graduate orientation program.
Johns Hopkin's Senior Director of Education and Practice Amy Deutschendorf set up a new graduate orientation program with stair-stepping responsibility. Each week has a focus, with key competencies. The approach is structuring the precepting sequence on hierarchical needs. New graduates must conquer equipment and environment before they can handle critical thinking in regard to complex patients or delegation. In this program, basic core behaviors are identified and must be demonstrated before the orientation is finished. Initially, the new graduate is required only to recognize and communicate an abnormal finding to the health care team rather than anticipate how the care will be altered. For example, the new nurse must be able to note and call the physician about a new respiratory rate of 40/minute, even if the nurse does not anticipate an order for intravenous furosemide. An overview of the program looks like this:
During week 1, the new graduate does not give medication and cares only for one to two stable patients. The goal is to master the environment, from the location of the crash cart to the documentation forms. During the second week, the focus is exclusively on medication, without patient care. Future weeks gradually add quantity and complexity to the assignment. The focus of the additional teaching and support throughout the entire first year is on high-risk areas. These include medication, falls, skin ulcer, documentation, concepts of managed care, and delegation.
Deutschendorf also suggests during the first 2 weeks, when the most teaching takes place, that the preceptor and orientee together have a reduced assignment. As mastery is achieved, the pair takes a regular assignment. By the fourth week or so, one mentor can actually supervise two new graduates (a practice routinely used and extended by nursing faculty up to 10 students at a time).

9. Are there other considerations for the orientation?
- Provide consistency in precepting to maintain a continuum of experiences and constant evaluation.
- Document concisely and completely to ensure that all competencies are covered.
- Give regular feedback to tell what is being done right and to provide clarification as necessary.

10. How can I guarantee that my new graduate employee won't leave after orientation?
Unfortunately, you can't. Some facilities contract an employment requirement with student nurses in exchange for tuition monies, but it is reported that up to 10% buy out their obligation and leave. Most new graduates experience some form of "reality-shock" within the first 6 months of working in a real-world environment. While the national RN turnover rates are around 14%, about 20% of new RN graduates leave during their first year of hospital employment. Anecdotally, it is as high as 50% at some hospitals.

Some orientation programs provide extended departmental support up to 1 year to ensure that the new graduate has a support system. A mentor resource can provide the new graduate with alternative perspectives and solutions to deal with the existing problems, other than leaving employment.

BIBLIOGRAPHY

1. Deutschendorf A: Managers Forum: Preparing and compensating preceptors. J Emerg Nurs 27(3):291–292, 2001.
2. Marett BE: Emergency nursing in perspective: Mentoring, sharing, supporting. J Emerg Nurs 26:401–402, 2000.
3. Oermann M, Garvin M: When coaching new grads. Nurs Manage 31:26–27, 2001.
4. Sturt P: Generational theories: "We never acted like that." ENA 1999 Scientific Assembly, Washington, DC, 1999.

16. STAFF HIRING

John Vicik, MSIR

Interviewing is like driving; the longer you do it, the worse you get.

Author unknown

1. What is the most efficient way to recruit staff?

Plan ahead. Hiring under pressure, or in a continually reactionary manner, is frustrating and many times results in poor hiring decisions. Greater lead time allows managers the opportunity to see more candidates and, as a result, be more selective. You want to avoid settling for someone you know is really not suitable; it only creates new problems.

While this certainly sounds desirable, turnover and labor shortages may make that seem unrealistic. However, managers should look down the road and anticipate staffing needs. Who may leave in the next 6 months? Who may request to go part-time? With an idea of what the future staffing needs will be, managers can work with others in their organization to always be on the lookout for possible replacements. Recruitment should be an ongoing process to find the best possible candidates.

2. Where is a good source to find employees?

One of the most effective sources for new employees is through employee referrals. Research has shown that employees who are referred by an existing employee tend to have higher than average retention rates. This may be due to the fact that they already have a realistic understanding of what the company and position are all about.

In addition, referral bonuses are a good way to spread the word that you are interested in, and will reward, employee referrals. Equity concerns are minimized with referral bonuses because it's the existing employees, not the new employees, who are receiving the bonuses.

3. Any other sources?

Recruit where people are when they are not at work. Community programs and locations that involve children and family activities are a good source for prospective health care employees. Ask churches or social organizations in your community, in which you know nurses or nursing assistants are active, to post a recruitment flyer or allow a presentation on the opportunities you have available. One hospital had increased success placing their want ads in the lifestyle, rather than employment, section.

4. Are job descriptions important?

Absolutely. A well-developed, current job description is critical in defining the qualifications and requirements for a position. It should contain the mental and physical requirements of a position, which can be useful for determining possible Americans with Disabilities Act (ADA) accommodations.

A job description is useful for recruitment, selection, performance evaluation, training, pay decisions, and regulatory compliance. Without a job description, hiring decisions become more subjective and have tendency to be based more on personality and chemistry than on an objective matching of position requirements with a candidate's qualifications.

Candidates appreciate receiving a current and appropriately detailed job description; offer it during the job interview. In addition, an assistive personnel's job description helps clarify for nurses which tasks can be delegated.

5. Do applicants need to fully complete an employment application if they have already submitted a resume?

Yes, if you hire them. It may seem like an extra burden to ask someone to complete an application after they have just handed you a resume. But they need to sign and verify that the information they provided is correct. People can misrepresent information on a resume. On a resume there is no signed statement that information provided is accurate. The application's signed statement to this effect could prove legally useful should the facts be different upon further investigation.

6. How long should you keep applications and resumes?

Generally speaking, 1 year for most employers and 2 years for educational and state and local governments. In many organizations, resumes and applications are centrally maintained in the Human Resources department.

Managers should understand that receiving a resume or application carries a responsibility that it will be considered should a suitable position open. Misplacing or not considering previously received resumes or applications for an appropriate position that becomes open could be the basis for a charge of employment discrimination. For this reason many organizations announce that their policy is to accept and keep applications or resumes only for currently open positions. I recommend returning the unsolicited applications.

Managers need to know their organization's policy of handling applications or resumes. They should also inform applicants on just how long they will retain applications or resumes on file before they are discarded.

7. What are some of the red flags you should look for in a resume/application?

While this may seem like judging a book by its cover, the truth is you can to some degree. If an application is incompletely filled out, this may be an indication that someone lacks attention to detail. Writing that is sloppy or illegible could indicate a lack of concern for the quality of their work. Misspelled words could indicate a potential for carelessness.

Sometimes these will not be the correct assessments. Each step in the selection process is an indicator of some trait or characteristic of a candidate that should be considered and weighed in the totality of all the information obtained.

Additional red flags to consider are the following:
• Unexplained gaps in employment history
• Frequent job changes or multiple short stays at previous jobs
• A downward spiral of jobs with less responsibility
• Abrupt career changes
• Being clearly overqualified for the given position
• The stated reasons why he or she left previous jobs
• Insufficient education or experience for the given position

8. With all the laws that affect hiring and human resources, what is the most important one to remember?

There certainly are numerous laws protecting the rights of employees in the workplace. The most familiar one is Title VII of the Civil Rights Act. This law states that employers should not discriminate against employees on the basis of race, color, national origin, religion, and gender in all terms and conditions of employment. Title VII underscores the basic intent of all employment laws to ensure that decisions affecting employment are not discriminatory but are job and business related.

9. What other laws are critical to know about for the hiring process?

A few of the more critical federal laws, in addition to Title VII, that affect hiring are the Age Discrimination in Employment Act (ADEA), ADA, the Pregnancy Discrimination Act, and the Immigration Reform and Control Act (IRCA).

- **ADEA**—Prohibits discrimination in employment for persons 40 years of age and older.
- **ADA**—Prohibits discrimination against a qualified individual with a disability because of the individual's disability.
- **Pregnancy Discrimination Act**—Prohibits discrimination on the basis of pregnancy, childbirth, or related conditions. This law requires employers to treat pregnancy the same as any other temporary disability.
- **IRCA**—Prohibits discrimination against foreign-looking job applicants and establishes penalties for hiring illegal aliens.

All managers would be well advised to become familiar with the specifics of these critical employment laws. In addition, there are various state laws that support equal employment opportunity and may provide additional protection to employees beyond what the federal laws require.

10. How can I avoid asking illegal questions in an interview?

- *Keep your questions job-related.* If a question has no connection to a person's ability to do the job; don't ask it. For example, "Where do you live?" or "Do you have children?" While these might be acceptable in a social setting, they have no relation to a person's ability to do the job. Concerns about availability due to religious or other obligations must be phrased in terms of job requirements. For instance, it is not acceptable to ask the applicant if he or she is a practicing Jehovah's Witness believer, but it is permissible to indicate that the job requires administering blood products and to clarify that this would be something he or she could do.
- *Consistently ask the same questions of all candidates.* If you ask a question that may not be completely job-related, at least make sure you ask it of all candidates. An example is clarifying childcare to be assured of the employee's reliable availability. However, most questions of this nature are usually only asked of female candidates and therefore have been found to be discriminatory. Discrimination is asking only some people certain questions.

11. Talk about the interview process and setting.

- *Arrange a proper location.* Ideally an interview should be conducted in an area where the candidate feels a sense of privacy.
- *Greet the candidate in a friendly manner.* The more comfortable a candidate feels, the more information he or she will be willing to share.
- *Initiate social conversation.* Allow time for the candidate to warm up. Talk about the weather or other "safe" areas of small talk. However, remember that the actual interview begins from the moment you greet the candidate. Does he or she appear professional? Does he or she make eye contact with you? Did he or she greet you in a friendly manner? You need to know whether this person can do the job, wants the job, and will fit in the institution's culture.
- *Describe the organization and position.* Begin in any manner you feel comfortable with. Be careful not to spell out in detail all of the qualities you are looking for in a person, or the interviewee will simply repeat back what you want to hear.
- *Ask prepared questions.* Determining some questions in advance will be a great assistance in keeping you on track during the interview. Feel free to take notes. However, take notes on a separate piece of paper, not on the application or resume, so they remain private.
- *Allow the candidate to talk.* While that seems so obvious, it's amazing how many times interviewers error by talking too much. The goal in an interview is to have the candidate do 75% to 85% of the talking. Remember the old saying: you can't learn anything with your mouth open.
- *Indicate the next steps to the candidate.* Make sure that the interview ends with the interviewee clearly understanding what the next steps in the hiring process will be and when he or she should expect to hear from you.

12. What are the different types of interviews?

There are many types of interviews. There are brief prescreening interviews that can be done over the phone or in person to judge prequalification factors, and there are more in-depth interviews used to make hiring decisions. Types of in-depth interviews include the following:

- Structured interviews (asking every applicant the same questions)
- Patterned interviews (asking every applicant similar questions)
- Stress interviews (how applicants will perform in high-stress positions)
- Nondirective interviews (asking open-ended, nondirective questions)
- Behavioral interviews (how the candidate previously handled specific situations)

Structured interviews, asking the same questions of each candidate, tend to produce the most reliable results. This consistency helps to ensure that similar information will be gathered from each candidate for objective comparisons. In addition, consistency helps avoid the potential for discriminatory questions of certain candidates.

One approach that works well is a semistructured approach. Formulate questions prior to the interviews for a specific position and then write them on a sheet of paper with space after each question to take notes on the candidates' answers. Make enough copies of this question sheet so you have one for each interview.

For each candidate, follow the questions on the sheet and record your answers and impressions. You then have documented comparable information to consider after you have completed all of your interviews.

13. What exactly is a behavioral interview?

Behavioral interviews have become a popular form of interviewing. They are believed to provide better insight into a candidate's creativity, abilities, thinking process, and work style than traditional interview questions.

A behavioral interview focuses on how candidates handled previous specific situations. The interviewer already has an opinion on how he or she feels certain situations should be handled. The interviewer asks the candidate to describe a situation or task, the action that the candidate took, and the result or outcome. The interviewer then evaluates the candidate's behavior in light of what he or she was looking for.

The basic rule of hiring is that past behavior is the best predictor of future behavior. People tend to be somewhat habitual; how they have handled certain tasks and situations in the past is believed to be a good indicator of how they will handle similar situations in the future.

14. Give some examples of behavioral questions.

- "Tell me about a time when you had to deal with a difficult family member." (showing an ability to deal with realistic problems)
- "Describe a time when you were overwhelmed at your job and how you handled that." (assessing for honesty and ability to ask appropriately for help)
- "Tell me about a time you had to break the rules and why." (looking for appropriate flexibility)
- "What would you do if an irate family member asked to speak to the nursing supervisor?" (looking for offering of self/problem solving)
- "What did you do to improve patient care at your last job?" (assessing whether the person sees his or her work as part of the whole)

Some managers focus on skill-related questions, especially when interviewing new graduates. Examples include the following:

- "Tell me the steps you take when suctioning a patient."
- "What assessments would you make in a postoperative patient who is running a fever?"
- "What precautions do you observe when administering blood?"

15. How much should I describe about a position?

Be realistic. It serves no long-term goal to avoid stating the unpleasant aspects of the job. Withholding information will cause hard feelings down the road. The goal of an interview is to make the right fit. Determining the right fit is a mutual process, and both parties have to provide complete and honest information for the relationship to last.

Common areas covered include orientation requirements, patient assignments/staff ratio, scheduling (including holiday and weekend) expectations, mandatory overtime/on-call requirements, dress code, and/or mandatory certifications.

This is also a good time to stress the important values of the institution and/or department, such as customer satisfaction. Some managers have candidates sign a contract stating their understanding and agreement to uphold these core values. Sometimes candidates will withdraw the application if they do not share that same value.

It's always best to for someone to know up front. They are more likely to stick with you through the bad times and you can always remind them that you were honest right from the start. However, don't scare the candidate away. Every job has some unpleasant aspects. They can be stated in a professional, matter-of-fact manner which the candidate will respect.

Remember, a certain amount of salesmanship is involved in convincing a qualified candidate that accepting your position and organization would be a good move. Be sure to include your area's positive points too.

16. How does interviewer bias affect hiring decisions?

Studies have documented several forms of interviewer bias. It's important to be consciously aware of these tendencies and make sure they don't lead to discrimination concerns or poor hiring decisions. A few of the more common biases are

- *Hiring in the same image*—People tend to hire others who remind them of themselves. While that in itself may not be bad, rejecting others because they are not similar could result in discrimination.
- *Stereotyping*—This involves having preconceived opinions on how people of a certain gender, color, physical appearance, age, and so on will perform on the job.
- *First impressions*—It's been said that a person's opinion of someone else is formed in the first 4 minutes of making contact. Those types of snap judgments can be very powerful and hard to erase. This can certainly affect the objectivity of the interview. In an unstructured approach, the interviewer may just be asking questions to confirm their preformed conclusions.
- *Halo/horn effect*—This type of bias allows one or two positive or negative points to overshadow all other information. When a strong positive aspect of a candidate is dominant, this is called the *halo effect* and negative information may be overlooked. When a strong negative aspect of a candidate clouds any positive traits, it's called the *horn effect*.
- *Nonverbal bias*—This can happen when nonverbal behavior, appearance, or dress cause the interviewer to form opinions about a candidate without regard to the candidates' qualifications or potential job performance.
- *Contrast effect*—Rating the candidates only against each other rather than against the requirements of the position. Some candidates may appear more qualified than they really are when compared to weaker ones who were also interviewed.

Similar to performance evaluation, when people are making judgments on other people, it's very hard to avoid errors of bias. However, these errors can be minimized in the interviewing process by

- Being aware of the tendency to form errors of bias.
- Having a current and appropriately detailed job description.
- Asking consistent questions of all candidates and objectively comparing their responses against the position's requirements.

17. How can I tell if someone is professionally motivated?

One indicator is how the candidate spends his or her free time. What professional journals does he or she read? Does he or she have membership in any professional organizations?

18. How can I tell if someone is "burned out"?

Burnout can be difficult to discover in an interview. Warning flags include the following:

• *Frequent job turnovers.* People approach problems by blaming and changing environments rather than looking at themselves.

• *Poor knowledge of one's own limitations.* People experiencing burnout often are unable to set appropriate boundaries. Have the applicant describe his or her strengths and weaknesses. Although a familiar question, the answer can be revealing.

• *A strong need to be liked and approved of.* People get burned out going too far to be liked. Ask how they would handle a disagreement with a coworker.

• *A lack of emotional maturity.* People who have a difficult time dealing with frustrations can burnout prematurely. Take note if you sense a theme of anger.

19. How can I tell if someone is going to be inflexible?

Watch verbal and nonverbal behavior. Does the candidate appear open or closed as you describe any set demands, such as uniform dress code or holiday requirements?

If you sense during the interview that the candidate is the one setting the ground rules of the position, that may be an indicator that he or she will have inflexible expectations about how and when he or she will work.

20. How much weight should I put on my "gut feeling" about a candidate?

That's a tricky question. Most of the professional Human Resources information would suggest that hiring decisions should be based on a careful analysis of previous work performance, behavioral characteristics, and possibly even pre-employment testing results. The suggestion is that hiring decisions should be objectively based on a careful matching of requirements against qualifications.

Every day, however, people are hired more because something clicked between the interviewee and the interviewer. At the same time, candidates who have all the right qualifications and skills are rejected because something just didn't feel right with the interviewer.

Managers develop instincts about people through experience. Those "gut feelings" should not be ignored but can be an indicator of the need to probe deeper. This could be done though reference checking, testing, the impressions of others, or more extended interviewing. Don't ignore your instincts, but rather explore your concerns.

We know from years of experience that, qualifications and backgrounds being mostly equal, the person the hiring manager likes the best is the one who usually gets the job. That's not necessarily bad. The manager will want that person to succeed and will tend to put more energy and thought into helping this candidate to do that.

21. Is taking the candidate on a tour a good idea?

Yes. If time allows, walk the candidate around the hospital or the unit. It gives the opportunity to provide a more realistic understanding of the position. In addition, observe how he or she interacts with other staff members or possible patient contact. Does the candidate appear comfortable in that environment?

22. Is pre-employment testing a good idea?

It depends on the type of test. There are Equal Employment Opportunity concerns surrounding pre-employment testing. The general guideline for testing is the same as for every step of the selection and hiring process—the test must be nondiscriminatory. The test must be reliable, valid, and job-related.

• *Reliable* means that consistent results are obtained from the test.

• *Valid* means that the test actually measures what it is intended to measure.

• *Job-related* means there is a clear link between what the test is measuring and future job performance.

Examples are a drug dosage and solution math test or rhythm interpretation test (for critical care). This is fine as long as the tests are required of all candidates for the position.

23. Are reference checks important?

Absolutely. Try to make personal contact with someone who has worked with the candidate, such as a previous supervisor or coworker. However, it is important to ask the candidates' permission to contact references. Candidates have the right to keep their job search confidential.

One question that can be revealing is, "What would your supervisor say about you?" You're likely to get a fairly honest answer from candidates because they assume you will be contacting their supervisor.

Written reference verification forms usually do not result in much more than a confirmation of employment dates. Personal character references, whose names candidate provides, generally do not provide information of any real value.

24. What is important to remember about company public relations in the hiring process?

It's a small world, especially in health care. How an applicant is treated will get around. If an applicant is not treated with courtesy and respect at any point in the hiring process, other prospective candidates will hear about it and may avoid your organization. Likewise, if the hiring process was a pleasant experience, that will make a lasting impression on an employee, which will also be shared with others.

It's important to make sure candidates are given clear information on what the hiring process will be and when they should expect to hear from someone else in the organization. If there is any change in the plan, the candidates should be contacted and given updated information. A simple telephone call can make all the difference. Candidates will appreciate your consideration of the need to know where they stand.

This is true even if you plan to reject them. It's not uncommon to hear candidates complain about how they applied and even interviewed for a position never to hear what happened with it. That leaves a poor impression. Make it a point to be sure at least every person you interviewed is contacted one way or the other.

25. How is the workforce changing?

The workforce is getting older. In fact, 52% of the workforce in 2000 are considered to be Baby Boomers. The first of those Baby Boomers may begin to retire in 2011. Who will fill those vacancies, especially in health care, where there is already a shortage of workers. For nurses there are two primary sources: immigration of foreign nurses and retaining older nurses.

There are a lot of myths surrounding the value of older workers. It's primarily these myths that should be retired and not the older workers. The truth is that older workers bring experience and a strong work ethic.

Older workers may need a few special considerations, such as more time for training, better explanation of the reasons behind change, or flexibility in working hours. Inflexibility in work scheduling options is the greatest barrier to retaining older workers. Part-time work options are critical for retaining older workers. But it is well-worth making these considerations.

The traditional workplace approach has been to provide training to younger workers, more than older workers, since it was assumed the younger workers will stay on the job longer and return the investment. In reality, this no longer true. In fact, it's more likely that an older worker will stay at one workplace longer than the younger workers.

26. What can I do to help with the labor shortage in health care?

Every person you come in contact with might be, or might know of, a great candidate. Remember, every time you go to a store or eat at a restaurant you are observing or coming in contact with people who are providing a service. If you observe that someone seems to truly enjoy working with people, that person might be interested in an entry level career in health care. Many people are unfamiliar with health care and have no idea how rewarding the experience can be. Ask people to come by for a visit. Who knows, one may go on to become an RN or a doctor. It's happened before. All it takes is a little encouragement and a step in the right direction.

One of the problems health care is struggling with is a poor public relations image. Rather than being seen as a respected industry, many current workers are talking prospective workers *out* of a career in healthcare. If we can't or won't sell our own occupations to others, we are going to be working short for a long time to come.

BIBLIOGRAPHY

1. Bell AH: The Complete Manager's Guide to Interviewing: How to Hire the Best. Homewood, IL, Business One Irwin, 1989.
2. Commerce Clearing House: Equal Employment Opportunity Manual for Managers and Supervisors, 2nd ed. Chicago, Commerce Clearing House, 1991.
3. Cook M: Human Resource Director's Handbook. Englewood Cliffs, NJ, Prentice-Hall, 1984.
4. Gomez-Mejia LR, Balkin DB, Cardy RL: Managing Human Resources. Englewood Cliffs, NJ, Prentice-Hall, 1995.
5. Judy R, D'Amico C: Workforce 2020. Indianapolis, IN, Hudson Institute, 1998.
6. Ledvinka J: Federal Regulation of Personnel and Human Resources Management, 2nd ed. Boston, Kent Publishing, 1991.
7. Milkovich GT, Boudreau JW: Human Resources Management, 6th ed. Homewood, IL, Richard D. Irwin, 1991.
8. Mitchell O: As the Workforce Ages. Ithaca, NY, ILR Press, 1993.
9. Sherman A, Bohlander G, Chruden H: Managing Human Resources. Cincinnati, OH, South-Western Publishing, 1988.
10. United States of America Federal Government: Uniform Guidelines on Employment Selection Procedures. Washington, DC, Federal Register, 1978.

17. ORIENTATION AND SOCIALIZATION OF NEW EMPLOYEES

Camilla L. Jones, RN, BBA

Six essential qualities that are the key to success: sincerity, personal integrity, humility, courtesy, wisdom, charity.

Dr. William Menninger

1. Why do new employees occasionally leave just after orientation?

Socialization of new employees is *crucial* to retention. The most common behavior observed in new employees "settling in" is that of seeking acceptance. According to Maslow's Hierarchy of Needs, the "sense of belonging" falls just after food, water, shelter, and safety. If a new employee does not feel accepted, he or she won't stay.

2. What can I do to make sure that the new employee is accepted?

The manager is responsible for two important initiatives to facilitate socialization of new employees:

1. Selecting a candidate who fits the job or work environment
2. Molding the culture to support and mentor new employees

3. What can I do to make sure I have correctly matched the candidate and the work environment?

- Spend quality time in the interview process.
- Ask open-ended questions.
- Encourage the candidate to ask questions.
- Have a group interview, using employees who will orient the candidate.

4. What specific benefits does a panel interview provide in matching the candidate to the job?

It provides the candidate with a multidimensional view of the work environment. Workers never see the workplace in the same light as the manager. The candidate may feel more comfortable asking potential peers questions. Most importantly, participation promotes ground level buy-in with peers. When peers are involved in the selection process, there is an automatic sense of responsibility to help the selected candidate succeed.

5. Is there a downside to using a panel interview process?

Participating employees must understand the associated labor laws and should interview only appropriate prescreened applications. The manager will consider the panel's input, but the final selection is made by the manager in light of both the initial interview and panel information. Minimize problems associated with panel interviews by having a defined structure to the process and by providing training for all participants.

6. How does a nonsupportive culture begin and survive?

New nurses have become disenchanted with the "eat their young" stigma that has chased the nursing profession for years. It is ironic that nurses who are critical of new employees are the very nurses who now complain that the unit is never staffed. It is also the writer's opinion that this behavior probably comes from an effort to build one's own self-esteem. The culture self-perpetuates if workers are never exposed to anything other than nonsupport: "I paid my dues. They have to pay theirs." It is an understatement that this "insider" or "club" mentality does not facilitate a welcoming environment.

7. **What is the manager's role in curbing non-support?**
   • Do not allow nonsupportive cultures to flourish.
   • Lead by example.
   • Set clear expectations to staff.
   • Address nonsupportive behaviors.

8. **Identify some nursing unit nonsupportive behaviors.**
   • Minimal orientation or assistance
   • Subjective or critical commentary
   • Isolationism
   • Lack of assertive friendliness
   • Withholding vital information
   • Territorialism
   • Failure to mentor
   • Active resistance to new employee input

9. **What else can I do to facilitate a culture that supports socialization of new employees?**
   Unhealthy organizational behavior survives only if it remains covert. This means that healthy organizational behavior must be addressed in a public forum as an organizational expectation. Communicate expectations that *staff* are responsible for the successful integration of the new employee. The new employee will be only as good as the orientation he or she is provided.

10. **Name specific actions to make sure I help, rather than sabotage, the socialization.**
   • Avoid endearing proclamations, such as "the candidate is perfect." It can set the employee up for failure and you could lose credibility if the candidate doesn't work out.
   • Introduce the new employee to every staff member or doctor available every time they are on the unit, even during the interviewing process. This action provides early familiarity and can increase comfort levels.
   • Choose a preceptor who wants to mentor a new employee.
   • Evaluate the orientation progress at regular intervals (recommended weekly) for early identification and intervention for any problems.

11. **What do I do if my new employee appears to be self-sabotaging?**
   New employees can sometimes exhibit behaviors that do not endear themselves to staff members. Some of these behaviors come from an effort to quickly prove competence or gain credibility, and some are due to insecurity in a new environment. These behaviors include the following:
   • Trying to take charge
   • Referencing their last workplace
   • Territorialism
   • Overenthusiasm
   • Failure to respond to suggestion
   • Self-isolationism
   • Hesitancy to participate
   • Lack of initiative
   • "I'm the expert" syndrome

12. **Any suggestions for handling this?**
   All new employees have a period of proving competency to gain credibility. If these behaviors start to crop up, they should be brought to the new employee's attention and discussed

in private. These behaviors can indicate that the new employee is having difficulty feeling accepted. Explore specific areas of concern and provide appropriate encouragement. However, also reinforce performance expectations specific to teamwork.

13. How do I decide if a new employee needs a formal preceptor?

All new employees should be assigned a designated preceptor. Even contract personnel must have a core orientation prior to working independently. Any new employee (no matter how experienced or short the orientation) needs a resource to ensure adequate orientation and compliance to facility policy and procedures.

14. When should I assign a preceptor?

The preceptorship usually begins once the new employee arrives on the unit. However, the most effective method is to assign and introduce the preceptor during the final hiring process. Some units have the preceptor participate in the final interview. In addition, providing an orientation overview to the new employee at the time of the final hiring is very beneficial.

15. How long should orientation with a preceptor last?

Orientation is determined based on the new employee's prior experiences, familiarity with the institution, and individual ability to learn. Most orientation programs are designed on a three-tiered matrix containing plans for new employees with little or no experience, 1 or more year's experience in a related field, and extensive or recent experiences in a related field. Some critical care units require additional classes and competency testing.

16. How do I pick the best preceptor?

It is always tempting to use the most competent clinical nurse. Preceptors should be selected based on their ability to communicate, educate, delegate, and evaluate progress. The most effective preceptors are able to combine roles of both clinical and social resource.

17. Do preceptors need special education?

Some people are certainly natural-born educators. However, providing structured expectations and resources will produce a consistent standard orientation. Selected preceptors should be very familiar with organizational policies, procedures, and competency tools. Some organizations have formal preceptor training. Elements usually include the following:
• Role of the preceptor
• New employee socialization
• Concepts of adult learning
• Goal setting
• Evaluation techniques
• Providing feedback
• Troubleshooting during the orientation process
• Documentation

18. Should I let someone precept a friend whom he or she recruited?

All preceptors should meet the defined criteria. Some companies believe that those persons who have a friend at work will have improved satisfaction and retention. The downside is that the objective evaluation process is usually sacrificed. In addition, other contacts and socialization efforts can be affected. This is not a "never" situation. Small towns with small hospitals may be in a situation where there is only one primary preceptor. If someone is precepting a friend, the manager should monitor the activities at regular intervals.

19. Can I mix and match preceptors or should I just select one?

It is always more effective to select one preceptor for the entire orientation process for continuity. It becomes difficult for the new preceptor to pick up where the last preceptor left off, even if the documentation is excellent. Less experienced employees can actually be set back in their orientation process if the precepting is too fragmented. A manager may be able to allow adjustments if the new employee is very experienced, if that experience is recent, or if the new employee is transferring within the same facility.

20. How do I make a clinical assignment for an orientee with a preceptor?

All clinical shifts should be assigned for the new employee based on the preceptor's schedule. The assignment should follow the matrix and should not be overwhelming or increased based on "two" persons doing the job. If anything, consideration should be given to reducing the assignment, especially in the early part of the orientation process.

21. But what if I'm short-staffed?

It's a mistake to depend on orienting personnel to fill vacant shifts. Using new employees to fill shifts prior to adequate orientation can place the hospital, the charge nurse, and the manager in a position of extreme liability. Staff member expectations change when a new employee is off orientation, even if the orientation is aborted. All personnel who are off orientation are to "pull their own load." If the new employee is not oriented adequately, he or she will not be as effective, which frustrates staff and the new employee.

22. My nurses don't like to precept. How do I motivate them?

Precepting is difficult and wrought with responsibility. If multiple resources exist, rotate precepting responsibilities. Consider compensation, including preceptor differential, clinical ladder advances, educational opportunities, or bonuses.

23. How do I know my new employee is ready?

The orientee should have competency objectives to meet prior to the completion of orientation. The clinical goals and objectives should reflect the competency documentation tool that is used by the facility. Most new employees will be able to complete the orientation process during the designated time frame. Occasionally, an orientee will require additional time, which is acceptable as long as the new employee is making adequate progress. It is helpful to have a formal system of anecdotal notes that are kept by both the preceptor and the new employee. The employee and the preceptor should meet with the clinical manager at least weekly to discuss concerns and progress.

24. What are the preceptor's responsibilities if the new employee is failing to progress or is not compliant?

The preceptor's responsibilities are to objectively document concerns or problems and to immediately bring them to the manager's attention. Remediation activities are usually agreed upon between the manager and the preceptor. The preceptor should not be involved in any termination processes.

BIBLIOGRAPHY

1. Deutschendorf A: Managers Forum: Preparing and compensating preceptors. J Emerg Nurs 26(5):496–498, 2000.
2. Meinecke J: No nurse is an island. Nurs Manage 31:35–36, 2000.
3. Moorehead G, Griffin RW: Organizational Behavior. Boston, Houghton Mifflin, 1995.
4. Oermann M, Garvin M: When coaching new grads. Nurs Manage 31:26–27, 2001.

18. STAFF SCHEDULING

Polly Gerber Zimmermann, RN, MS, MBA, CEN, *and Mark Ambler,* RN, BSN, CCRN

The great rule of moral conduct is, next to God, to respect Time.

Johann Kaspar Lavater

1. What is ratio staffing?

Ratio staffing involves specific RN to patient ratios, such as 1:2, in which one nurse is assigned to two patients. Ratio staffing has been the main staple of RN staffing but is confining because it does not allow for acuity.

2. Tell me about legislated staffing ratios.

In October 1999, California became the first state to enact mandatory staffing ratio legislation. This legislation requires minimum, specific, licensed nurse-to-patient ratios for all acute care hospitals. Previously, similar ratios existed in California only for hospital intensive care units and operating rooms.

The bill was sponsored by the California Nurses Association. It was seen as the culmination of nurses' concern over adequate staffing reaching the public to force staffing changes for the better. Since then, more than 34 bills regarding staffing-related initiatives have been introduced in various state legislatures.

3. What ratios are hospitals using?

In a nationwide 2000 survey, the average in medial surgical units is one RN for 5.7 patients on the day shift and 7.4 patients on the night shift. The range of RN-patient ratios reported was from 1:4 to 1:11 on the day shift and 1:4 to 1:13 on the night shift. A problem identified is that many patients are not sleeping on the night shift, which makes the upper end of this range a large load for nurses. California is currently narrowing in on a 1:5 ratio. In critical care, on average, RN-patient ratios were 1:2 on both the day and night shift.

4. I see the hoped-for benefits. List some criticisms of legislated staffing ratios.

- Staffing levels are being determined by the government, away from the bedside.
- Needed changes will be slow and cumbersome because they must go through legislation.
- A fear that the minimum levels will become the standardized maximum.
- A difficulty in achieving agreement even among various nursing organizations as to what the optimal staffing level should be.
- This is a misguided focus. The emphasis should not be on mere numbers but on patient outcomes.
- Having mandated staffing ratios does not guarantee the outcome of adequate staffing. Staffing needs can change instantaneously as a patient rapidly deteriorates.
- A nurse is not a nurse. Staff characteristics, such as experience level, influence the patient load that a specific nurse can adequately handle.

5. What is patient-focused staffing?

Patient-focused staffing considers the total care needs of the unit's population. This model of staffing requires a change in process. It requires forethought, an autonomous nursing staff, and independent ancillary staff. The nurse must now look away from thinking "I can only care for x number of patients" to "I can only provide x amount of care."

Management and the bedside nurses must review the unit's care needs, then divide that care fairly among the staff. "Seasoned" staff may have the larger patient volume, but also have more ancillary assistance. Novice staff may have a smaller assignment and less ancillary assistance. The unit's staff must work well together and provide a unified, not just individual care, team effort.

6. What are the scheduling issues with these types of staffing?

Both of these care models creates schedule dilemmas. With ratio staffing, you must staff the unit with the minimum staff, then flex up or down as patient numbers allow. With patient-focused staffing, you must have a full view of the unit's typical activities to make proper staffing decisions. You may be able to trend your staffing, but for the most part, staffing decisions are made by each and every shift. Most units plan their staffing needs on the presumption that all of their beds will be full with the typical level of acuity.

7. What other factors can influence the best staffing level besides the number of nurses?

Influencing factors are related to the characteristics of the patients, the staff, and the system. See also the chapter on staffing budgets.

8. Tell me more about patient factors.

Some patient factors are acuity, turnover, volume (particularly a fluctuating census), need for instruction, family/emotional needs, or language/educational concerns. For instance, a Russian-only speaking patient who is a new diabetic on insulin and is going home tomorrow probably requires more nursing interventions than a stable 3-day postoperative English-speaking hysterectomy patient.

9. Describe staff factors.

Staff factors include the level of experience of the nurse, his or her specialty, competency, turnover, and skill mix. For instance, a float nurse, agency nurse, and new graduate nurse could not handle the same unit assignment as two senior, experienced RNs with an LPN. Potential problems exist when the staffing on a unit is composed of 25% or more temporary workers (either from a float pool or an external agency).

10. List some system factors.

System factors include the location of support areas (e.g., drug cart, dirty utility room), support personnel, support services (e.g. delivery of drugs, collection of lunch trays), and physician practice patterns. For instance, many EDs report that after renovation that increased square footage, it took more time to give care to the same number of patients because of the increased distance to essential areas, such as the narcotic supply.

Another factor to consider is documentation, since up to 30% of the RN's time is taken up with that task. Consultant Holly A. DeGroot found that one hospital's ED nurses spent 6.8 full-time equivalent (FTE) hours per day doing the required documentation. Streamlining this process could free up the current nursing staff to provide more nursing care.

11. What shift length should you use?

Shift length is usually determined before your arrival as a manager, and staff should be consulted before any major change. Eight hours is traditional, but 10- or 12- hour shifts are popular. Many units use a mixture of all three. Four-hour shifts are useful for peak activity times and part-time staff.

Most managers find it easier to make a schedule with 12-hour shifts than with 10-hour shifts. It is also usually easier to find coverage for a sick call on a 12-hour shift, which can then be divided in half. However, both nursing and physician studies have indicated that working 8-hour shifts, rather than 12-hour shifts, improves patient care, especially if there is shift rotation.

12. What is the best start time?

Circadian expert Martin Moore-Ede, MD, PhD, indicates that in general it is difficult to get out of bed before 6:00 AM or to sleep past 1:00 PM. However, a workforce older than 45 years of age may prefer an early start time because older people tend to wake up earlier. As a whole, he recommends a shift change between 7:00 and 8:00 AM and does not recommend any shift ending in the middle of the night.

A new trend, especially in departments with a wide census fluctuation, is atypical start times. For instance, one ED uses the shifts of 800–1800, 400–1400, 1400–12 midnight, 1600–200, and 1800–400. This arrangement is popular because staff members can be available for their school-aged children, and no nurse has to work the entire traditional night shift.

13. Our hospital requires shift rotation. Is there a best way to schedule that?

Studies report that a days-evenings-nights rotation is easier on your circadian rhythm than a nights-evenings-day rotation. One week at a time on each shift gives your internal clock time to adjust. Experts recommend not working more than three night shifts in a row. Realistically, these recommendations are often not feasible, but it can be worthwhile to follow them as much as possible.

14. How do you begin to make a schedule?

Nationwide, 80% of acute care nursing units have decentralized staffing schedules. Most managers start by penciling in the following:
- Weekend requirements
- "Requests"
- Holiday and vacation days

Then they pencil in the hired shifts for staff, usually in blocks of 3 or 4 days in a row. However, you do have to keep in mind the various individuals' experience level. You don't want all new graduates staffing the unit just because the rotation works out easily.

Most managers give preference for the desired staffing patterns or day shifts to the full-time staff (since they have a higher commitment and must work more often), then to the part-time staff, and finally to float-pool registry staff to "fill in the holes." Sometimes what happens, however, is that the registry must receive priority because of their limited availability and the department's need.

The advantage of this type of schedule making is that it allows maximum flexibility for the individual staff member in making requests for specific days. The disadvantage is that it can easily take a manager 12 to 16 hours to prepare a 4-week schedule.

15. There seem to be so many possibilities.

Most staff have some kind of personal preference. One nurse likes one day on, one day off. Another nurse wants long stretches so she can have 5 days off in a row without using any vacation time. "Rewarding" good nurses with their preferred scheduling pattern can be a powerful retention tool and contributor to employee satisfaction.

I also have found that nurses, as a whole, are understanding of the need to occasionally rally and work a less than desirable shift or pattern. The key is to ask the person ahead of time as a favor rather than just arbitrarily assigning it.

16. What is a set, or master, scheduling pattern?

Historically begun in production/manufacturing industries, this system assigns each employee a set pattern of scheduled days that does not vary from schedule to schedule. In one survey, 64% of the responding hospitals report using a master schedule in at least some units. For instance, one unit has a 6-week repeating cycle established for the next 3 years. Any requests for exchanges must be negotiated between the staff.

The advantage is that it takes less time to make the schedule and each nurse knows the schedule in advance and can plan accordingly. Some units even found it was a good recruitment tool. The disadvantage is the loss of easily obtained accommodations for unique needs.

17. Give some examples of more unique set schedules.

One hospital uses 12-hour shifts of three-on, three-off. Staff work three weekends in a row (assuming Friday is a weekend day) and then have the next three weekends off. It is popular because there are 8 days off in a row (a "mini-vacation") every 6 weeks:

Week 1:   work Friday/Saturday/Sunday
Week 2:   work Thursday/Friday/Saturday
Week 3:   work Wednesday/Thursday/Friday
Week 4;   work Tuesday/Wednesday/Thursday
Week 5:   work Monday/Tuesday/Wednesday
Week 6:   work Friday/Saturday/Sunday

Another hospital uses a pattern of 10-hour shifts, 7 days on, then 7 days off. Within the 2-week pay period, the nurses work 70 hours and take 4 hours paid time off (a combination of vacation and sick benefits). (The hospital provides full-time benefits for staff working 64 hours or more.) The staff like the long stretches of off-days. The holidays that each employee will work rotate as a result of a yearly one-time, 2-week schedule of 40-hour weeks of 8-hour shifts.

18. Are there any examples of a financial advantage to having a cyclic, set schedule?

Besides the saved schedule-making time, some established patterns have resulted in a financial gain. One hospital hires all staff to work one of two distinctive cycles of 12-hour shifts: 2 days on and 2 days off, 4 days on and 6 days off (2,2,4,6), or 2-6-4-2.

Staff are paid for 4 additional hours per week (8 hours per pay period) of their base hourly rate only if they had no call-offs (sick day, absence), paid time off (vacation, holiday), education time, or tardies within that week. Clocking in *even 1 minute late* disqualifies the staff member for all incentive pay in that period.

This established schedule and incentive pay became such a powerful recruitment tool that the hospital filled all of its vacant nursing positions. Tardiness became a thing of the past. And the hospital's incidental overtime fell to less than 20 hours per month, since nurses were voluntarily willing to stay a little extra for emergency needs.

19. What is the Baylor Plan?

There are many variations, but the Baylor Plan basically involves having some designated staff who work every weekend and some staff who work only weekdays. The weekend staff is usually rewarded with some type of pay premium but fewer benefits. Often a contract is signed so that the employee commits to this schedule for a set period of time, such as 6 months.

The advantage is that staff like it and it aids recruitment and retention. Nurses with children prefer the weekdays; nurses in school often prefer the weekend. The disadvantages are that it usually costs more staffing dollars in the budget and the weekend group can feel isolated.

20. What other factors should I consider as I plan the schedule?

Monitor the support staff and services as closely as the nursing staff. DeGroot advocates focusing on the percentage of time that nurses actually spend with patients rather than on the total number of nurses. She found in one hospital, for instance, that the ICU nurses with a ratio of 2:1 were actually spending less direct patient time than nurses in other units with lower staffing ratios. The reason was that the ICU lacked necessary support systems, such as a unit secretary and a drug delivery system.

21. I manage an emergency department. Every now and then, we get a sudden surge of many high-acuity patients that overwhelm the department. How can I staff to deal with that?

It is impossible to staff for unusual times when unexpected volume or acuity overwhelms a patient care department. With overcrowding becoming a more frequent occurrence, EDs are starting to look at some type of emergency plan to marshal additional resources. Aspects include the following:

- Calling in additional staff/floating in-house staff to the ED
- Calling in additional ancillary staff, such as laboratory or radiology personnel
- Holding orders on nonemergency patients until all emergency patients are cared for
- Admitting ED patients to the in-patient unit even though the admission work-up has not been completed
- Using other areas for the additional patients, such as after-hour preoperative/recovery rooms or out-patient clinics.

Hospitals are also developing plans to deal with an unexpected, institution-wide saturation when volume, acuity, bed availability, or staffing issues arise. Possible actions include limiting elective surgeries, denying direct admissions, or working with physicians for accelerated discharges of qualifying patients. One hospital even cancels all management meetings while all nursing administrators help out on the patient floor units.

22. When an employee is absent (called out sick, vacation) from a regularly scheduled weekend or holiday, should I require a make-up weekend or holiday?

It depends. First realize that you must have a universal policy. Requiring make-ups discourages abusive use and removes any need to judge whether the person was *really* ill. Disadvantages are that it is sometimes difficult to appropriately schedule in these make-up days and the compliant staff get punished.

One manager has the policy that make-up is expected "contingent on the needs of the department." Many managers choose not to have routine make-up obligations and then deal with any abuse under the ordinary disciplinary rules.

23. How do you cover holidays?

Holiday coverage is a sensitive issue with most employees. "Old school management" used to schedule the new employees on the holidays to show appreciation to the long-term employee. However, this practice usually does not meet JCAHO's standard for consistent patient care. Possible solutions include the following:

- Self-scheduling
- Every-other year (e.g., work Christmas this year, off next year)
- Optional choices within requirements (e.g., two of the five "major holidays"— Thanksgiving, Christmas Eve, Christmas, New Year's Eve, New Year's Day, and two of the four "minor holidays"—Easter, Memorial Day, July 4th, Labor Day).
- Narrowing the choices to key prime shifts with fewer requirements (e.g., one of the six prime shifts of evenings on Christmas Eve, nights on Christmas Eve, days on Christmas, evenings on New Year's Eve, nights on New Year's Eve, days on New Year's day).
- Every-other-holiday within the same year (e.g., off on Thanksgiving, work on Christmas; off on New Year's Day).

In my experience, most employees have one or two important requests with flexibility on the others. For instance, as long as they have off on New Year's Eve and Day, they don't care about Thanksgiving or Christmas.

24. Any tips for making it a smoother process?

In my experience, you should initially insist that employees commit to their regular shift for their required worked holidays. Otherwise you can have an evening shift nurse assuming a day shift on Christmas Eve to fulfill the holiday obligation. I also do not allow holiday requests in the request book; these are a unique situation all their own. Negotiation among staff is always a possibility.

Keep detailed records of the assignments and rules so each employee knows what to expect next year. You may also want to address this topic in hiring interviews so there are no surprises.

25. Should I schedule fewer staff on holidays so more can enjoy the day off?

Unless you know for a fact that you will have a decreased census, you must keep the same safe, consistent level of staffing. Patient needs don't change just because it is a holiday.

I do not schedule myself on holidays because I sometimes become the last resort for a sick-call or crisis.

26. How do you cover vacations?

Try to meet most plausible vacation requests. Employees need time off to rejuvenate and prevent burnout. But you need to control staff numbers during high request times, typically the summer and December. Communicate any stipulations about the number of employees who can have vacation at the same time. Options for granting vacation time include:

- First come, first served in a request book
- Group bidding by seniority
- Limits to only so many summer weeks, regardless of the accrued time
- Sharing nurses from the same type of unit within a hospital network to cover unusual needs

27. What is the manager's role in a leave of absence (LOA) under the Family Medical Leave Act (FMLA)?

You are only the facilitator. When an employee requests a leave of absence, you can inquire why but then direct that employee to the proper department. Do not try to interrogate the employee, insinuate it is excessive, hint at disciplinary actions, or discuss the employee's situation with anyone but your appropriate hospital contact. If other employees ask why, only respond that the employee will be off. Any deviations could become a legal issue. However, when an employee does not work his or her weekend shifts because of the leave, the manager is allowed to require make-up weekend shifts.

28. Describe a float pool and how it is used.

This is a broad term used to describe many different concepts. Approximately 71% of surveyed hospitals have an internal float pool, which is a type of institutional registry or resource team, and 46% said the option worked well for them. This is a decrease from previous years. The reason provided is a difficulty in recruiting enough qualified staff for the float pool. More nurses are opting to work part time as part of a unit rather than being in the float pool.

Nurses in a float pool are not affiliated with any unit and agree to be assigned to where they are most urgently needed. They are usually classified for or limited to units in which they have established experience, training and competencies, such as critical care (ICU, ED) or maternal-child (labor and delivery, postpartum, nursery). Hospitals vary in whether these positions receive benefits.

Lawrenz Consulting found that hospitals also had float pools for LPNs (64%), nursing assistants (71%), and unit clerks (58%). Having other types of personnel, besides RNs, in the float pool prevents using a nurse for a need that could be met by someone with lesser training.

In addition, many hospitals or specialty units will have a PRN pool (also sometimes called per diem/casual) of nurses who commit to work for their unit a certain number shifts per schedule. The number of hours they are scheduled is not usually guaranteed but will fluctuate depending on the unit's needs.

29. Should I use mandatory overtime to cover my needs?

Most managers consider mandatory overtime unsafe. At the time of this writing, professional organizations, unions, and legislative action are growing toward preventing this.

30. Discuss how you flex up or flex down staffing levels.

Flexing down staff means eliminating an employee when there is an unanticipated drop in patient care needs. It is not as simple as it sounds, however. It is usually done by asking an employee to leave work early for no pay, with or without accrued time off. There should be some type of department process determining who is asked to leave first and whether or not it is optional.

In my experience, if asked, most staff do not mind leaving. However, if an employee wants to complete the shift, I allow it even if he or she had worked an extra shift earlier in the week. It shows the appropriate consideration to the nurse because he or she helped you out earlier by working that extra shift. Rejoice than an employee wants to work! Then ask the next person in line.

You may also offer the opportunity to float and help other units in the hospital. Remember, nursing as a team is working for all patients, not just this unit.

Flexing up on a short-term basis involves scheduling additional people for a planned "surge" in need, calling them on an as-needed basis or according to an on-call system. For further discussion, see the chapter on on-call systems.

31. No matter what I do with the schedule, I am always finding staff looking at it and making comments.

This common behavior was difficult for me to get used to when I first started making schedules. I assumed it meant dissatisfaction. Now I realize the schedule is just an interesting, common topic for discussion (like the weather) because it does affect everyone's lives so much. I do not worry about any actions or behaviors about the schedule unless a person is concerned enough to approach me directly.

BIBLIOGRAPHY

1. American Association of Critical-Care Nurses: Maintaining Patient-Focused Care in an Environment of Nursing Staff Shortages and Financial Constraints. AACN Public Policy, 2001.
2. American Organization of Nurse Executives: Patient Care Redesign. Chicago, Health Forum, Inc. 1999.
3. Bowden C: Managers Forum: Unique schedule patterns. J Emerg Nurs 2002 [in press].
4. Cavouras CA: Nurse staffing levels in American hospitals: A 2001 report. J Emerg Nurs 28:40–43, 2002.
5. Lawrenz Consulting: Annual Survey of Hours: Perspectives on Staffing and Scheduling. 19(3):1–6, 1999. *www.lawrenzconsult.com*
6. Stone S: Managers Forum: Unique schedule patterns. J Emerg Nurs 2002 [in press].
7. Thomas H Jr, Schwartz E, Whitehead DC: Eight- versus 12-hour shifts: Implications for emergency physicians. Ann Emerg Med 23:1096–1100, 1994.
8. Weiss DH: Fair, Square, & Legal, 3rd ed. New York, American Management Association, 2000.
9. Whitehead DC, Thomas H Jr, Slapper DR: A rational approach to shift work in emergency medicine. Ann Emerg Med 21:112–120, 1992.
10. Zimmermann PG: Managers Forum: Staffing standards benchmarking. J Emerg Nurs 27(2):179–181, 2001.

19. SELF-SCHEDULING

Mark Ambler, RN, BSN, CCRN

When you prevent me from doing anything I want to do, that is persecution; but when I prevent you from doing anything you want to do, that is law, order and morals.

George Bernard Shaw

1. What is self-scheduling?

Self-scheduling puts the staff in charge of both daily scheduling and their *own* schedule according to agreed-upon rules. Employee "buy-in" is usually high because they feel more in control. However, there is no perfect world in which everyone is 100% satisfied. One unit with an established self-scheduling program estimates they meet about 80% of the first-round requests.

2. Who is in charge of the schedule?

Ultimately the manager of the unit is responsible for all schedules, but you can delegate some authority to coordinators or a scheduling committee. It is best to have a minimum of two people involved to allow for more visibility, to provide a "checks-and-balance" system, and to decrease burnout.

3. How can signing up for shifts with self-scheduling be handled in a fair and consistent manner?

One solution is that the coordinators create a "skeleton" schedule. This schedule will show requested days off and required needs for each day. Usually stringent weekend assignments are required, with the option to exchange after the schedule is finalized. Employees then fill in days, as they want, while monitoring each day's total need.

A common solution is to have employee groups that take turns in signing up, as follows:

Group 1: Top priority (almost always get their choices)

Group 2: Limbo group (somewhat guaranteed to get their requested schedule)

Group 3: Gatekeepers (used to fill in staffing needs).

The staffing coordinators usually have authority to move the third group as needed to fill unmet needs.

Most use groups with a mixture of full-time and part-time employees. The groups, as well as the order of the employees inside the group, are rotated with each new skeleton schedule.

Each group usually contains staff from all shifts. However, some coordinators allow the full-time evening and night staff to sign up first. This is their "perk" for taking an undesirable shift and also results in the rest of the staff working fewer of these shifts. Others always allow full-time staff (from all shifts) to sign up first, followed by part-time and then registry/agency/PRN staff. Overtime opportunities can be offered to the entire staff after all groups have signed up, or be available on the same group rotation.

4. It seems that this could create more problems than solutions. Any tips?

Those experienced with this system recommend establishing group ground rules from the beginning that include the following:

- Requirements for weekends and holidays.
- How vacation and "absolute needs" (e.g., a wedding) will be handled, including a maximum number.
- Deciding when the skeleton schedule will be posted. Make it during daytime hours. One ED had nurses lining up at midnight to be the first to sign up!

- Deadlines for each stage of the scheduling process.
- Mandatory sign-up for the shift(s) the individual was hired for. For instance, someone hired for the 12-hour night position cannot sign up for 8-hour day shifts.
- Provisions for scheduling someone who is out of town when the skeleton schedule is posted.
- Determining whether or not you will allow phone-in requests for filling in the schedule.
- How agency/float pool/registry personnel will be handled.

5. We just started self-scheduling and have some problems. Are we doing something wrong?

Most successful programs counsel to allow 6 months for an adequate trial. It takes at least 1 year (sometimes 2) until the system flows smoothly because staff must become proficient in negotiating. Allowing ample trading (provided that trades are equal and do not affect the staff's balance) is the key to success.

Persistent problems can usually be resolved by establishing an appropriate ground rule. Some units even have a scheduled meeting every 6 months to specifically deal with self-scheduling review and resolution.

BIBLIOGRAPHY

Zimmermann PG: How we do it: Self-scheduling in the emergency department. J Emerg Nurs 21(1):58–61, 1995.

20. ON-CALL STAFFING

Mark Ambler, RN, BSN, CCRN

Hope for the best, but prepare for the worst.

English proverb

1. What is an on-call system?

On-call scheduling manages unforeseen staffing needs as the census, acuity, or length-of-stay dramatically changes by "calling in" the unit's employees on an as-needed basis. Employees sign up for extra shift(s) or day(s) on the schedule as "on call." The employee is usually paid a nominal wage (usually $2–$3 an hour) during unneeded time and regular or overtime wages during clock-in time. There is usually a minimum amount of time, such as 2 or 4 hours, for which the employee will be paid for coming in, even if the employee was needed for a shorter period. A newer trend is to use this system for areas that can have unexpected fluctuating census, such as emergency departments or intensive care units.

2. What should I consider if I am thinking about starting an on-call system?

- *Verify that your staffing level is adequate and resolve attendance issues.* On-call scheduling is not intended to substitute for staffing vacancies or abusive patterns of sick call. Other factors are probably involved if on-call staffing will be needed more than two to three times a week.
- *Obtain administrative approval.* This system involves a pay scheme for nonproductive time.
- *Consider staff response.* Initial staff buy-in is a delicate matter, since staff members were hired without this understanding. Resistance is more likely from single parents without childcare options or those who have a significant commute. Present the new system as a positive change for safe patient care and allow a period to make arrangements.

Also consider whether it would be beneficial to have assistive personnel on call instead of, or in addition to, nurses.

3. What other factors need to be decided for an on-call system?

Allowing staff to make decisions about these types of issues often helps acceptance. Factors to be determined include the following:

- Shifts/rotations for on-call (8 hours? 12 hours? 24 hours?)
- Days designated for on-call staffing? (7 days a week? only weekends?)
- Process of notification? (phone? beeper?)
- Response time (30 minutes? 1 hour?)
- Who has the authority to activate (charge nurse? nursing supervisor?)
- What criteria will be used to activate (volume? acuity? transport?)

4. What criteria for activation of on-call staffing do other hospitals use?

Most recommend not using the on-call nurse for sick-call or vacation coverage. This can lead to an abuse of the system, since the mentality of a "spare" person develops. Besides, then there isn't the extra person when the need arises, the very reason the program was established in the first place.

Departments with fluctuations must define what being "overwhelmed" will mean. A generic description is that the situation is not expected to improve on its own in a timely manner. Some definitions include the following:

- A monitored transport that will take an RN away for more than an hour
- Having five or more urgent ED patients waiting more than 30 minutes to see a physician

- Having two or more unexpected 1:1 patients
- Holding four or more in-house admissions in the ED
- A community "disaster" involving a sudden influx of seven or more serious patients at one time

5. What are suggestions for maintaining an on-call system?

Institutions with well-established systems offer these recommendations:

- *Limit on-call shifts to 12 hours or less.* There will be days when you will need someone for the complete 24 hours. Having the same individual on-call for the entire day does not make that possible.
- *Have a peer committee oversee the system.* Staff often respond better to peer pressure.
- *Restrict staff from working full shifts before or after the on-call time.* It is feasible and convenient for staff to have 4 hours on call before a regular 8-hour shift. But you cannot allow staff to be on call for 12 hours (on the assumption that they won't be needed) before their regularly scheduled 12-hour shift.
- *Allow staff to exchange on-call shifts, similar to what is allowed with assigned shifts.* Many institutions also allow staff to "give away" on-call shifts, since the exchange does not affect benefits or budget.
- *Responsibility for activation should remain with someone in a clinical role, such as the charge nurse.* That person will be in the best position to judge the true need.
- *Clearly identify your on-call expectations with future staff in the hiring interviews.* Prevent surprises.
- *Use the same discipline approach for any problems with staff compliance with the on-call system, such as not responding when called or not signing up.* It signals the importance of this responsibility.

BIBLIOGRAPHY

1. Lawrenz Consulting: Annual survey of hours. Perspect Staffing Scheduling 19(3):1–6, 1999; *www.lawrenzconsult.com*
2. Zimmermann PG: How we do it: On-call staffing for emergency departments. J Emerg Nurs 19(6):529–531, 1994.

21. ONGOING STAFF EDUCATION AND PROFESSIONAL DEVELOPMENT

Mary E. Fecht Gramley, PhD, RN, CEN

A teacher affects eternity: he can never tell where his influence stops.

Henry Adams

1. Describe the qualifications that the clinical nurse specialist (CNS) or unit educator should have.

The CNS should hold a minimum of a master's degree in nursing. The baccalaureate degree is the foundation for the profession; the master's level demonstrates advanced study and preparation. The CNS should have clinical experience and advanced knowledge in the specialty area. In addition, the individual should demonstrate leadership and professionalism. Selection of the appropriate individual is crucial.

2. Talk about the role of the CNS/unit educator.

The CNS/unit educator position should meet needs of staff, manager, physicians, colleagues from other disciplines, patients and significant others, and the community. This is not a small undertaking, but it is a very rewarding one. It is difficult for the CNS to be a valuable resource if the hours of the position are limited, or the CNS is considered part of the routine unit patient-care staffing. Some of the multiple role functions include the following:

- Be a resource and support person for staff
- Assist the manager during preparation for regulatory visits (e.g., JCAHO)
- Design, develop, and deliver a variety of educational programs (e.g., required competency skills), regulatory (e.g., age-related, pain) and new policies and procedures
- Serve on departmental and hospital-wide committees
- Participate in community activities
- Provide expert consultation
- Research (e.g., promoting research utilization, identification of researchable clinical problems, or data collection)

3. What can a manager do when there is no unit educator to assist with the development and maintenance of staff skills?

- *Use the current experienced staff to design programs.* The manager may need to teach the staff members adult education principles, program design, teaching, and evaluation methods. But the investment can be worthwhile. Staff members will grow professionally as they prepare the program and can become valuable resources for your unit. Designated staff educators describe enhanced job satisfaction. A side benefit is that staff now gain a greater appreciation for the amount of time and effort necessary to develop and present a quality program.
- *Guest speakers.* Use colleagues from other disciplines. Members of community organizations are often willing to share their expertise. A CNS from another specialty or institution will frequently agree to present something from their expertise or unit.
- *Send staff to external programs.* Attendance at an external program provides not only new information but also opportunities to network with other professionals. It sometimes validates that your practice or experience is in line with that of other facilities.
- *Journal articles.* Assign continuing education unit (CEU) credit articles in the specialty's journals to cover new developments or review the basics.

• *Contribute to the development of an institution-wide education program.* Use the system's e-mail or videos with quizzes to meet requirements and earn continuing education hour credits.

4. How do you measure competency?

Former JCAHO surveyor and consultant Ann Kobs clarifies that competency can be validated by two possible methods: actual observed behavior and the absence of error. To meet the JCAHO requirement, it is only necessary to formalize a process in which a supervisor documents these two points after observing the individual's day-to-day performance.

5. I am not required to verify competency of temporary agency nurses, am I?

Yes. An individual nurse's competency must be validated regardless of the length of employment, even if it is only one 8-hour shift. However, this verification can be a simple checklist completed by a supervisor or charge nurse.

6. How do I meet the requirement that staff maintain age-related learning competencies?

This JCAHO requirement can take considerable time to accomplish. The best way is to develop an institution-wide system that is easily accessible, short, and to the point. The goal should be to minimize the time required to complete the education requirement and to maximize the convenience for the staff.

One method is to provide a monthly e-mail reading and quiz. Develop a monthly reading of no more than two pages followed by a quiz of 10 questions pertaining to the reading. Examples of topics include health promotion for school age children, pediatric pain management assessment tools, or physical assessment: respiratory function in the elderly. The quiz is graded and recorded and then returned so nurses can learn from incorrectly answered questions.

7. How do I deal with staff who make significant spelling errors when documenting?

Consult with the person and suggest a remedial spelling course or spell checker. Sometimes people do not believe spelling matters; you may need to reinforce that it does. If the situation continues to be a problem, incorporate spelling into the evaluation process.

8. Describe how to maintain staff interest in educational programs.

Nothing hinders attentiveness more than a small, cramped, overheated room with too few chairs. Educational presentations are often held in the staff lounge, which was intended as a break room for a few people. Staff will be more cooperative and interested if they witness an effort to accommodate their comfort and schedules. Strategies include the following:

• Design games, such as Jeopardy or Trivial Pursuit. One manager plays "Who Wants to Win a $100,000?" and awards a 100 Grand candy bar.
• Invite other department colleagues to discuss "hot" issues
• Enlist staff to research a topic and report back.
• Communicate by mail on a regular basis. This provides time for staff to digest information and formulate questions or suggestions.
• Provide food. When there are limits to hospital-provided food, staff can take turns or a vendor can provide treats.
• Rotate the meeting times, with multiple options.
• Reserve a large enough, appropriate room.

9. What other techniques are there besides the traditional lectures or videos?

Nursing schools have been successfully incorporating a number of cooperative learning techniques that require participative techniques, such as using unfolding case studies. Present a patient situation and stop. For instance, "You have a 2-day postoperative diabetic patient who had a colon resection. Today he is complaining of increasing pain. What do you need to assess? What do you need to consider?"

• *Have a group discussion.* Include what could be happening, what data is still needed, or what immediate action is needed.

- *Think, pair, and share.* After the scenario, have 1 minute of silence for thinking and then staff, in pairs, come up with the answers.
- *Round table:* Pass a notebook around the table. Each person must write something related to the situation, with subsequent participants allowed to build on their input. Go around the table at least twice.

The advantage of using evolving case studies is the obvious application, the broadening of perspectives, the involvement of everyone, including the quieter members, and the realization that everyone has something to offer.

10. How long should an orientation last?

Each employee is unique and will require different levels of information and support. For this reason, it is difficult to set an absolute time frame, although many units and hospitals have a standardized plan. Many provide 6 to 8 weeks for a new graduate or a new specialty and 1 to 2 weeks for an experienced nurse.

Reasonable expectations should be set, and a fair, objective assessment of the progress of the employee made at several points. The preceptor should seek input from other staff and professional colleagues and consult with the manager.

If an employee needs additional orientation time, the goals and time frame must be clearly set with the manager, staff person, and preceptor. Reasons for not extending an orientation and terminating the position can include the following:

- Unacceptable personal work habits or attitudes (slovenly appearance or statements such as "You mean you expect me to be on time every day?").
- Severe deficit of basic nursing knowledge (e.g., unable to do a simple dosage calculation, failure to recognize patient has ventricular fibrillation).
- Failure to accept responsibility to rectify deficiencies (e.g., the orientee continues to believe he or she is excellent and any problems are the result of the preceptor).
- Lack of progress (e.g., still performing at the same level after 6 weeks). This is sometimes a problem when a new graduate is overwhelmed in a critical care area. (Time in a medical-surgical unit might be needed first to develop basic organizational skills.)

11. Who makes the best preceptor?

Good preceptors are pivotal in developing satisfied, competent employees and ensuring that there is completed paperwork for the regulatory visits. Some hospitals develop their own formal preceptor training classes. Topics include characteristics of adult learners, learning styles, and giving constructive feedback. Some also have regular preceptor group meetings to discuss concerns with an education specialist.

A preceptor should be an experienced, seasoned staff nurse who is capable and willing to work with new employees on the unit. One recommendation is a nurse with at least 2 but less than 5 years of experience. That way there is still the ability to share one's expertise at a level in line with the trainee's current ability.

Johns Hopkin's Senior Director for Education and Practice, Amy Deutschendorf, looks for preceptors that demonstrate core behaviors, rather than length of experience. Their first essential requirement is that the person wants to be a preceptor. Other essential behaviors are someone who is safe (follows policies or procedures), is independent (though knows when to confer with a resource), and can think critically.

The preceptor does not need an advanced degree to perform this function. (You have a unit CNS/educator for the advanced role). What is more important is that the preceptor is patient and has an ability to simply explain things. The preceptor should have a concerned, nurturing attitude toward new employees and the ability to recognize that each employee is unique.

12. Name some compensations that could be given to a preceptor.

- List the role/title on the annual evaluation.
- Integrate it as part of a clinical ladder program.

- Pay for certification courses (such as ACLS).
- Grant an extra educational day.
- Send to a nursing convention.
- Recognition affairs, such as an annual preceptor luncheon.
- Time off. One hospital gives a 12-hour vacation day after the preceptor has completed 500 hours; another gives one 8-hour compensation day after 20 shifts of precepting.
- Provide goodie "perks." Items such as car wash tickets or dinner at a local restaurant can be donated by volunteer services.
- Financial compensation. One hospital provides $0.50 an hour.

In the end, however, many preceptors indicate that the biggest rewards are being valued, contributing to the future, and the challenge of relearning. After all, he who teaches learns the most.

13. Give an example of a financial reward for preceptors.

One hospital provides financial incentives on a four-level and longevity (retention) basis. Level I nurses work with student nurses during a routine clinical experience. This is considered normal professionalism and receives no reward.

For a Level II reward, the nurse works with a senior student nurse who has no on-site instructor supervision (e.g., leadership rotation). A $50 gift certificate is awarded on the student's successful completion of the rotation.

At Level III, a nurse assumes full responsibility for the orientation of an RN who has a minimum of 1 year of recent, relevant experience in the delivery of acute care. This includes identifying learning needs, mutual goal setting, collaborating with colleagues to meet the goals, and providing ongoing/final evaluation. The primary preceptor receives a $100 gift certificate and 12 hours of choice time (e.g., paid time off at a time mutually agreed on with the manager). A second RN serves as an off-shift, secondary preceptor and is eligible for a $50 gift certificate and 6 hours of time off.

At Level IV, the orientee has less than 1 year of recent, relevant experience. The primary preceptor receives a $200 gift certificate and 24 hours of choice time, and the secondary preceptor is eligible for a $100 gift certificate and 12 hours of choice time.

The longevity bonus is given to the primary preceptor of a Level III or IV preceptorship on each of the first three annual anniversaries of the precepted employee. To qualify for the $200 gift certificate each year, the precepted employee must have remained on staff, without interruption, in a regular part-time or full-time position, and have a satisfactory evaluation.

14. How would needs vary for these two orientees in a critical care unit: a new graduate but previously a paramedic and a nurse with 5 years' experience in home health?

The new graduate who was previously a paramedic probably has honed assessment skills. Beware, however, that you do not assume this individual is a "well-oiled" professional nurse based on the previous prehospital experience. A paramedic is accustomed to caring for one patient in the short-term under the direct supervision of the medical director of the emergency medical services system. The hospital environment is different.

The nurse with 5 years' experience in home health should be a seasoned practitioner. Even though the setting is different, the nurse has had 5 years to practice nursing skills and procedures and plan, evaluate, and revise nursing care. More complex procedures are being performed in the home environment today, including central line medication administration. This nurse is probably well versed in practicing independently and knows the importance of conferring to problem-solve. See also the chapter on preceptors.

15. List ways that I can encourage staff to exhibit professionalism.
- Promote and model it yourself.
- Encourage participation in professional organizations.
- Provide opportunities to network with other positive role models.
- Work to maintain dress code policies that support professional appearance.

- Support and promote education for staff.
- Reward positive, "can do" attitudes and behaviors.
- Give credit where it is due.
- Demonstrate appreciation and respect for staff who have proven their loyalty, reliability and skills.
- Avoid activities that staff may perceive as insulting. For instance, one hospital had a fresh out of college non-nurse consultant present a program to teach nurses how to "be nice to patients." The average nurse, in the mid-40s, is well-versed in therapeutic interactions.

16. Should I promote certification in my specialty for all staff?

Certification by no means guarantees that a staff member is the ultimate expert in the field. However, the attainment of certification does show that the individual studied, prepared, and achieved a set of criteria. Attainment of certification is a means of seeking excellence in one's profession. A study of 19,452 randomly selected nurses from 23 certifying organizations found that 72% of nurses reported one or more benefits of certification, including enhanced professionalism, and almost all reported that certification brought about at least one change in their practice. In addition, staff certification has been used as a negotiation advantage for managed-care contracts.

17. List ways to recognize staff who achieve certification.

Recognition is important to showcase those staff as role models. Some medical auxiliary organizations may provide financial support. Recognition methods include the following:
- Annual evaluation criteria
- Pay raise
- Reimbursement of testing fee
- Paid education hours for the test time
- Publishing the accomplishment in the hospital's newsletter
- Having a unit wall plaque with photographs or engraved names of certified staff
- Recognition luncheon

18. I have three staff interested in providing tours of our nursing unit for community groups (e.g., scouts). How do I choose the most appropriate one?
- *Consider whether all three staff can participate at different times.* Chances are they will not all be available each time.
- *Consider the personal appearance of the individual.* The public has a preconceived notion of how a professional nurse should look. Once I watched a nurse dressed in mismatched scrubs, with dried blood on her shoes and fly-away hair, give a terse, hurried tour. It seemed to leave the visitors confused.
- *Consider the ability of the staff member to communicate in a positive manner.* No unit is nirvana; improvements can be made. However, there are still positive aspects to emphasize, such as the new equipment or that all staff have ACLS certification. It is poor judgment to share problems with visitors, for example, that radiology is slow or there is often no time for staff lunch breaks.

19. How do you encourage staff to participate in community health-related activities?

The hospital often has a vested interest in some community activities and needs individuals to participate. Make staff aware of opportunities. Some possibilities include Safe Kids, Community First Aid, Walk for Breast Cancer, community cardiopulmonary resuscitation classes, ENCARE (Emergency Nurses Cancel Alcohol Related Emergencies), Cancer Survivors Days, or Prom Night.

It will require time on the part of the staff for instructor courses, planning, or carrying out the activity. Staff may be reluctant to participate unless they are paid, and pay may be required if the amount of time exceeds the regularly scheduled hours of work. Negotiate with administration for appropriate funding. One manager's medical tent labor and supply costs were $8000.

Some institutions incorporate community involvement as part of the annual evaluation or clinical ladder. Most staff will agree that they receive personal satisfaction from teaching health-promoting behaviors, raising funds for worthy organizations, and networking with other committed individuals.

20. A staff member recently took a national standardized course that included a skill station, taught by a local instructor, and was unsuccessful. This staff member blames the instructor for the failure. Should I approach the instructor and discuss the performance of this staff person with him?

It might be most informative to ask the staff member about his or her personal preparation strategy. Most courses will allow a retake of an examination or a skills station. Perhaps with a review of materials, the individual staff member will be able to succeed.

The instructor has an obligation to prepare material, present it in an organized manner, and fairly evaluate the participant. Consideration can be made for participants who may have learning disabilities or personal difficulties at a particular time. However, the instructor is not responsible for guaranteeing success for all participants.

It is the responsibility of the participant to come to the course prepared. Most national standardized courses provide a textbook and specific directions as to what must be done to be successful. This includes reading the textbook, studying areas where the information is new, and asking questions to clarify information.

In one course's instructor-given survey, 60% indicated they had read less than half of the material beforehand. Many nurses mistakenly assume they will be spoon-fed the test's answers.

There are ethical, if not legal, obligations to maintain confidentiality that you should consider before becoming involved. Direct the participant to discuss the performance with the nurse instructor if there is confusion about the reason for the failure. If the participant believes an objective third party is needed, perhaps someone not directly related with this staff member's ongoing performance and evaluation, such as the director of the education department, can become involved.

21. What is the key to success in preventing errors in patient care when students are on the unit?

Communication, communication, communication. Working with students should be a positive experience. They are the staff of tomorrow.

First, it is crucial to provide a thorough faculty and student orientation to the facility. It should include the policies and procedures, equipment, emergency responses (e.g., fire, code), documentation forms and expectations, and computer usage.

Second, clarify the student arrangement with both the nursing staff and the clinical nursing instructor. Consider the term that is used throughout the communications—"student nurse" versus "nursing student." "Nursing student" indicates that the individual is a "student" who is studying nursing. On the other hand, the use of "student nurse" suggests that the primary role is a nurse who happens to be a student. (For example, a resident is a physician, although he or she is still under supervision.)

It is a distinction between primary role (noun) and the description (adjective) that some suggest helps to clarify the student's role. The choice might affect the staff's expectation. Sometimes (even subconsciously) more is expected of a "student nurse" than a "nursing student," whether those added expectations are realistic or not.

22. How should I describe the arrangement between the staff and students?

Student nurses are guests of the host institution, through a contract between the school of nursing and the hospital. The instructor's license allows the students to practice under the supervision and direction of the instructor. Students are responsible for their own practice and faculty are accountable for selecting appropriate learning experiences.

A helpful analogy is how unlicensed assistive personnel (UAP) are used. Appropriate assignments must be made by the RN, and the UAP is accountable for completing it. But the UAP practice must take place under the direction and supervision of an RN.

Similarly, a student is not licensed as a registered professional nurse and does not have that scope of practice. Therefore, either the faculty or an assigned registered nurse preceptor must supervise this student's (unlicensed personnel) practice too. This is why the RN faculty, the RN preceptor, or the RN assigned to the patient must cosign for the patients' medications, nursing notes, and professional treatments.

23. What is the best way to handle it when a learning opportunity arises for the students?

When a learning experience arises, such as inserting a urinary catheter, the staff should communicate directly with the instructor. The instructor is then responsible for assigning (and supervising) an individual student with the task, if the task is appropriate for the students. The instructor has a responsibility to communicate and rectify any personal unfamiliarity with the policy or procedure to supervise the student.

Should time not permit, then the staff nurse should complete the procedure (with the student observing). It is unethical to put the patient in jeopardy or delay treatment because a student wishes to learn a new technique or the instructor is not familiar with a procedure.

24. Do nursing school clinical instructors have any thoughts on this topic?

One experienced instructor for generic associate degree nursing students indicates the following:

- *Amen to channeling through the instructor.* The instructor knows the student's capabilities to safely handle this responsibility. Students currently failing theory are still allowed to complete all concurrent clinical experiences.
- *Continue to help oversee the student's work.* The instructor has up to 10 students and may miss something. A common student error is to correctly assess and chart something important (e.g., temperature spike), but then not follow through with a report and an intervention. Ultimately the staff nurse is responsible for the patient; the instructor is responsible for the student.
- *Keep your teaching with students to clinical basics, related to diseases.* Students must be taught the ideal before the real. It doesn't help a beginning student to be told how to argue with a physician or the laboratory's idiosyncrasies. It does help the student to be shown a classic jaundice presentation or to listen to wheezes.
- *Be honest with the instructor about a student's performance.* Weaker students will often "hide" from, or even lie to, instructors but will be up-front with staff. You are not doing anyone a favor by protecting a student exhibiting incompetent behaviors or lack of follow-through. The instructor needs to know to help the student.
- *Let the instructor pick the patients.* Well-meaning staff want to give either the hardest patient or the "interesting case" to the student. It is not a learning experience to care for something never studied (e.g., a head injury needing a Glasgow Coma Scale score when the theory work is on the gastrointestinal symptoms) or is not even part of the curriculum (e.g., malaria). Beginning students need routine textbook cases to reinforce the normal findings for this condition before being able to appreciate the unusual.

25. What actions can help a smooth working relationship between the nursing instructor, students, and staff?

- The instructor should arrange a meeting with the nurse manager, and possibly several staff, members prior to the beginning of the clinical experience. A list of subjects and skill labs completed by the students to date can be reviewed.
- Post a printed list of skills that students are allowed to perform, and responsibilities they will assume (such as charting, bedside glucose monitoring, intravenous medications)

each and every day that the students are on the unit. There may be new, floating, or agency staff working on any given clinical experience day who may not be familiar with arrangements for students.

- Ensure periodic check-ins between the nursing instructor, nurse manager, and staff throughout the school period. A lack of communication can result in an unresolved issue creating misunderstanding and ill will.
- The unit should feel free to request that students not be present for a unique event time, such as when a JCAHO accreditation visit will occur. The presence of students may be stressful, and staff needs to focus on the activities related to the visit. The instructor can arrange an alternative student experience for that week.
- A presentation by the institution's nurse recruiter can describe and explain employment opportunities available to students. This gives the students first-hand information about job opportunities and the application process.

BIBLIOGRAPHY

1. ANA Code for Nurses. Am J Nurs 100(7):70–72, 2000.
2. Bracken LJ, Martinez RR: Education. In Jordan KS (ed): Emergency Nursing Core Curriculum, 5th ed. Philadelphia, W.B. Saunders, 2000, pp 751–764.
3. Cary AH: Certified Registered Nurses: Results of the study of the certified workforce. Am J Nursing 101(1):44–52, 2001.
4. Joint Commission of Accreditation for Healthcare Organizations: Hospital Accreditation Standards. Oak Brook, IL, JCAHO, 2000.
5. Leftridge DW, et al: Improve communication in a shared governance system. Nurs Manage 30:50–51, 1999.
6. Marrett BE: The power of perception: President's message. J Emerg Nurs 26:93–94, 2000.
7. Pickering TC: Incorporating age specific criteria in ED skills stations. J Emerg Nurs 25:321–323, 1999.
8. Proehl JA: Relight your lamp: President's message. J Emerg Nurs 95:75–76, 1999.
9. Taylor K: Tackling the issue of nurse competency. Nurs Manage 31:35–38, 2000.
10. Zimmermann PG: Managers Forum: Precepting. J Emerg Nurs 26(5):496–498, 2000.
11. Zimmermann PG: Managers Forum: Verifying staff competency. J Emerg Nurs 27(5):495–496, 2001.

22. CLINICAL LADDERS

Camilla L. Jones, RN, BBA

If the shoe fits, you're not allowing for growth.

Robert N. Coons

1. What is included in a clinical ladder program?

It depends on the program goals and objectives. Examples of areas included are

- Staff education
- Preceptorship
- Mentorship
- Performance improvement
- Community outreach
- Operational projects
- Customer satisfaction
- Patient follow-up
- Certifications
- Higher education
- Leadership
- Worker flexibility
- Expense reduction
- Research
- Case management
- Improved attendance
- Improved workplace safety
- Emergency preparedness coordination
- Employment longevity
- Professional development

2. How can a clinical ladder program assist in recruiting or retaining nurses?

Clinical ladder programs can provide powerful incentives and concrete rewards for accelerated performance or professional growth. Most provide opportunities to advance in job grade, pay, responsibility, and certification or skills. They can support autonomous practice, professionalism, and empowerment. They can also provide a clear direction for nurses to know how to grow and learn in their profession within their own organization and to improve their own marketability.

3. Talk about the basic framework of a clinical ladder program.

Most programs have multiple layers, each with its own criteria and indicators that will identify the person's achievements and function at that higher level. The overall goals of the program can be translated into indicators (objectives) within each level of the program, with specific behavior options identified. For instance, the leadership requirements may be fulfilled by functioning as a charge nurse on a unit at a lower level, precepting new employees or hospital committee membership at an intermediate level, and creating or translating a form, serving as an officer in a professional association, or performing community service at an advanced level. Behaviors are assigned point allocations and then totaled to identify the level of the nurse's performance.

Most programs involve some type of monetary reward between the different levels. Some programs are set up to increase base rates of pay. Others assign a point value to every desirable behavior and reward bonuses based on point accumulation. The monetary value might be varied between types of positions within the hospital based on market analysis, but the method of evaluation should be the same for all job levels participating in the program. Any combination of methods can work. The key is to determine what you want to accomplish.

4. How do I make sure the process is fairly applied?

It is crucial that the program guidelines are followed and that evaluation processes are objective or the program will be invalidated. Most programs require the ladder candidate to provide supporting documentation of his or her achievements. This gives the candidate and the manager something concrete to evaluate. Be sure to provide a structured tool that assists the candidate in logging his or her achievements to facilitate consistency. Complex tools that depend on narrative recollections are generally more subjective and less effective.

5. How does the pay increase or bonus process occur?

At designated times, usually annually, the employee is evaluated using the clinical ladder tool. In some cases, the clinical ladder tool is the same as the performance evaluation tool. Examples include the following:

1. A minimum score on criteria to remain at that clinical level
2. Meet all criteria or be excluded from the level
3. Accrue point(s) assigned to each criterion, which then represents the clinical level and/or monetary accumulation.
4. Assigned differentials for each clinical level

At this author's hospital, all nursing (and some technical) staff in the hospital are hired based on their experience, desire, and ability to meet the criteria within 6 months of employment. The nurse/tech is required to meet at least an average score on all indicators or he or she must step down a level. In the RN clinical ladder program, there is a $1.50 per hour spread between each clinical level. When the nurse steps up a level, the differential is added to the base rate; when he or she steps down a level, it is removed.

6. Which clinical ladder system is the best?

Each has pros and cons. The point system (rewarding productivity) is viewed as equitable and works well for self-starters. And, if the employee does not have a lot of initiative, it might be used as a platform for limited or selective production. A complaint sometimes raised with this concept is that there can be too many required "extracurricular" activities. If the staff nurse is to provide good in-patient care, why must the nurse perform uncompensated additional community service to achieve an excellent rating?

The performance evaluation option allows the manager to include baseline criteria for every clinical ladder level, then build upon those minimal requirements for higher clinical levels. However, criteria must be carefully selected so as not to exclude very productive, capable workers who can't meet all of the criteria (i.e., the nurse who can't attend every staff meeting because he or she is attending school or has child care issues).

Another issue is whether the nurse's educational program should be part of the requirements. Some institutions require a bachelors (or masters) degree in nursing at the higher levels. Others believe the clinical ladder should reward current performance regardless of the nurses' educational background.

7. How do you decide what level to hire a candidate into?

Most programs take into consideration the new-hire's previous experience and desire and/or ability to work within a leadership role. There is often one level for a new graduate and a higher level for a nurse with work experience in that specialty. It is also general practice to require at least 1 year of nursing practice in that specialty prior to allowing a new graduate nurse to be promoted to a higher clinical level. However, if a new-hire experienced nurse comes in at a higher level, the program must have a built-in assessment opportunity of the nurses' performance in meeting that level's criteria.

Some programs require every new employee to hire in at the lowest clinical level, with a re-evaluation in 6 months. This provides an opportunity to validate a nurse's actual performance and ongoing service in the institution's activities (committees) and goals. However, this approach can deter recruitment efforts.

8. Name areas that are evaluated.

The department's and/or the organization's mission, goals, and values should always be the basis of all objectives and criteria. Common themes include flexibility, mentorship, case management/cost savings, performance improvement or quality control, leadership, and professional growth.

9. **Mention some indicators or criteria of flexibility.**

They usually measure willingness or work ethic, such as the following:
- Floats or covers shifts in a pinch
- Expands case load as needed
- Expands responsibility or job set
- Adjusts schedule
- Works different shifts/signs for on-call
- Participates in emergency preparedness activities

10. **Name some criteria to evaluate mentorship.**

These commonly focus on service. For example, the nurse serves as a
- Preceptor to orienting employees
- Resource to students
- Mentor to new graduates/for career shadowing
- Trainer in educational or inservice programs
- Educator for community research

11. **List some clinical ladder criteria for evaluating case management or cost savings.**
- Facilitates appropriate length-of-stay (LOS)
- Assists in post-hospital placement and/or home health implementation
- Eliminates unscheduled sick time or absences (usually excludes bereavement)
- Develops and implements a cost-saving project
- Participates in or designs an inventory control process
- Coordinates or develops a revenue-producing project
- Documentation reflects no variances that cause payment denials
- Reviews records to validate charges
- Participates in staff education to promote compliance

12. **Give some clinical ladder criteria to measure performance improvement or quality control.**

This objective usually requires performance improvement participation, such as the following:
- Committee work
- Data collection, evaluation, and/or research
- Guest relations program
- New product evaluation and/or pilot program
- Outside agency review process

13. **What are examples of leadership criteria?**
- Clinical or administrative charge duties
- Coordinates daily (monthly) staffing
- Participates in annual performance review process
- Contributes in annual budgeting process
- Serves on an interdisciplinary committee
- Chairs a committee or task force
- Functions as an educator for required hospital inservices
- Implements or facilitates guest relations program
- Acts as an advocate to patients, physicians, peers
- Consults in area of expertise to the hospital or the community
- Participates in a community-based activity or effort

14. **Indicate criteria for professional growth.**
- Maintains pertinent certifications
- Obtains a bachelors or masters degree

- Completes all required pertinent clinical education
- Attends national conference in clinical specialty
- Participates in legislative effort
- Submits article for participation

15. Do you have any other tips to make a clinical ladder program successful?

When setting up a program, immediately identify and include any mandatory organization core competencies. Then include representative staff members to provide additional meaningful criteria and promote buy-in. They will be instrumental in selling your program. Be prepared to use their suggestions, or declining morale and program failure can result.

16. List some criticisms about clinical ladders.

- *Differences in self-perceptions.* It can be difficult to view oneself objectively. This can set up discord rather than motivation. As one anonymous boss said, "After listening to my employees, I have to conclude that I have only three types of people working for me: Stars, All-Stars, and Superstars! How is it possible for all my people to be above average?"
- *Inconsistency in evaluation.* Managers differ in interpreting what they reward. Is attending inservices "part of the job," or something to be commended? Do you reward a job well done, or only those duties beyond the normal job expectations?
- *Top-heavy departments.* In promoting retention, you might end up with most of the nursing staff at the top, which can affect the staffing budget.

BIBLIOGRAPHY

1. Wright C: Tallahassee (FL) Memorial Regional Medical Center Professional Nurse Advancement Program. ED Manage 4:Supplement, 2000.
2. Zimmermann PG: Managers Forum: Clinical ladders. J Emerg Nurs 27(4):380–381, 2001.

IV. Directing and Controlling

23. ISSUES OF DAILY MANAGEMENT

Kirsten Johnson Moore, RN, MSN

Our grand business is not to see what lies dimly at a distance, but to do what lies clearly at hand.

Thomas Carlyle

1. Why is day-to-day management so important? Isn't it the vision that matters?

Clinical managers have a tremendous effect on the work environment and the teams that they manage. In light of the fact that we are entering a period in which experienced personnel are at a premium, it is imperative that strong leaders create an environment that makes people want to stay. Influencing the components of daily management of a busy department is essential in your success as a manager.

2. How do you staff your department to meet seasonal fluctuations?

Start with the creation of a good operational budget. Pull your admission data for the previous year to reveal the number of patients admitted per day in relation to the day of the week to identify your high-volume days and times.

Based on the resulting numbers, you may decide either to add full-time equivalent staff (FTEs) or to create an on-call system for the identified times. This may look like an additional 11 AM to 11 PM shift Saturday, Sunday, and Monday, or an individual on-call from 5 PM to 1 AM each day.

The goal is to plan prospectively, not just chronically react to a crisis. Remember, though, that you may need multidisciplinary care, such as a registered nurse (RN), aide, radiologist, or physician. Many emergency departments (EDs) report that only adding a nurse results in minimal impact on patient waiting time. For more information on this topic, see the chapter on staff scheduling.

3. How have you incorporated non-nursing caregivers into your department?

The use of non-nurse caregivers, in light of the current job market, may be inevitable. Employ the following strategies to maximize the success of such a role in your department:
- *Develop a job description.* This should include input from the nursing and medical staff, hospital administration and policies, and the local and state regulatory boards.
- *Identify the qualifications needed for the role.*
- *Delineate the tasks of the position.*
- *Design a competency-based orientation and continuing education.*

4. List some of the most common tasks departments typically include in a non-nurse caregiver job description, after appropriate training.
- Vital signs
- Telemetry monitoring
- Phlebotomy
- Specimen collection
- Diagnostic procedures (electrocardiography, pulse oximetry, bedside blood glucose, urine pregnancy, guaiac testing)

• Procedure assistance (suturing, lumbar puncture, casting)
• Stocking supplies
• Miscellaneous roles (transporting, responding to institutional emergencies)

5. Our department has expanded rapidly over the past several years, making communication difficult. How have other departments overcome this challenge?

Challenges in efficient communication in a large department include linking patient care areas, communicating within the department, and connecting with other departments, such as laboratories. Solutions include two-way radios, cellular phones, and pagers.

6. Tell me more about the use of two-way radios.

Each staff member can carry a radio, or you can designate a team leader for isolated areas. Consider linking support services, too.

The benefit of compact radios is that they are inexpensive and easy to use, they dramatically decrease the need for overhead paging, and they do not interfere with telemetry. Practical issues include having spare radios, extra batteries, and charging space. You may want to agree as a group on your radio etiquette, such as to limit unnecessary chatter.

7. Can you use cellular phones within the hospital?

Many departments provide cellular phones to each nurse (and physician). Support services or physicians can just call the nurse's number directly, or the call can be transferred by the unit secretary to the nurse.

They do not incur the traditionally costly air time and avoid interference with telemetry systems when connected with the facility's main system. Benefits include decreasing the number of calls managed by the unit clerk, the "on-hold" phenomenon, or waiting by a phone for a return page. It is also helpful for staff to find each other in a large unit.

The downside includes the cost of the devices, the placement of antennas in the department, and potential repair cost for damage and loss. There is also the requirement of space for storage and charging when not in use. In addition, you may need to monitor the number of personal calls made with the devices.

8. Talk about the use of pagers as a method of communication.

The use of alphanumeric pagers can be a viable, nonverbal method of sending a cryptic message to staff. Requirements of this type of system include software, a modem or network system, pagers, and strategically placed computers.

Benefits include the ability to directly reach an individual, to communicate information without verbal interaction, and a decrease in departmental noise. (Staff also appreciate having a method for their own families to access them directly.) One department that uses this process saw an immediate 30% reduction in phone calls. The disadvantage is that these components can become very expensive for the department: approximately $150.00 per beeper.

Some departments with known waiting periods (ED, intensive care unit [ICU], surgery) have provided beepers to family members. This allows the family to freely roam within the hospital but be easily accessible when needed.

9. What methods of communication do you provide for patients and families in your department?

For a family who has just experienced a traumatic injury or devastating diagnosis, the ability to reach significant others for support is essential. Traditionally, this has been done through the use of a centrally located phone within the department or waiting area. Privacy and confidentiality are nearly impossible in these situations.

Many hospitals are addressing this need by placing a phone (and sometimes a modem line) in each room. Just be sure to define your calling area. However, if your facility is a tertiary referral center, you may need a method to allow families to call outside the local region.

10. Discuss the role of case managers.

Case management is defined as a collaborative process that assesses, plans, implements, coordinates, monitors, and evaluates options and services to meet an individual's health needs to promote quality cost-effective outcomes. The role of the case manager in the department can include the evaluation of patients with recurrent visits and development of a plan of care that can link the patient with community health resources outside of the institution. Other roles the case manager may fill include insurance consultant, discharge planner, and facilitator (admission to and discharge from pathways). Even many EDs are using case managers to help their patients with home services and appropriate follow-up care. Although the individual in this role often reports to another department, the manager works closely with him or her in ensuring quality patient management for the patients' needs.

11. Tell me about the role of a child life specialist.

A child life specialist works with the hospital caregivers to make the environment more child-friendly. This person can be a consultant in the design of your waiting and treatment rooms, as well as in the purchase of activities for the patients. During a difficult procedure such as PICC line placement or bone marrow aspiration he or she can be dedicated to distracting the patient through the procedure. Examples of ways to make the environment more child-friendly may include the placement of diversions (radio/cassette players, books, VCR and Nintendo machines, hand-held games), room décor (fish, characters from children's literature), and use of nontoxic blowing bubbles to "blow away" pain. The person in this role often reports to the nurse manager.

12. Describe a stat nurse.

A stat nurse is an experienced nurse who floats among the hospital's units, wherever most urgently needed. For example, within one shift, a person in this role could assist with stabilization of a ED critical patient, facilitate the admission of a postoperative patient to the ICU, perform the admission nursing assessment on a unit with census fluctuations, or respond to a cardiac arrest. This position has been successful in reducing some hospitals' external agency use; one program saved $120,000/year. Proper unit use of the nurse in this role is part of the manager's responsibilities.

Successful programs indicate that the nurse selection is key. The individual must be an experienced in-house nurse, independent, and flexible. There must also be clear criteria of how the nurse will be used. An administrative concern is downtime, although one program demonstrated a consistent use of more than 95%. Have some tasks (callbacks, chart audits) available to fill downtime.

One institution created a SWAT (smiling, willing, able, and talented) team for as-needed help 24 hours a day, 7 days a week. During seasonal fluctuations, a second nurse and a nursing assistant were added to the team. The SWAT nurse is also trained for some hospital-wide procedures, such as PICC line placement.

13. Talk about the role of sexual assault nurse examiners (SANEs)

Forensic nursing programs in the United States train individuals in the management of sexual assault victims in the ED. Their role consists of performing an examination and evidence collection in such a manner that it is admissible in criminal cases. Other services that are sometimes offered include pregnancy testing and prophylaxis, sexually transmitted disease prophylaxis, HIV testing, and referrals to follow-up therapy. The implementation of this role has standardized the care victims receive, especially in large teaching institutions, and helped increase convictions.

14. How do you manage patient flow within your department?

Computerization and communications technology are the foundation of an efficient patient care department. The elimination of a paper patient chart and conversion to an electronic medical record is inevitable. The patient's computerized record would function as a tracking system within the facility, such as following the patient from the preoperative clinic, through the operating room, to the postanesthesia care unit, to final admission to the patient care unit. The process can begin with registration and continue through order entry, nursing and physician documentation, discharge instructions, and prescriptive writing. One benefit of a computerized system is the ability to order entry and review patient care charts from various locations within the organization. In many institutions, this record can be accessed by satellite facilities, as well as by referring and primary physicians. When exploring what system will work best for your department, it is important to create a multidisciplinary group with information systems input that will guide the evaluation and implementation phases of the projects.

15. Communicating with my large staff is very challenging. Do you have some suggestions?

Nine elements have been identified that play an integral role in communicating effectively:

1. *Vulnerability.* Self-confidence and the courage to be vulnerable are essential in creating, growing, and strengthening relationships.

2. *Openness.* Avoid defensiveness and explore all the possibilities.

3. *Positive listening.* Accurately hear what the person is saying and feeling, avoiding interruptions and finishing sentences for others.

4. *Kinesics.* Pay attention to and sometimes look beyond the body language the person is exhibiting.

5. *High expectations.* Make sure every member of the staff and the role they perform feel significant

6. *Avoiding judgments.* Do not focus on the weaknesses of the individual or characterize the individual based on the behaviors of the group.

7. *Reinforcement.* Recognize and reward the strengths of the employee and find ways to enhance their development.

8. *Caring.* Treat each person as an individual and challenge the policies, practices and systems that do not allow you to do so.

9. *Integrity.* Without integrity, the individual lacks credibility. Without the perception of integrity and credibility, there will be no effective communication.

16. Name some common causes of communication breakdown.

- Failing to see the person as an individual
- Using value statements and clichés
- Giving false reassurance
- Not clarifying your responses.

Avoid these by conveying empathy, using open-ended questions to facilitate the conversation, and taking time to reflect on the information given. Creating an environment of effective and open communication takes time and attention and is a group effort.

17. List some easy daily techniques to help promote unit communication.

- Spend time talking to the staff informally.
- Be visible on the unit.
- Pay attention to shift changes (a transition time is usually a higher risk for problems).
- Compliment staff in writing.
- Post notes of praise to the staff or department in a public place, such as a "kudos board."

18. What are the qualities that you look for in an individual before you place him or her in a charge nurse role?

I look for clinical competence and leadership potential. This individual is the manager of the shift and therefore needs to use many of the same tools that the department head uses. The role requires consulting about clinical care issues, prioritizing problems, delegating, and multitasking. None of these skills are innate. Therefore, it is important for the manager to develop capable charge nurses by mentoring through role modeling, individual counseling sessions, and structured educational sessions.

19. How do you cope with difficult personnel?
Every department has a cadre of difficult employees, including the gossiper, the constant complainer, the problem partners, and the occasional abusive consultant. Some basic techniques that you can use to turn these colleagues into allies include the following:
- Identify the positive intent in what the person is communicating and respond to that point.
- Don't be afraid to admit that you may be wrong.
- Focus on the other person's accomplishments.
- Ignore hostile or threatening questions.
- Clarify the message you are hearing by repeating it back to the person.
- Let the individual know exactly what you need from him or her.
- Follow up attentively on the issue being discussed.

20. Give some communication techniques for dealing with coworkers who have chronic attitude problems.
- If you are repeatedly interrupted, resume your point from exactly where you left off in the conversation.
- Don't be afraid to use silence, especially if you feel the comments or conversation is inappropriate.
- Draw the person out after an attacking or inappropriate remark, challenging the person to explain or justify his or her statement.
- When all else fails, you can make peace with a difficult person by identifying and praising his or her strengths.

See also Chapter 25, Coaching and Disciplining.

21. We have a lot of conflict on our unit. Does that mean something is wrong with the unit?
Conflict is present in all organizations. This is especially true in hospitals because of the complexity of the institutional relationships, interactions among the staff, and their dependence on one another. Poorly managed conflict is the problem. It can result in distrust among employees, ultimately effecting the quality and efficiency of patient care. The goal is to reach a win-win outcome for the parties involved.

22. What are the predictable processes of conflict?
- The situation or condition that created the conflict
- The perceptions or feelings of the individuals involved
- The behaviors they exhibit due to the conflict
- The resolution or suppression of the conflict
- Evolution of new attitudes and feelings between the parties as a result of the conflict

23. List approaches for managing conflict.
- Encourage staff to first deal with the conflict directly.
- Maintain boundaries of appropriate behavior.
- Bring the involved parties together and function in a mediation role.
- Intervene when appropriate.
- Be realistic regarding the potential outcome.
- Educate the staff regarding conflict resolution.
- Model effective behaviors of conflict resolution

24. Name some specific conflict management techniques to use during the process.
- Protect the self-respect of the parties involved.
- Avoid placing blame for the problem on either participant.

- Allow open discussion of the problems from each party.
- Make sure both parties listen to each other.
- Identify the key theme in the discussion.
- Assist the parties in developing alternative solutions.
- Select a mutually agreeable solution.
- Schedule a follow-up meeting on the progress of the plan.
- Give positive feedback to both participants regarding their roles in resolving the conflict.

25. I don't know where to start with performance appraisals of my employees. Can you help?

Create an accurate appraisal tool (or tailor the existing one) to include not only the basics (e.g., clinical competency, attendance) but also aspects you consider important, such as initiative, critical thinking skills, or team work. The appraisal tool should reflect the job description, have measurable behaviors, and have similar core actions for all RNs in a given position throughout the hospital. Meet with the employee throughout the year to share your perceptions about meeting these goals. See also the chapter on discipline and coaching.

Key actions for a successful appraisal meeting include the following:
- Prepare for the evaluation by reviewing the previous evaluation and goals identified.
- Make arrangements for employee input. This can be achieved by self-evaluation, chart review, clinical exemplar, and educational record.
- Obtain peer input, either in verbal or written form.
- Place the person at ease.
- Make it clear that the goal of the performance review is to help the employee do the best possible job.
- Review the ratings with the employee and cite specific examples of behaviors.
- Ask the employee for his or her perspective of the evaluation, then listen, accept, and respond to him or her.
- Decide together some ways in which the employee's performance can be strengthened. These should be documented as goals to reach during the next year.
- Express your confidence in the employee and his or her performance.

26. What are some tips to remember when counseling employees?

Keep these guidelines and behaviors in mind during your counseling session:
- Gather the facts before acting.
- Do not act while angry.
- Discipline employees in private.
- Clearly explain the offensive act and explain why the behavior cannot continue.
- Indicate the disciplinary action that you are taking and the justification for it, and then document it and provide the employee with a copy.
- Agree on the specific steps to be taken to solve the problem and then document them.
- Do not let the discipline become personal.
- Conclude by assuring the employee of your interest in helping him or her succeed.

27. I spend my day stamping out fires. Is there a better way to solve problems?

You can approach many problems using eight basic steps:
1. Define the problem.
2. Gather information.
3. Analyze the information.
4. Propose solutions based on the important aspects of care.
5. Consider the consequences of implementing the solution.
6. Make a decision.
7. Implement the solution.
8. Evaluate the solution.

It is important to communicate the findings and to carry out an ongoing reassessment and improvement of the solution. See also Chapter 33, Quality Management and Process Improvement.

28. I want to start focusing on leading and not just managing on a daily basis. Any ideas on how to do that?

Begin by assessing your leadership skills. Leaders influence others to accomplish both their individual and departmental goals. Characteristics of a good leader include insight into self and others, risk-taking, problem-solving behaviors, flexibility, adaptability, enthusiasm, and strategic thinking.

Motivate individuals to go beyond their scope of responsibility to achieve a common vision or mission. Leadership by expectation is one style that may work for you.

29. Describe leadership by expectation.

Simply put, it means to become what we expect. Staff create mutually agreed-upon goals; you anticipate the best from them, hold them accountable for results, and reward performances that contribute to the achievement of departmental goals. It takes courage to lead by expectation, because you must be ready to take risks, to change attitudes, and to challenge the status quo.

It is the legacy of managers to develop individuals who could move into their position. The authority of true leaders comes from the examples they set daily, not from their title.

BIBLIOGRAPHY

1. Johnson Moore K: Strategies for successful management. AirMed J 18:28–39, 1999.
2. Gebelein S, et al: Successful Manager's Handbook. St. Paul, MN, Personnel Decisions International, 2000.
3. McGuffin J: The Nurse's Guide to Successful Management. St. Louis, Mosby, 1999, pp 83–116.
4. McKay JI: The emergency department of the future: The challenge is in changing how we operate. J Emerg Nurs 25:6, 1999.
5. Sullivan E, Decker P: Effective Management in Nursing: Nature of Goals and Their Importance Conflict. Menlo Park, CA, Addison-Wesley, 1988, pp 513–521.
6. Toropov B: Manager's Guide to Dealing with Difficult People. Paramus, NJ, Prentice-Hall, 1997, pp 135–170.
7. Walsh KM: ED case manager: One large teaching hospital's experience. J Emerg Nurs 25(1):17–20, 1995.
8. Zimmermann PG: Use of "stat" nurses in the emergency department. J Emerg Nurs 2(4):335–337, 1995.

24. MOTIVATING AND EMPOWERING STAFF

Kathleen Lezon, RN

> *Men are born to succeed, not to fail.*
>
> Henry David Thoreau

1. What is motivation?

Webster's dictionary defines *motivation* as "that which provides motive" and *motive* as "something that prompts a person to act in a certain way, or determines volition; incentive."

2. What is meant by motivation in the workplace?

Motivation in the workplace refers to conditions that we as managers put into place to inspire our staff to do the job that we would like them to do with the quality and enthusiasm that we would like them display.

3. Is motivation really the manager's job? Doesn't motivation comes from within?

In the workplace, the manager's job is to get the work of the business accomplished through people. We can do that by providing motivation to get the job done. In our business of health care, it is even more important that the work get done correctly and safely within a variety of constraints.

Most experts agree that to get the best out of people, it is imperative to understand human nature and how it applies to work. True, motivation comes from within, but it is often influenced by many external factors. The manager has control over some of these external factors and can have a major influence on how the employee feels about his work. There are many theories about what motivates people, and the wise manager picks and chooses to apply principles to individual situations and employees.

4. Motivational theory sounds so "textbook." Is it really applicable to the day-to-day operations of a nursing unit?

Yes, motivational theory can actually be put to practical use. Understanding theory helps us to develop better practice, and to gain a better understanding of the people around us. It's also important to remember that almost no theory works in every situation, and some should not be used at all.

Think back to some managers in your past. You may be able to recognize theories in action and make some decisions about what does and doesn't work, and why.

5. Tell me about Theory X and Theory Y.

Theory X is based on Sigmund Freud's work. It seems that Dr. Freud thought very little of human ability to accomplish independently. At the heart of this theory is the belief that people are lazy, avoid work, have no ambition, take no initiative, and avoid taking any risk. Theory X managers believe that all their employees want is job security, and they must be coerced, rewarded, intimidated, and punished in order to produce. The role of the manager is seen as policeman, constantly watching, correcting, punishing, and prodding.

In contrast, *Theory Y*, developed by Douglas McGregor, describes the desire to succeed as an inherent employee trait. Theory Y managers believe that people want to learn, and that work is the natural human way of developing self-discipline and higher skills. In this model, the employees are primarily seeking the freedom to do difficult and challenging work, rather than monetary reward. Theory Y mangers tend to seek opportunities for their employees to grow.

6. What do Maslow and other theorists say?

Abraham Maslow, a developmental psychologist, described the human hierarchy of needs and commented on how work helps to meet those needs. Work helps to meet safety and security needs by providing pay, which can help to provide food, shelter, and clothing. Once the lower level needs are met, Maslow believed that humans would strive for self-esteem and then self-actualization. Maslow taught that "Hard work and total commitment to doing well the job that you are called to do..." is one of the bricks on the road to self-actualization, or "being all that you can be."

Finally, many other (and more widely accepted) theorists, from Frederick Herzberg, to Chris Argyris, to Rensis Likert, to Fred Luthans, believed that a more realistic approach to motivation includes a combination of all of the above factors and a manager who can recognize how and when to act appropriately.

7. How do I pick the theory for me to apply?

No two employees are alike, but there are seven general strategies for helping your staff really want to do the good job that they are able to do.

1. Positive enforcement
2. Effective discipline and punishment
3. Treating people fairly
4. Meeting employees' needs
5. Setting goals
6. Involving employees in decision making
7. Effective communication

© Lezon, 2000

8. My good people know they're doing a good job. There are not many medication errors, and there are no patient complaints. Isn't that positive reinforcement?

To the employee, positive reinforcement does not mean not getting in trouble. As managers, we spend so much time problem-solving and dealing with substandard behaviors that sometimes the good performers don't get as much of our attention as they should.

Everybody likes approval, recognition, or praise. Once a year at evaluation time isn't enough. Providing those positive "strokes" needs to be an ongoing, everyday part of your life as a manager. Staff who do their job well may develop a "Why bother, I don't care attitude" if the only time they hear from you is when there's a problem.

For instance, when you audit patient records, you certainly make an effort to point out deficiencies to someone in the hopes that they'll do it right next time. But do you stop and tell the nurse with the great documentation how good her notes are? Mention it as soon as possible after you notice it. Even better, be sure to say it within earshot of other people.

9. How do you give effective verbal praise?

Be short, be specific, be sincere. For instance, "Sue, I know that was a tough admission history on Mr. Jones. Your documentation is great; the specifics on how he was treating his leg ulcer will be of real value to the wound team. Thank you."

Positive reinforcement can be written. It's a nice idea to document the incidences of performance "above and beyond the call of duty." Copy not only the employee, but also your supervisor, the individual's employee file, and any one else who might be relevant. We take time to carefully document disciplinary actions. Why not take time to write down the good stuff too.

10. Does positive reinforcement really affect the way employees feel about their work?

Think back to a time when you really worked hard, gave your all, and it seemed like nobody noticed. How excited were you to behave the same way the next time you were faced with a similar situation?

Positive reinforcement is an easy thing to do. Make it part of your everyday routine. It makes your staff (and you) feel good. The experts say that positive reinforcement works, but I am even more convinced by my own personal experience.

11. Give an example of positive reinforcement.

I was hired as a manager of a busy progressive care unit in a large inner-city hospital. The workload was difficult, and the hospital had undergone a variety of organizational changes in a short period of time. I had an excellent staff who cared about their work and their patients. I realized that I didn't always tell them how good I thought they were. After reading about positive reinforcement, I made a point of addressing the good job that they were doing.

- Once or twice a week, I wrote a short note of praise to one of my staff members. Just a few lines of praise and a "thank you," placed in the employee's mailbox. It may have been about a positive comment that I heard from a patient or a coworker, the completion of a project they had been working on, or coming in to work an extra shift.
- I constructed a "Wall of Fame" in the staff lounge. I hung evidence of achievement, such as the picture of one of our staff who received the hospital's monthly customer service award or copies of the certificates of our nursing assistants who completed a telemetry tech course. When our performance data showed improvement in a particular area, the data were displayed for everyone to celebrate (remember, praise can be individual or collective).
- I hung a bulletin board in the main corridor of our unit next to the nurses station. Positive notes from a patient or family about a specific employee or the entire staff were hung for all to see (removing any confidential information). I also sent copies of the letter to my division director and vice president and to the employee's personnel file. Anyone who came onto our unit could see firsthand that positive things were being said, and written, about the staff.

12. Did this make a difference?

I knew it was the right thing to do, but I wasn't convinced that it had made a difference to my staff until a few things happened.

- One nurse came to pick up her paycheck, accompanied by her children. She brought them into the staff lounge so she could show them mommy's picture on the wall. As she told them about her work, it was obvious that she felt good.
- Another nurse who had floated to the unit was reading the bulletin board full of patient cards and letters. One of the regular staff stopped and said to her, "See? You're working with the 'A Team' today!"
- During an exit interview of a relocating nurse, she said, "Kathy, you probably don't remember this, but about a year and half ago you wrote a note to thank me for doing a good job. I found it in my mailbox at the end of long shift, and it really made a difference. No other boss has ever done that for me before, and I wanted to thank you. I still have the note."

13. How is effective discipline a motivational tool?

At first glance, it seems a little strange to think of discipline as a motivational tool unless you subscribe to Dr. Freud's theory. However, a manager who is light on holding people accountable doesn't help anyone, not even the employee making the errors. There is little more demotivating than working your hardest and seeing someone else continually delivering substandard work without it being dealt with. After a while, most hard-working employees in this situation develop a "why bother" attitude.

A manager who fairly and consistently administers effective discipline addresses the issues of unacceptable performance and helps employees come "up to speed" (or find somewhere else to practice). Holding everyone to high standards, and reinforcing high performance expectations, helps everyone to excel and feel successful.

14. Treating people fairly should be a basic principle in the workplace. Explain how it effects employee motivation.

It's true that fairness seems to be one of the simple "rules of the road." However, fairness its not always easy to implement. We think about fairness in terms of discipline, but also consider it in terms of other opportunities.

When you need help with a new project, whom do you choose? We all tend to recruit our "old reliable" employees for special challenges because we know they'll get the job done. This is unfair. First of all, are your "old reliables" burdened by the extra workload that these new projects present? Secondly, by your choosing the first person that comes to mind, does someone with the talent and ability to be successful in this endeavor lose the opportunity to excel? Does everybody have the chance to do well and be recognized?

A manager who is not always fair in both ways loses credibility. When employees perceive that they will receive a "fair shake," they are more likely to feel good about the place they work and the person they work for.

15. My staff are always concerned about money. I have strict guidelines and a tight budget for annual raises. What can I do?

Money is a concern for all employees (although studies show more so for blue collar workers than white collar workers). Otherwise, we'd all lie by the pool drinking piña coladas all day! But there are factors that are more important than salary. Deming believes that most people are driven by the desire to do a good job. Other influences on job satisfaction include the following:
- Job security
- The ability to work independently
- The opportunity to be creative and contribute ideas
- A sense of growth
- Being recognized for contributions to the greater good
- Camaraderie

If these things are in place, then there is less concern for big dollars. The key to non-monetary rewards is to know what is important to the employee to choose something that will be meaningful.

16. What kinds of non-monetary rewards can I provide? I don't have a big budget.

Think about what is important to the employee. A title that they can be proud of? The chance to teach others? A flexible schedule? The ability to influence processes at work? Consider the following:
- A change in responsibility and title (charge nurse? preceptor? safety representative?)
- An opportunity to learn a new skill (cross-training?)
- A chance to be on an important committee
- An opportunity to help interview potential new employees
- A paid day to attend a continuing education program
- Arranging for coverage to attend a family function

17. What can I give as non-monetary rewards on a day-to-day basis?

When an individual, or group of individuals, has done an exceptional job, consider the following:.
- Lunch tickets to the cafeteria
- Ordering pizza or some other meal
- A luxury item, such as a radio or coffee maker for the staff lounge
- A pair of movie tickets
- An interesting continuing education program during work hours (with appropriate staffing so people don't have to leave the program to check their patients)
- Cups, mugs, pens, T-shirts (check with your marketing department, pharmaceutical, and equipment reps)

• Praise in writing to the employee and to your boss
• A chance to go to lunch with senior management
• An extra day off

18. You mentioned earlier about meeting employees needs. My employees have the staff and equipment they need. Is this enough?

When motivation theorists talk about employee needs, they refer not only to the tools employees need in the workplace to do a good job. It is the need to be recognized as an individual, with professional and personal goals. Showing people you value them as individuals with special talents and needs helps them feel good about the part they play when they are at work.

Do you know what goals each individual has for his or her professional life? Show your employees you care by helping them find work that they love. This may mean facilitating further training/education, scheduling around a college schedule, helping them assume a slightly different role (preceptor, mentor), and even, although we hate to lose our prize employees, helping them find a position in the department that they really want to transfer to.

Do you know what is happening in your employees' personal lives? You're not Dear Abby, but if someone's performance is slipping or they seem distracted, do some detective work. Are there childcare/elder care/transportation problems? Can you assist by adjusting schedules or making them aware of resources in the workplace? Has someone's spouse or child just achieved something wonderful? Can you help the employee celebrate the event by passing the word on to coworkers or granting time off for a particular event?

19. Is that all there is to meeting employees' needs?

Employee needs are varied and dynamic. More things that you can do to meet a variety of needs include the following:
• Provide sufficient materials and equipment nurses need to keep up with technology and workload.
• Illustrate to your staff how their contribution fits into the organization's goals.
• Educate staff about new procedures, technology, and equipment.
• Encourage nurses to ask questions and share experiences; recognize and value your internal experts.
• Give timely, honest feedback about nurses' performance; people want and need to know how they're doing.
• Be available as a resource or when your staff needs to come to you with a problem.
• Develop teamwork among nurses.
• Articulate clear expectations for staff members; set goals for individual and group performance.

20. How does setting goals influence motivation?

Work-related goals give the employee direction. How can you be inspired to achieve if you don't know what you're supposed to get done? Goals give us a target for performance, as well as something to celebrate when the goals have been met. Doesn't a little celebration make everyone feel good?

21. Does my department need a complex list of goals?

Work-related goals don't need to be complicated. They may be as simple as having all orthopedic patients ready for physical therapy by a prescribed time, a threshold for medication errors, or achieving compliance with patient documentation.

Goals can also be developed with individual staff members, related to performance. For example, one nurse may be striving to become proficient in a procedure that is performed on your unit. Another may be working on assuming the role of charge nurse. Still another may be working on documentation or communication skills.

The guidelines for goals for the employee are exactly the same as for our patients. Goals must be specific, realistic, and measurable. People need to know what you expect of them, they must be able to achieve them, and you must have a way to determine that the goal has been met.

22. Who decides what our goals are?

The best and most achievable goals are those developed collaboratively. Certainly, you have organizational expectations. Bring them to your staff to discuss together and develop a plan for achieving them. Maybe the employees have ideas about what should be accomplished, by whom, how, and when. By involving employees in goal setting, you create a commitment to reaching or exceeding the goals.

Goals set for individuals are doomed to remain unmet unless you and the employee come to an agreement on the validity of the goal, the steps toward achieving the goal, and the time frame for completion. If the goal that you wish to set with your employee is unacceptable to the individual but crucial to the smooth functioning of your department, then perhaps the employee is working in the wrong place. Your role may be to simply help him or her find a work situation where the work goals are in line with his or her personal agenda.

23. What about involving employees in other decisions?

Excellent idea, although it takes a lot of energy, commitment, and communication. Again, if your employees are involved in planning and implementing a change, they have a stake in its success.

24. Describe what kind of decisions employees should be a part of.

Not every decision can and should involve employees. However, using guidelines, collaborative decision-making can be useful in areas such as hiring, equipment acquisition, scheduling, systems changes, and even budgeting. For instance:

- Involve a staff member in the selection, orientation, and socialization of a new employee.
- Ask the end users about equipment that you are planning on purchasing.
- Have staff members work together to develop the staffing schedule.

When change is inevitable, as in merging of departments or changes in vendors, work design, staffing patterns, or hospital systems, involve the people most affected by the change in planning and implementation. This increases your chances of success. Don't you feel better about a transition that you have been a part of, rather than one that has been dropped in your lap? The feeling of having control over your work situation does wonders for motivation.

25. Doesn't involving employees in decisions involve a lot of meetings?

It can, but consider this time well spent. Meetings can be short, with decision making broken up into phases, much like the nursing process:

- *Assessment:* Is there a problem or a change that needs to happen? What decisions need to be made?
- *Planning:* Gather input. Brainstorm. Listen to ideas. Then formulate a plan. Who will be involved, and what will their roles be? Set a goal.
- *Implementation:* Do it! Interview the new employee, change how scheduling is done, revise the shift routine.
- *Evaluate:* After a specified time frame, try to determine how things are going.
- *Revise:* Are adjustments needed in implementation? Have you discovered new problems (go back to assessment). Have you reached your goal?

26. Tell me how communication plays a part in this whole process.

Communication is the cornerstone not only to employee motivation, but also to good management in general. Regular, consistent communication with your staff, both for positive reinforcement and for discipline, allows you to routinely practice the seven strategies of motivation. Subtleties in your communication, such as your tone of voice, or the timeliness with which you address an issue, may effect how you are perceived.

To truly understand your employees' needs, you must talk with them. Not *to* them, *with* them. Communication is a two-way street, and your responsibility is to receive messages as they were intended, as well as to skillfully send messages.

27. What about talking to staff about "high stress" issues, such as budget, cutbacks, and personnel issues?

It doesn't take long for the rumor mill to take over when change is in the air. Chatter and speculation over workplace issues distracts people from their true purpose on the job. It creates an atmosphere of uneasiness and distrust, especially when things like job security are at risk. The best rule of thumb for discussing such topics is to keep your people informed. Tell them what you know (to the extent that you don't divulge proprietary information), and tell them as soon as you are able.

Be truthful. Tell them what you are able to tell, but don't feed into rumors with speculation. If you don't know an answer, say so and do your best to find out and report back to them. Even if you are sharing bad news, your employees will appreciate the respect you show them by "keeping them in the loop." If you don't talk with your staff, they will talk anyway. The rumors that develop and the misinformation that circulates can create far more panic than the truth.

28. Do you have any quick tips for communicating with employees?

Over the years, I have found some tried and true principles for helping to be sure communication runs smoothly:

- Be clear about the message that you want to send; think before you speak.
- Use plain language. Avoid technical jargon, which may be confusing or misinterpreted
- Confirm that what you said is what the other person understood.
- Clarify any fuzzy points.
- Take time to listen, rather than just waiting your turn to speak.
- Reiterate what you have heard to be sure that you understand.
- Communicate routinely, be consistent, and remember, "practice makes better."

29. How often I should try to motivate?

Employee motivation is not a periodic exercise; it is an ongoing practice. Consider that almost every action you take, any communication that you have has potential effects on how inspired your staff is to do a stellar job.

Applying the principles of motivation does not happen overnight. As with all other managerial skills, it requires forethought and planning, attention to your behavior, and practice, practice, practice. With time, however, these strategies become almost automatic, and you can feel responsible for helping your employees and your department achieve wonderful things.

BIBLIOGRAPHY

1. Cook M: Ten Minute Guide to Motivating People. New York, Macmillan Spectrum, Alpha Books, 1997.
2. Drucker PF: The Frontiers of Management. New York, Harper & Row, 1986.
3. Dunn-Cane K, et al: Managing the new generation. Nurs Manage 69(5):930, 933–936, 939–940, 1999.
4. Heyman R: Why Didn't You Say That in the First Place? How to Be Understood at Work. San Francisco, Jossey-Bass Publishers, 1994.
5. Lezon KM: Satisfaction in the Workplace. What Do Employees Want? Fort Pierce, FL, Healthcare Education Resources, 2000.
6. Manning M: Leadership Skills for Women. Achieving Impact as a Manager. Menlo Park, CA, Crisp Publications, 1995.
7. Porter-O'Grady T: Celebrate the loss of loyalty. Nurs Manage 29(9):5, 1998.

25. COACHING AND DISCIPLINING

Barbara Pierce, RN, MN, and James Noland, RN, MSN, CRNP

Never doubt that a small group of thoughtful, committed citizens can change the world: indeed it's the only thing that ever does.

Margaret Mead

1. What is the difference between coaching and disciplining?
Coaching is the process of facilitating development through the use of advice, encouragement, education, hands-on experience, and immediate, constructive feedback. It is a skill used to motivate and a proactive action to help develop staff, often focusing on anticipated needs. Disciplining involves coaching principles but involves specific actions when performances have failed to meet basic expectations, rules, or policies.

2. I have difficulty with coaching sessions for my staff. What is the best way to handle these sessions so that the staff is receptive?
Coaching is a learned skill. It is one of the best ways to build a team with the desired performances.

First, believe in the employee and that individual's value. Often the employee senses your honest interest and will respond to that.

Second, find at least one thing you honestly admire in each employee. It may be a clinical skill, but it can be something as basic as the knack to organize the unit's social events. When you show regard for what they already do well, people are usually more receptive to your thoughts on what could be done better.

3. I have a nurse who is a real star. Should I coach her in leadership skills?
Leadership roles are obviously not the best fit for everyone. Discuss it with the nurse and clarify that management is only one option for career advancement.

It is interesting to consider the example of Federal Express Corporation (FedEx), which has a leadership development program. They identified nine core attributes in their successful leaders: charisma, individual consideration, intellectual stimulation, courage, dependability, flexibility, integrity, judgment, and respect for others.

FedEx has a formal 8-hour class to help employees explore the challenges and frustrations (as well as the rewards) that are faced by managers. The three key challenges the class addresses are the increased workload, the unrelenting sense of obligation, and the headache of responsibility for other people.

Interestingly, only 20% of the people who take the class end up assuming a management role. But FedEx found that those who move to management do so knowing what to expect and usually end up more satisfied and successful.

Consider discussing these things with the nurse. Why not allow the nurse to try some managerial tasks, such as scheduling, to see if that type of work, with the concurrent human element, is enjoyable to him or her.

4. What is the best way to enforce policies?
Use these basic steps:
- *Involve staff in the development of the policy.* This improves buy-in to the changes and results in greater understanding of the policy.
- *Distribute the policies, explaining the reasons or need for the policies.* Many units have staff sign off that they have read the policy.

- *Clarify the repercussions for failing to follow the policy.* Listen to staff concerns, but behavior expectations must be articulated and acted upon consistently.
- *Enforce the policy.* You may allow a learning curve, with friendly reminders, but be sure an effective start date is mandated.

Use each step as an opportunity to teach, counsel, and reinforce the expectations. Most employees are not as worried about being fired as they are of falling out of favor. Personal and peer pressure can accomplish a lot.

On the other hand, be sure to compliment and reward compliant behavior. Mark your calendar to remind yourself to give feedback to employees who are improving their performance.

5. Administration has implemented some very unpopular policies. How do I enforce them when I don't believe they are right?

When faced with implementing difficult or unpopular policies that you don't support, such as a change in skill mix or dress code, follow these steps:

- *Clarify your concerns.* Understand how this policy affects the entire organization. In these trying times, an organization has to sometimes take risks and try new things.
- *Discuss your concerns only in private conversations with those who can maintain your confidence.* To be successful, staff must see you as totally supportive.
- *Orchestrate the presentation of the policy to the staff.* Consider having an administrator at the meeting to personally explain the policy. Discuss its challenges but also why it is important to the organization.
- *Include the benefit for staff, such as the answer to the basic "what's in it for me."* For instance, "The hospital needs to make its bottom line to give raises and to buy capital equipment we need to care for our patients." Collect staff's ideas.
- *Implement it to the best of your ability, being a daily cheerleader.* Give support, listening to staff concerns. Some experts recommend that you increase your visibility twofold during times of upheaval.

6. What if I am asked to implement a policy that violates my own moral or ethical values?

First ask yourself some questions.

- *Is it legal?* The hospital compliance officer or legal consult may be a resource.
- *Is it safe?* The hospital risk manager or safety officer may be a resource.
- *Is it good for our patients?* Network through your professional organization or do a literature search to see what, if any, results are known from others who had a similar situation.

After you have answered these questions, meet with your boss to discuss your concerns. If the bottom line is that the organization cannot make an exception, you must implement it. You may then have to consider whether this leadership role is the right choice for you.

7. What do I do about an employee with a bad attitude?

Negativity decreases productivity, work satisfaction, and teamwork. Once started, it can run rampant throughout a unit like a cancer. Too many managers ignore the problem, thinking that an employee is just having a bad day. But ignoring the patterned response only empowers the negative person. Our patients and team members deserve better.

Address the negativity. Counsel employees with specific examples, such as incidents of inappropriate whining, backbiting, or constant public complaining.

Sometimes an employee feels that a lack of complaining reflects a lack of awareness of the problems. What may need changing is the person's approach through reassurance that knowledge of the problem is there and what is needed are efforts toward the solutions. One manager posts a sign in her office, "I understand what bothers you. What steps are you taking to fix it?"

Some units have the staff develop a set of behavioral expectations. The rationale is that you can't change attitudes, but you can change behaviors. All staff sign off indicating their commitment to adhere, similar to a contract. The contract is publically displayed to remind peers of their mutual agreement. This contract is also used during the interview process.

8. Can you give examples of non-negotiable factors that a unit may have in their expectations for behaviors?

- Engaging in gossip at work
- Noncompliance with dress code
- Noncompliance with acceptable phone greeting
- Overuse of phone to make personal calls
- Eating food outside of designated eating areas
- Use of profanity in the workplace
- Being late for one's shift without calling
- Refusal to problem solve
- Responding to any patient need with "It's not my job."
- Failure to attend a minimum of eight staff meetings within 1 year
- Inappropriate use of furniture
- Reading of nonprofessional material in a work area

What is key is not always what is on the list, but that everyone participates in writing up these behaviors. Some even update them yearly. That way the staff have buy-in and assist in the enforcement.

9. What are some steps I can take to prevent negativity on my unit?

- Engage and empower staff in the decision-making process for change in the the units.
- Develop a culture of positive feedback. Reward in public; counsel in private. Life is full of 6-second compliments and 60-second complaints.
- Be approachable and available to listen to concerns.
- Be a good role model. Maintain your own positive attitude.
- Involve peer pressure to prevent negative attitudes from taking hold. Encourage staff to confront coworkers first and come to managers for help with mediation only if unsuccessful.
- Involve staff in the hiring process to help hire the compatible people who will agree to these standards.
- Train staff in conflict management skills.
- Refer staff to the Employee Assistance Program as needed.
- Employ stress-reduction techniques.

10. What is the best process to use to discipline an employee?

Most hospitals have progressive discipline plans that assist both the supervisor and the employee. They generally follow these steps:

- *Verbal warning:* An informal session reminding the staff member about the performance expectations. This warning may or may not be written and is generally not put in the employee's permanent file.
- *Written warning:* A formal action that specifically outlines the policy violation and what must be corrected. A copy of this warning is given to the employee and one is put in the employee's permanent file.
- *Suspension:* Removing the employee from the work area, usually without pay. This is intended to get the employee's attention and serve as a "last chance" to change his or her ways. Some institutions require the employee to come back with an action plan on what he or she will do differently.
- *Termination:* Loss of employment. Involve Human Resources prior to this step. You must make sure all obligations have been met and that the action will hold up to a legal challenge.
- *Sentinel events:* Behaviors that are so severe that the normal progression is waived and the employee proceeds directly to suspension or termination. Examples could include deliberately hitting a patient or stealing drugs to sell.

11. How do I handle the overall good employee who just can't seem to get to work on time?

Everyone has the occasional emergency, but a pattern of tardiness must be addressed. The issue must be dealt with in a timely and consistent manner across the department.

Meet with the employee to see whether there is a new issue, such as an ill child or transportation concerns. In extenuating circumstances beyond the employee's control, you may want to consider adjusting the start time. For instance, an employee must drop off a parent with Alzheimer's disease at the day care center and is always 15 minutes late because the center doesn't open early enough. Obtain the employee's permission to discuss it with the team so others understand why an exception has been made.

Also consider allowing staff to negotiate flexibility between themselves to leave early and arrive late (as long as the exchanges remain equal). And don't forget to acknowledge those who are on time.

12. What about tardy employees who have no extenuating circumstances?

In many cases, the employee often fails to accept responsibility to change necessary actions. One employee actually said, "The problem is the public transportation service reliability. I always take the same bus and every day I am 15 minutes late!" Another commonly reported response is that the employee does not believe that being late is a significant problem.

It is not the manager's responsibility to assist employees in organizing their personal lives. The focus must remain on the mandatory expectation to be on time, with failure to do so handled as any other disciplinary action.

Some managers include an assessment by a clinical nurse specialist in mental health or a representative from the Employee Assistance Program who will objectively and independently meet with the employee to identify personal issues. Lateness can be one symptom of issues such as domestic violence or substance abuse. Others will offer a family or medical leave if the individual is clearly jeopardizing his or her job.

13. The number of sick calls is going up as we get busier. How do I handle absenteeism?

Two major causes for sick calls (besides illness) are job dissatisfaction and generous sick time programs that employees see as their due. Measures to prevent sick leave abuse include the following:

- *Work on the causes of job dissatisfaction.* Are there too many days without breaks or too long of stretches on the schedule?
- *Build a strong team.* Staff is less likely to unnecessarily call in if they feel committed to the team that would now work short.
- *Have a large PRN pool that staff can use for special needs.* If staff can easily arrange their own coverage for their needs, they will be less likely to call off. Allow trading days as long as there is no overtime.
- *Reinforce that sick pay is for illness only.* Having a program that allows staff to cash in banked sick days helps avoid the "use it or lose it" mentality.
- *Look for patterns of absenteeism.* A common one is Fridays or Mondays with a weekend off. Promptly, specifically address these.
- *Have management personally take all sick calls.* Speak directly with the employee, not the family member, and ask, "What is wrong?" Keep a record.
- *Consider requiring a doctor's excuse for employees with patterns of frequent sick calls.* Consult with Human Resources, but some managers build this in as part of the progressive discipline.
- *Develop rewards for good attendance.* Set a good example yourself.

Besides the managerial irritation to try to find coverage, absenteeism affects the remaining staff that, at times, is left working short or with less experienced staff. One novel approach is to give them a choice. A replacement can be used (often a float or agency nurse who is not as familiar with their unit's routine) or they can work short one person and divide up that salary among themselves for the day. (This assumes, of course, that staffing is still at a safe level.) This at least compensates those left short for their extra efforts.

14. Disciplinary sessions don't seem to help. How can I get different outcomes?
Two areas that traditionally need improvement are clearly communicating the needed changes and providing ongoing follow-up feedback. There should be no surprises at an evaluation meeting with an employee because of all the previous frequent feedback that had been given to the individual. To try for an improved response, do the following:
1. *Ask the employee to recite back what he or she has understood from the meeting.* Include behaviors that need to change and an action plan for improvement.
2. *Summarize in writing the meeting's key points and expectations and have the employee sign a copy.* Give a copy to the employee and put one in his/her file.
3. *Repeat the critical messages a minimum of three times.* Employees are often nervous and may not absorb all that was communicated.
4. *Give ongoing feedback on a regular schedule.* Make reminders for yourself.

15. Some of my employees are just mediocre.
There are some people who do their job only well enough to get by. As J. Bronowski said, "The world is made of people who never quite get into the first team and who just miss the prizes at the flower show."
What can be doubly irritating is that sometimes this type of individual tends to be vocally critical of you and the organization but will not exhibit any desire or willingness to initiate or to participate in positive changes.
Try to get at the possible origin of this individual's behavior by asking some questions:
• Is this person bored with the job?
• Is this an intelligent individual who needs more challenge?
• Is this a long-term employee who is stagnant?
• Is this person "borderline" in knowledge and skills and seeks to hide it through avoidance?

16. What can I do to motivate the mediocre employee?
Each individual is different. Discuss your observations with the employee to try to understand the specific needs in this case. Suggestions include the following:
• If it is boredom or lack of stimulation, try cross-training, mentoring, or teaching responsibilities. Seek the employee's advice.
• If they just feel like one of the crowd or unappreciated, assign them an area for which they are responsible for becoming the unit's "expert" or assign a special project. Give more public recognition or rewards.
• If ability is the possible reason, consider having a clinical nurse specialist (CNS) or nurse educator work with them to help identify the specific problem area. They may need more training, but it may be something like organizational skills or self-confidence that is lacking rather than nursing knowledge.
However, if the behavior continues, give accurate performance appraisals relative to the clearly articulated job expectations. Some staff need a fear of consequences before they will change or leave. Managers have had the experience of some nurses, when pressed, admitting they are overwhelmed and transferring to a different environment (e.g., from intensive care unit to out-patient clinics).
Using peer evaluations may help the employee see how his or her behavior is perceived by their colleagues. One emergency department (ED) found that it was effective to have peer review scores count 12% toward the merit-based compensation increases.

17. What if the employee honestly does not have the same perception of the offensive behavior?
At times, it may become fruitless to argue over the details as different people do have different perceptions. You have three different patient complaints; the employee says he or she

was not rude and all the patients are prejudiced. Indicate that you may have to agree to dis-agree on this and leave it. But then focus on ways to achieve the results you expect: fewer patient complaints.

18. I get so nervous before a disciplinary action session. How can I better prepare myself?
- Make an outline of the key messages you want to convey.
- Hold a practice session with a mentor. Ask for and accept constructive feedback.
- Consider asking for assistance from Human Resources personnel. They can often sit in on the sessions.

19. List some points to remember about a successful disciplinary session.
- Handle the issue in a timely fashion, the sooner the better.
- Maintain the respect of the individual at all times. Discuss behaviors; don't attack the person.
- Listen. Allow the employee to tell his or her side of the story.
- Hold strict confidentiality at all times. Have the session away from the unit in a private office. Do not discuss the disciplinary action with any other staff member. Do not write the words "suspension" or "termination" on work schedules.
- Consider including a witness at the session. Besides back-up for you, it signals that this is important. The witness should be another nurse manager or someone from Human Resources, not one of the staff.
- Inform employees what steps they can take if they disagree with the disciplinary action.
- Complete any required forms prior to the session and have them ready for signatures.
- Allow the staff member a break away from the unit to think and to compose himself or herself before returning to patient care.
- Clarify the timeframe before the personnel record is cleared from any disciplinary action.

20. What is the best way to handle a termination session?
All avenues should be exhausted before taking this serious step. There are four steps to follow:
1. *Explain the facts and the reason for the termination.* Give specifics.
2. *Explain the termination process.* You may want a Human Resource representative present to answer questions about unused benefits, insurance coverage, or future references.
3. *Allow the employee to give input.* However, keep the focus on facts.
4. *End the meeting on a positive note.* Wish the employee future success. Have the employee leave the hospital after the session.

21. How do I handle it when staff asks me about a team member's termination?
Terminations have an impact on the unit beyond the affected individual so it is normal to have staff questions arise. But management must respect the terminated employee's confidentiality and never discuss any aspects of the termination. Simply state that the employee does not work here any longer and we wish him or her the best in the future.

Sometimes, the confidentiality issue is specifically raised during the disciplinary session. Both the employee and management can agree to "mutual non-disparagement." This phrase means that neither of you will speak ill of the other. It is, of course impossible to control any individual's off-the-cuff comments, but the request sends a message of legal proprieties. But in the end, you must remain silent even if the terminated individual is telling very different stories to other employees.

A termination may set off other staff's fears about their own job loss. Meet with the good members of the team to give positive feedback about their performance to lessen any paranoia.

22. You hear so much about disgruntled employees who become violent. What are special precautions I should take?
- Have a witness, from Human Resources or another administrator, at the termination session.
- Place yourself so that you are nearest to the door, not the employee, who could then block your exit.
- Notify security when a termination is taking place.
- Ask the employee to immediately return keys, parking pass, identification badge, and any other items that are hospital property before leaving.
- Remove the employee's access from the computer system right away (even before the session) to avoid the potential for sabotage.
- Consider changing the codes or locks if the employee does not return keys or access items.
- Take any actual threats seriously and immediately report them to the local police agencies and hospital security.

23. We are using many "travelers," that is, nurses from an external agency who have signed a 3-month commitment, and nurses from an external agency working just one shift. I'm not responsible for verifying their competency, am I?
You have a responsibility to verify a nurses' competency on the job regardless of the length of employment. The external agency role is to be a screener, similar to most hospital's human resource departments, and does not judge nursing ability. However, this verification of competency can be a simple process by two possible methods: actual observed behavior and the absence of error. Most institutions formalize the process by a simple checklist that can be completed by a supervisor or charge nurse after observing the individual's performance.

24. I have a psycho boss. Help! What can I do?
Stress in the workplace is affecting everyone. Turnover, increased workload, and financial pressures have affected some individuals so that they exhibit erratic and irrational behavior. Their own insecurity causes them to micromanage, have unrealistic expectations, or communicate ineffectively. Realize that their behaviors stem from their own issues and not necessarily from your performance. Some steps to help are as follows:
- *Take care of yourself.* Eat right, get your rest, and exercise.
- *Avoid running around the organization venting your frustrations to everyone.* Find one person who will protect your confidentiality and share your story.
- *Continue to meet face to face with your boss on a regular basis.* Avoiding the boss is not the solution.
- *Clarify expectations with your boss frequently.* End meetings by restating agreements.
- *Document everything.* Put agreements and deadlines in writing.
- *Consider including a third party in meetings.* It can signal accountability while also providing you with confirmation.
- *Get feedback from others about your performance to help you keep an objective perspective.* Reaffirm your own confidence and competence.
- *Stay on the high road.* Do not burn bridges or lower your standard of performance.

BIBLIOGRAPHY

1. Addesso P: Management Would Be Easy...If It Weren't for the People. New York, Amacom, 1996.
2. Huff D: Managers Forum: Changing bad attitudes. J Emerg Nurs 24(5):434–444, 1998.
3. Kobs A: Managers Forum: Verifying staff competency. J Emerg Nurs 27(5):495–496, 2001.
4. Manion J: Everybody's a coach: The leader's role in developing others. Presented at the Nursing Management Congress, September 19, 2000, Phoenix, AZ.
5. Marquis BL, Huston CJ: Management Decision Making for Nurses, 3rd ed. Philadelphia, J.B. Lippincott, 1998.
6. Podesta C: Self-esteem and the Six-second Secret. Newbury Park, CA, Corwin Press, 1990.
7. Row H: Managers Forum: Mentoring future managers. J Emerg Nurs 25(5):413, 1999.
8. Umiker W: Management Skills for the New Health Care Professional, 2nd ed. Gaithersburg, MD, Aspen Publishers, 1994.

26. THE IMPAIRED NURSE

James Noland, RN, MSN, CRNP

Never cease loving a person, and never give up hope for him, for even the prodigal son who had fallen most low, could still be saved.

Søren Kierkegaard

1. Are drug and alcohol problems new for nursing? I don't remember talking about it years ago.

Chemical dependency among nurses is not new. What is new is the awareness. Research validates that
- The nursing profession lacks specific knowledge about the disease of addiction.
- Boards of nursing are reluctant to implement diversion programs because of their lack of understanding about chemical dependency.
- Schools of nursing devote very few hours to the study of chemical dependency.

The goal then is to educate nurses, nurse managers, and nursing leaders about chemical dependency. One Vice-President of Nursing has a hospital-wide staff education program on the topic every 6 months.

2. Isn't the incidence rare in nurses?

It is thought that approximately 10% of the general population has an addiction problem, with probably a higher percentage present in the "helping professions." This means that at least 10% of any nursing population could have such a problem. As one Vice-President of Nursing said, "You have to wonder where are the impaired nurses in our organization and are they getting help?"

3. List things to consider that would pose a high risk for addiction.

Characteristics that can help create a situation conducive to drug or alcohol addiction include a high stress area and easy, frequent access to controlled substances.

4. What do you mean by a high stress area?

Emergency departments (EDs) and critical care areas are definitely areas of high stress. One study reported that nurses in these two areas are likely to abuse marijuana or cocaine. It has also been hypothesized that nurses working in these two areas tend to have sensation-seeking personality traits and may be more predisposed to addiction.

5. Describe what you refer to as an area of frequent access.

Postanesthesia care (PACU), EDs, labor and delivery, oncology, surgical, and orthopedic units are all areas where narcotics are frequently administered. A nurse will have ready access without arousing any suspicion.

6. How do the signs and symptoms of addiction differ depending on the substance of abuse?

The physical signs of alcohol abuse and narcotic addiction are listed in the tables below. The impairment or hang-over from alcohol represents the more "traditional" signs. Nurses addicted to narcotics, on the other hand, are often the "best" workers, with good attendance and frequent overtime, in order to have access to the drugs. However, many addicted nurses will use both narcotics and alcohol.

Physical Signs of Alcohol Abuse

SUBTLE	OBVIOUS
Deteriorating appearance	Slurred speech
Weight loss	Tremors
Coughing	Unsteady gait
Decline in hygiene	Lethargy
Frequent use of mints	Smell of alcohol on breath
Unexplained bruises	Frequent trips away from the work area
Irritability with peers; abrasive with others	Isolation
Mood swings	Frequently late or tardy

Signs of Narcotic Addiction

Arriving at work early and staying late

Volunteering for additional shifts

Often volunteering to be in charge of the medication keys or to administer the medications

Preferring shifts where there is less supervision

Rapid mood swings

Frequent bathroom breaks

Dilated or constricted pupils

Sloppy documentation

Frequent spills, breaks, or wastes

Signing out more narcotics than other nurses

Giving the maximum dosage of medications ordered

Disappearing into the bathroom directly after accessing narcotics cabinet

7. I suspect a colleague is using drugs, but I am afraid to say anything because I don't want the nurse to lose his or her license. What should I do?

Every nurse has ethical and legal obligations to protect patients from harm. Knowingly allowing an addicted colleague to practice is unethical and might subject you to disciplinary action if you were covering up for an impaired colleague who injured a patient.

Early intervention in the addict is key, but hard to accomplish. To safeguard patient care, however, it is critical to identify the addicted nurse as soon as possible and remove him or her from patient care.

It is a myth that the nurse's license is always immediately revoked. At least 20 states now have programs set up through the state regulatory agency, such as the State Board of Nursing. These programs assist nurses suffering from drug and alcohol addictions to get into rehabilitation. This, of course, assumes that no patient harm occurred and there was no criminal activity (such as stealing the drugs to sell on the street). The possibility does exist that the employer may choose to terminate the nurse, but early intervention and increased understanding can help prevent that.

More important, untreated addiction is a progressive, fatal disease. There are many success stories of recovered nurses. In the end, you must remember the lives of that nurse and patients are at stake.

8. Who can I talk to at my institution?

Most institutions have policies dealing with the chemically dependent employee. Contact your Employee Assistance Program. Other possibilities include a social worker, chaplain, staff psychologist, the psychiatric clinical nurse specialist, or even other nursing personnel who are recovering from chemical dependency.

The institution's attitude will be a key factor. Hopefully the message will be that its desire is to help addicted nurses get treatment and remain (if able) in the profession.

9. How should I approach the nurse?

Have a frank, open, honest, and direct conversation about what you observe. Point out the facts and don't make accusations. Describe the behavior you see and address performance issues. Remain positive, sympathetic and sensitive. Let the nurse know that help is available and that he or she can recover. Convey to the nurse that he or she is not alone; many other nurses suffer from chemical dependency.

10. How do most impaired nurses respond to confrontation?

Expect the nurse to deny the problem at first. Nurses think they can control their addiction. This denial is the prevailing defense mechanism. It is not a simple matter of lying or willful deception, but rather a psychological mechanism operating unconsciously to protect the "self" by avoiding reality.

As the nurse accepts his or her addiction, he or she is often consumed with guilt, shame, remorse, and regret. The nurse is fearful of losing his or her livelihood and profession. There is a risk of suicide at this point. It is important to be prepared to immediately get the nurse into treatment.

11. What if the nurse continues to deny everything?

You may need to involve others for a more pivotal confrontation. It is important to have a good deal of evidence to break through the denial. Studies show that the chance of treatment and recovery is improved by involving the employer.

12. How should a nurse who returns from treatment be handled?

If the state regulatory agency offers an impaired nurse assistance program, there will most likely be contract stipulations for a period of time. Contracts will differ but have some similarities.

- *Definition of the conditions under which the nurse may work.* The nurse is often restricted from practicing in unsupervised positions, such as home health, travel nursing, or agency work. Some hospitals require the day shift to ensure that regular supervision is present.
- *Restriction from administering narcotics for a defined period of time.* This may mean the nurse must transfer to an area that does not have access to narcotics, such as quality assurance.
- *Submission to random urine drug screens.*
- *Involvement with the peer assistance program.*
- *Attendance at a weekly support group, such as Alcoholics Anonymous.*
- *Maintaining satisfactory professional performance.*

There may also be stipulations about notifying new employers of their contract conditions if they chose to change jobs during this period.

13. Should the recovering nurse tell other staff about the situation?

One experienced administrator encourages returning nurses to tell peers that they have been in treatment and would appreciate their support. Without divulging the gory details, it prevents resentment from other staff for what could be perceived as preferential treatment. Most nurses find acceptance through their honesty. It also communicates to everyone that this administration gives help, rather than judgment or punishment, to those who have needs.

But usually the decision is left up to the nurse. The nurse should have some prepared response for when coworkers ask about their sudden absence. Offer to role-play that situation with the nurse.

14. What should I do as the manager?

It is important to remember that the nurse needs support. The nurse could still have feelings of anxiety, shame, guilt, remorse, and particularly embarrassment at this point. Therefore, your role is to help facilitate a smooth transition back to work. Remember, you are helping to save a life.

BIBLIOGRAPHY

1. Pullen LM, Green LA: Identification, intervention and education: Essential curriculum components for chemical dependency in nurses. J Contin Educ Nurs 28(5):211–216, 1997.
2. Sloan A, Vernarec E: Impaired nurses: Reclaiming careers. RN 64(2):58–64, 2001.
3. Sussman ED: Combating the Hidden Enemy. N J Nurse 25(8):2–3, 1995.
4. Trinkoff A, Storr C: Substance use among nurses: Differences between specialties. Am J Public Health 88: 581–585, 1998.

27. LEADING AND MANAGING
A DIVERSE WORKFORCE

Linda S. Smith, MS, DSN, RN

Keep out of ruts; a rut is something, if traveled in too much, becomes a ditch.

Arthur Guiterman

1. What is culturally competent leadership in nursing?

Culturally competent leadership (CCL) is the ability to work efficiently and effectively with workers at all levels of diversity. These levels or layers of diversity include the following:

- Personality
- Internal dimension, including age, gender, ethnicity, physical ability, physical size, and sexual orientation
- External dimension, including income, habits, religion, geographic location, and marital status
- Organizational dimension, including seniority, union affiliation, management status, and classification

Thus, diversity includes differences in learning style, education, job description, and more. CCL means that all workers are supported and encouraged to develop to their full, creative potential.

2. Who is the "average" registered nurse?

The largest group of health care providers in America is registered nurses (RNs). The latest available data from Health Resources and Services Administration indicated approximately 2,558,874 RNs with current practice licenses. Of these, 59% were working full-time. Salaries, age, education, and ethnic and gender diversity are increasing; hospital practice is decreasing. Additional data include the following:

- 10% ethnic or racial minority
- Average age of 44.3 years
- 5.4% male
- 58.4% with less than a baccalaureate degree in nursing
- 6.3% with formal advanced practice education; approximately 9.7% with master's degrees or doctorates
- 60% working in hospital settings; 17% working in community or public health settings
- Average full-time salary of $42,071; recruiters report that compensation levels for RNs jumped from 10% to 20% from 1999 to 2000 due to the shortages

3. What are the characteristics of the health care clients?

For the United States, racial and ethnic minorities make up about 27% of the working-age (18–65 years) population. For this working-age group, minorities are projected to total 38% by 2025 and 48% by 2050. Thus, diversity among clients and nonprofessional health care employees will dramatically increase.

4. What role do different languages play?

More than 300 languages and dialects are spoken within the United States, and at least 8.7% of the population is foreign born. The Civil Rights Acts of 1964 requires that institutions that receive federal funding make a reasonable attempt to provide interpreter services. Studies show that health care is affected for patients with limited English proficiency (LEP) and limited literacy. The lack of bilingual services includes the following:

- There is evidence of an unconscious bias creating undertreatment of pain. In one study of males with isolated long bone fractures, non-Hispanic white males received pain medication in the emergency department (ED) at a 2:1 ratio over Hispanic males.
- Only 53% of the patients with LEP reported that side effects of their medication(s) had been explained to them versus 84% of English-speaking patients.
- The number of follow-up office visits, prescriptions written, and prescriptions actually filled increased significantly when patients with LEP received consistent interpreter services.

5. Why is celebrating diversity among clients and staff so important?

Culturally competent corporations tend to be identified as superior performers. Diverse groups make better decisions and are at a competitive advantage. Diversity conveys respect for each individual. By celebrating diversity, organizations work effectively across diverse worldviews and serve as change agents in a diverse world. Thus, CCL directly leads to culturally competent client care.

6. Can you give an example of what you mean?

A non-Hispanic visiting nurse was doing diabetic teaching for a Hispanic patient. The patient had consistent weight gain despite his statements indicating he was adhering to the diet, particularly the restricted sample foods (e.g., concentrated sweets, pastas). Finally a Hispanic nurse, familiar with the culture, asked about ethnic foods. Only then did it come out that the client thought he could eat unlimited fried platanas, a starchy vegetable common in the Hispanic diet.

7. I believe I manage my unit's diversity. Isn't that enough?

The construct of CCL is very different from a mere cursory examination of affirmative action. CCL taps into the full potential of every worker. Every day, employees need to believe their contributions are valued. Viva la difference! That is the motto of multicultural work groups that celebrate differences and agree to share information in respectful, flexible, purposeful ways.

8. What can I do to best prepare myself for leading and managing a diverse workforce?

Make a personal and professional commitment to understand, rather than deny, differences. Appreciate that CCL is the direct result of an ongoing facility-wide diversification process. Understand also that you will model as well as implement CCL.

9. What are some activities that I can do to develop CCL?

Self-study CCL activities for personal methods of discovery may include the following:
- Attending cultural events where you are the minority representative
- Foreign travel
- Foreign language competence
- Reading and viewing good culturally relevant books
- Web sites
- Films
- Think/write about your personal history and heritage
- Consult with facility and professional cultural experts

10. As I learn to increase my culturally competent leadership skills, what is my most important first step?

It is important to recognize and celebrate your own diversity because most people view culture as someone else's perception. Self-discovery will help you identify your own personal assumptions, goals, values, and biases. By being aware of our personal perceptions and culturally dictated activities, we can then appreciate the beliefs and behaviors of others.

11. What questions should I ask in self-assessment?

Do I...:
- seek diversity-oriented experiences?

• take advantage of diversity-oriented learning opportunities?
• use culturally competent mentors?
• plan culturally-mixed social activities for my unit and facility?
• examine regularly my personal bias, attitudes, beliefs, and prejudices?
• assess conflict resolution skills?

12. Once I take this step, what should I do?
After a careful self-assessment, managers need to:
• Recognize and describe diversity as a strength
• Learn and teach about staff culture
• Respect and value all groups and diverse opinions
• Create work-place environments that help all staff interrelate socially
• Ensure representation of all groups at meetings
• Develop equal and fair growth opportunities for all employees
• Remove cultural barriers
• Participate in the formulation of fair and equal management policies
• Reward staff who demonstrate cultural competence
• Openly and aggressively seek resolution to culture-related conflict or problems

13. How will mentoring programs help me (and my staff) lead and manage a diverse workforce?
Mentoring culturally diverse workers in the political skills needed will help their organizational success and survival. Ideally, assign mentors from the same cultural group to new staff members for orientation.

14. Are there any special concerns for homosexual patients?
Author Jeffrey Zurlinden found several themes that lesbians and gay nurses would like other nurses to know.
1. *Avoid false assumptions.* Nurses often think they detect sexual orientation on the basis of looks or mannerisms and then tailor their responses accordingly in stereotypic ways.
2. *Behave and use language that allows every patient to be honest.* For instance, rather than asking a man wearing a wedding ring if he wants to call his "wife," ask if he wants to call "anyone."
3. *Understand that homosexual people seek health care unrelated to their sexual orientation.* Homosexual people have common conditions such as urinary tract infections or breast cancer, but nurses tend to focus only on HIV.
4. *Remember homosexual people may also be the parents of a child.* It is estimated that 6 to 14 million U.S. children are raised by homosexual people.

15. Any considerations for my homosexual staff?
Author Jeffrey Zurlinden heard several themes from his interviews with lesbian and gay nurses.
1. *Avoid different treatment.* Most still do not share much of their personal lives with coworkers because they fear discrimination.
2. *Keep assignments fair.* Those who come out report being expected to work more "family holidays" because they "do not have a family."
3. *Do not assume they should or want to take care of all of the homosexual patients.* Every nurse has a responsibility to treat homosexual patients with respect, dignity, and professional competence.

16. What special challenges do I face when working with an aging workforce?
The health care workforce is aging; society around us is aging. Baby boomers will start to retire in or before the year 2011; California predicts that 50% of their nurses will no longer be

practicing in the year 2012. Yet the population of those 82 years of age and older is growing at a rate that is six times faster than the rest of the population.

Health care facilities need to understand that gray matters. Managers should prepare now by establishing improved recruitment, support, and retention strategies for older nurses. Beyond improved recruitment procedures (which would include refresher courses for unemployed nurses), managers could

- Endorse an organizational culture that establishes experience as invaluable.
- Recognize the cultural value of an older workforce when caring for an aging population.
- Provide flexible shift scheduling such as 6- or 8-hour shifts (12-hour shifts can be difficult for older workers) and part-time options.
- Provide flexible between-work scheduling (three or four shifts in a row can take a physical and emotional toll).
- Support lighter duty options when available.
- Develop a career ladder that facilitates the movement of experienced nurses into alternative roles.
- Provide on-site elder care (aging workers often must care for dependent relatives).
- Discover ways (through focus groups) to make the facility more ergonomically helpful and efficient.

17. What special challenges do I face when working with people with disabilities?

The number of American workers with declared disabilities is increasing. The Americans with Disabilities Act (ADA) of 1990 was written and signed into federal law with the purpose of mainstreaming people with disabilities into American society, including the workplace. Adult workers with disabilities are to be respected and valued as individuals, just like any other employee. When working with persons with disabilities, managers should do the following:

- Speak directly to the person; speak as you would to any other worker.
- Respect the person's privacy.
- Respect the person's right to ask for reasonable accommodation.
- Consider that people with disabilities know themselves best of all; they know what they can and cannot do.
- Understand that labels can do enormous damage. The disability does not define the person. Do not say disabled person, victim, cripple, sufferer, or handicapped; better to say, "person with a disability."

18. What techniques should I use for my staff member who falls below the 8th grade literacy level in reading, writing, and mathematics?

Employees' ability to perform within the health care workplace depends on their ability to rapidly learn new skills. Training must be individualized, relevant, and effective. For the majority of health care workers, job training in English works well. However, when English is poorly comprehended because of low literacy levels or English as second language (ESL) issues, practical and creative approaches on the part of nurse managers are needed. These could include the following:

- Develop teaching/learning materials in other languages.
- Have visual-enhanced procedure manuals (graphs, pictures, drawings, photographs).
- Record procedures on video with corresponding manuals in English and other languages.
- Provide scaled-down versions (simple words, phrases) of policy and procedure manuals in other needed languages.
- Employ professional interpreters during training sessions (although training in the native language is better).
- Create training materials with side-by-side languages.
- Facilitate on-site ESL and mathematics classes.

19. Can you give an example?

A video of a common procedure can be cheaply made right on the unit. For example, the next time a blood spill needs to be cleaned, record a skilled employee completing the task while talking through the entire procedure. Your audio-visual department could duplicate the English version film and dub in other languages as needed.

20. Which Internet web sites might be most helpful to me as I learn and implement culturally competent leadership?

http://www.yforum.com The national forum on people's differences. An excellent site that offers open and free diversity dialogue.

http://www.aimd.org/resource.html A resource list on managing diversity compiled by the American Institute for Managing Diversity, Inc.

http://www.ala.org/diversity/resource.html Good collection of resources to help managers become more culturally competent. Resource categories include words, managing diversity, the work/communication, recruiting for diversity, retention of diversity, mentoring, and others.

http://www.nadm.org/ (Click "links" on the site top tool bar.) Outstanding list of accessible Internet resource links including health care, education, human and ethnic resources, government and public sector, foundations/scholarships/grants, resources for legal, disability, religion, gay and lesbian, women, and reference sites.

http://www.diversityrx.org/html/divrx.htm A web site designed to promote language and cultural competence to improve health care quality for diverse communities and groups.

21. Specifically, how do I promote CCL among staff and professional colleagues?

There are a number of ways. Nurse managers can
- Attend multicultural workshops and request help and support from CCL colleagues in other facilities and departments.
- Carefully review errors, complaints, grievances, incident reports, and exit interviews as potential signs of unsuccessful CCL.
- Hold on-site diversity potluck luncheons during work time. These could be scheduled monthly with a different staff-member volunteer bringing a specially prepared ethnic main dish. As food is eaten and shared, the volunteer describes traditions of food preparation, rituals, heritage, and health care custom.
- Confront cultural insensitivity facility-wide with one or two pre-agreed upon words. For example, a special word like "hurt" or "stop" could be used to signal a culturally insensitive interaction. This signal would immediately initiate a private meeting regarding the perceived insensitivity.
- Invite staff members to write articles about their backgrounds and publish these in your facility's newsletters. An on-going diversity column, devoted to these short pieces, would honor and recognize staff-authors.
- Put diversity concerns on your staff meeting agendas; promote the idea that the only "bad" question is the question not asked.
- Develop group cohesion by validating perceptions, clarifying misunderstandings, and formulating mutually agreed upon goals and unit norms.

22. What must I never do, whether in front of just one person or many?
- Intimidate by appearing uncaring, closed, frustrated, or indifferent
- Demonstrate in word or deed that questions are stupid, irrelevant, or time wasting
- Treat staff differently
- Disregard the importance of ethnicity in employee job performance
- Demonstrate intolerance to cultural or group differences
- Expect one person to speak on behalf of his or her entire culture[10]

23. How do I assess a culturally competent organization?

Measures of CCL come in many packages: quantitative, qualitative, and anecdotal. Some important ways to measure the results of implemented CCL include decreased Equal Employment Opportunity (EEO) complaints, decreased staff turnover rates, greater retention rates of minority employees, greater minority involvement in meetings, committees, and decision-making situations, and exit interviews that positively identify CCL efforts. Additionally, patient and staff satisfaction surveys, along with routinely scheduled staff focus groups, can be used if specific questions relative to CCL are addressed.

24. What are some ways to evaluate that?

Some evaluation measures you might include (Smith, 1999):
• Skills, creativity, and competency of all staff are enhanced.
• Cultural links with the community are established.
• Racism, sexism, and all other -isms are carefully identified and eliminated from all policies and procedures.

25. Do any organizations formalize diversity?

Yes. For instance, Brigham and Women's Hospital created a diversity mission statement. "[The hospital] is committed to creating an environment that values, supports, and respects differences. This includes, but is not limited to, race, gender, ethnicity, language, sexual orientation, age, physical or mental ability, and national origin."

In another example, one visiting nurses organization worked through their Massachusetts Nurses Association union to include diversity in the contract. Statements include, "The agency and the MNA agree that the nurses serving the geographic area covered by the Agency should reflect the population served."

BIBLIOGRAPHY

1. Animal and Plant Health Inspection Service (APHIS) Council on Managing Diversity: What is workforce diversity? U.S. Department of Agriculture, 2001. *http://www.aphis.usda.gov/mb/wfd/define.html*
2. Benedetti DA: Education, business and labor leaders share diversity strategies. Catalyst 7(1): 2001. *http://www.cde.psu.edu/catalyst/vol7no1/strategies.html*
3. Cohen J: Disability Etiquette (99-0212-002). Jackson Heights, NY, Eastern Paralyzed Veterans Association, 1999.
4. Davis PD: Enhancing multicultural harmony. Nurs Manage 26(7):32A–32H, 1995.
5. Frauenheim E: Gray matters. Nurs Week 2(2):16–17, 2001.
6. Health Resources and Services Administration, HHS, Bureau of Health Professions, Division of Nursing. Notes from the national sample survey of registered nurses 1999. *http://bhpr. hrsa.gov/dn/survnote.htm*
7. Population Reference Bureau: America's racial and ethnic minorities. Population Bulletin 54(3), 1999. *http://www.prb.org/pubs/population_bulletin/bu54-3/part3.htm*
8. Smith LS: Trends in multiculturalism in health care. Hosp Mater Manage Q 20:61–69, 1998.
9. Smith LS: Achieving and recognizing institutional cultural competence. Competence Matters 2(3):15–21, 1999.
10. Smith LS: Teaching to a diverse student group: Transcultural concepts. In Scheetz LJ (ed): Nursing Faculty Secrets. Philadelphia, Hanley & Belfus, 2000, pp 123–129.
11. Tompkins NC: Lessons in many languages. HR Magazine 41:94–96, 1996.
12. Zurlinden J: Gay and Lesbian Nurses. New York, Delmar, 1997.

28. MANAGING GENERATION X EMPLOYEES

Claire Raines, MA

*Focus groups clarified another source of intense stress: Baby Boomers conveyed nega-
tive perceptions of Generation Xers with whom they work.*

S.R. Santos and K. Cox

1. Who is Generation X?

People born in the years following the Baby Boom are generally called "Generation
Xers." They've also been known as the Post-Boomers, the Baby-Busters, and the Thirteenth
Generation (because they were the 13th generation of Americans after the Declaration of
Independence). In the early 1990s, a young Canadian, Douglas Copeland, wrote a novel
called *Generation X*. In that book, he asks that his generation be given an "un-label," and
that's where the X came from.

The post-World War II boom in births began in 1946 and lasted until 1964. Officially,
Xers are those born between 1965 and 1980. Some generational experts, though, say the
Generation X personality began with birth year 1960. Bottom line, these are your employees
currently in their 20s and 30s.

2. What does Generation X have to do with nursing?

Today, the average age for nurses, depending on the source, is 44 to 47 years. Many
nurses are, of course, older than average, making many of them members of the World War II
Generation. This generation is known for their dedication, hard work, patience, and respect
for authority. Even greater numbers of nurses are members of the Baby Boom Generation,
known for their idealism, team-orientation, and driven work ethic.

When these two generations were young, there were two basic career choices for women:
teaching and nursing. Think of the tremendous impact that had on our hospitals. The best and
brightest professional women, devoted to quality patient care, went to work in health care facilities across the nation.

Then along came Generation X. Not only was this generation smaller than the one before
it, but the Women's Movement had changed the way women thought about their professional
lives, adding a whole spectrum of new career choices. Gen X women—and men—were not as
attracted to health care professions, especially nursing, and they chose other careers. These sociologic changes contributed greatly to today's nursing shortage. Add in factors such as mandatory overtime, the increasing complexity of care, and decreasing nurse-patient contact, and you
have a critical business issue.[1] To thrive—even to survive—health care organizations must find
ways to attract and retain Generation Xers. Smart managers will learn all they can about
Generation X—how and why they're different, what matters to them, and, most important, how
to create work environments that satisfy them and bring out their best.

3. Why are Gen X nurses different?

They grew up in a different world. There's an Arab proverb that says, "People resemble
their times more than they resemble their parents." Think about the first 15 to 20 years of your
life. What was in the headlines? Who were the heroes? What was the mood of the time? What
music did you listen to? Generations share these historical and sociologic events and trends,
causing them to develop their own unique mindsets, values, priorities, and styles.

Generation X grew up amidst Watergate, the energy crisis, soaring divorce rates, and an
uncertain economy. At school, they watched the Challenger space shuttle disintegrate before
their very eyes. After school, 50% were latchkey kids who were on their own, playing

162

Nintendo and Atari and learning to be self-reliant. Contrast that era with the ones that shaped the Boomers and the WWII Generation, and you begin to understand how Gen Xers have a unique perspective.

Comparison of WWII Generation, Baby Boomers, and Generation X

	WWII GENERATION	BABY BOOMERS	GENERATION X
Defining events	WWII	Civil rights movement	Watergate
and trends	Great Depression	Vietnam	Divorce
	Patriotism	Woodstock	Uncertain economy
	Radio	Prosperity	Challenger
	The Silver Screen	Children in the spotlight	Energy crisis
Characteristics	Respect	Idealism	Self-reliance
	Discipline	Teamwork	Pragmatism
	Loyalty	Driven work ethic	Financial savviness
	Stability	Personal gratification	Balance
	Law and order	Health and wellness	Commitment reluctance
	Hierarchy	Youth	Nonauthority

4. List some of the defining characteristics of Gen X employees.

They are self-reliant; they tend to be pragmatic; they are financially savvy; they want balance in their lives; they're reluctant to commit; and they possess a casual attitude toward authority.

The Xers and the Boomers: 12 Delineators

XERS		BOOMERS
Job	1. Perspective on work	Career
Blunt	2. Communication	Diplomatic
Unfazed	3. Authority	Impressed
Indifferent	4. Approval	Seek validation
Scarce	5. Resources	Abundant
Mistrustful	6. Policies and procedures	Protective
Self-reliant	7. Reliance	Team-oriented
Balanced	8. Work ethic	Driven
Task and results	9. Focus	Relationship and results
Assimilated	10. Technology	Acquired
Merit	11. Entitlement	Experience
Survival	12. Perspective on the future	A better world

From Raines C, Hunt J: The Xers and The Boomers: From Adversaries to Allies. Menlo Park, CA, Crisp Publications, 2000., with permission.

5. Tell me more about the characteristic of self-reliance.

Gen Xers report they were often left to fend for themselves as children, and they learned to take care of themselves in the midst of uncertainty. As a result, they typically have little faith in organizations. They believe job security depends on their own resumes. Meredith Bagby of CNN Financial News quotes a survey that says more Gen Xers believe in UFOs than believe Social Security will be there for them when the time comes. As a result of this tendency toward autonomy, older managers often accuse Gen Xers of not being committed to the team.

6. Explain the characteristic of pragmatism.

Baby Boomers were told as children that their generation could change the world. Gen X children, on the other hand, were taught that it's a tricky world, and that you have to be on guard in order to survive. Typically, Xers don't see the world as optimistically as the generation before them. They're more practical; some even accuse them of skepticism and cynicism.

7. Discuss the characteristic of financial savvy.

As children, Generation Xers learned how far a dollar goes—and doesn't go. They were often given a check to pay the plumber or some cash to pick up some groceries after school. They speak the language of money. Today, they know they're needed on the job market—particularly in the health care industry—and they're sophisticated shoppers. They know what Hospital XYZ is offering in salary, schedule, and benefits, along with how it compares with what Company ABC has to offer.

8. Discuss the characteristic of balance.

Gen Xers watched their parents work weekends, bring work home in the evenings, struggle to get along with difficult bosses, and then get laid off. They accuse Baby Boomers of "living to work." They say they just want to "work to live." They report that work isn't necessarily their first priority. No generation has valued flexibility more than Gen Xers, who want time to pursue a life outside of work.

9. Tell me more about the characteristic of commitment reluctance.

Gen Xers know the traditional "lifetime" contract between employer and employee is irrevocably broken. Most of them are wary of layoffs, and they don't tend to give their loyalty to an organization. Some Xers become very loyal, but usually to a manager who cares about them, and then only with time.

10. Explain the characteristic of nonauthority.

As children, Xers saw the leader of the nation go down in disgrace. They watched on TV as Reverends Bakker and Swaggert crashed and burned. Many of them counseled a parent through an ugly divorce. As a result, they don't put leaders on pedestals. They tend to treat the CEO the same as someone their own age and rank.

11. It seems like Gen Xers aren't as loyal as older employees. And they don't seem to be willing to work as hard. Do others have the same experience?

There's a human tendency, when people are different than we are, to pass judgment on them—to decide we're right and they're wrong, even to decide we're good and they're bad. Generations tend to have their own frames of reference and their own work ethics. Look at a couple of the tables in this chapter and you'll see that you're not alone; others are making the same complaints, and more.

But, notice also, the other side of the equation. Baby Boomers complain about Xers, but Xers have some bones to pick with Boomers, too. We need to recognize that each generation brings unique contributions to the workplace, and that our differences are a good, not a bad, thing.

Boomers often accuse younger employees of "not being willing to pay their dues." At its worst, that translates to, "I was miserable for my first 10 years on the job, and it's not fair that you shouldn't be also." In today's job market, the concept of dues-paying is null and void. Effective managers don't expect young employees to "pay dues."

What Xers and Boomers Say About Each Other

WHAT XERS SAY ABOUT BOOMERS	WHAT BOOMERS SAY ABOUT XERS
They're workaholics.	They don't want to pay their dues.
They think a half-day means leaving at 5.	They think "job" instead of "career."
They thrive on office politics.	They're not loyal.
They talk the talk, but they don't walk it	They constantly ask, "why?"
They ask for our opinions, then do it their way.	They have no work ethic.
Their lives center around their jobs.	They're not team-oriented.

Adapted from Zemke R, Raines C, Filipczak B: Generations at Work: Managing the Clash of Veterans, Boomers, Xers, and Nexters in Your Workplace. New York, Amacom, 2000.

12. When will they change?

Sociologists tell us the frame of reference we develop in our first 10 to 20 years of life tends to be the one through which we see the world for the rest of our lives. People's basic values remain consistent throughout a lifetime. Generation Xers are starting their own families, building professional skills, gaining work experience, and moving into positions of power and control in many organizations. The way they see the world of work, however—their approach to the job, their view of authority, the type of work environment they prefer—will most likely *not* change.

What can change is the manager's approach. Successful managers will do everything they can to understand and empathize with Gen X employees and to adapt their management style to maximize the effectiveness of all their people.

13. What unique contributions do Gen Xers make to the workplace?

Generation Xers bring a fresh perspective to work with them. They tend to be pragmatic, results-oriented, creative, and open-minded. They grew up in the midst of change—many even lived in different neighborhoods on weekends and vacations—and they're more flexible than any generation before them. And, although many older associates have embraced technological advances, Gen Xers simply assimilated it; they're naturals when it comes to laptops, Palm Pilots, the Internet, and e-mail.

14. How do I manage them effectively?

Here are four principles widely endorsed by successful managers of Gen X employees, and by Gen Xers themselves. They are to develop their resumes, be flexible, lighten up, and appreciate them.

15. Tell me what you mean by "develop their resumes."

Many Generation Xers see themselves as free agents or contractors. They know their resume is their only ticket to job security. They want opportunities to make themselves more marketable—business results, numbers, and accomplishments.

Give them creative challenges. Mentor them, give them constant feedback, and teach them helpful information and skills. Help them get signed up for training and certification programs.

Keep in mind that their learning style may be different. They tend to respond best to fast-paced, interactive activities, role playing, games, and case studies, where they get immediate feedback and reinforcement.

16. Discuss the principle of flexibility in terms of Generation X.

Typically, Gen-Xers are committed to creating life-work balance. They saw the prices their parents paid for 60- and 80-hour workweeks—stress, poor health, divorce, neglected children—and they are determined not to make the same mistakes. Help them work out a schedule that allows them to pursue other interests—a young family, social life, hobby, or school.

Be sensitive about religious and cultural holidays. Ask your people to teach you about themselves, what it was like where they grew up, what's important in their family and culture. Make certain your staff feels that it's safe to speak up. Have an open door policy and honor it.

17. Explain the principle of lighten up.

Generation X is the first generation to consistently include "fun and informality" on their top five characteristics of the ideal workplace. Many feel that Baby Boomers take themselves too seriously. In the past 10 years, the Xers have changed the way we dress at work significantly; no longer is a person's professionalism judged on who designed their suits.

Fill an employee's workstation with balloons. Hire a juggler to come to a staff meeting and teach everybody to juggle. Give everybody a pair of Groucho glasses with nose and moustache. Ask everybody to wear their favorite baseball hats for a special occasion. Hold a Nerf basketball game.

18. Illustrate what you mean by the principle of appreciating them.

In interviews, Gen Xers consistently say, "If I just knew someone around here appreciated what I do, it would make a world of difference." Your employees today know they have a choice as to where they work. Show them how glad you are they choose to work for you.

Thank them privately and publicly when they do a good job. Write a card that is specific and genuine. Repeat compliments from colleagues and patients.

19. How can I communicate more effectively with Generation Xers?

One Nike ad says it this way. "Tell us what it is. Tell us what it does. And don't play the National Anthem while you do it." Gen Xers often feel the media—especially advertising— lied to them, and they've grown distrustful of any message that seems like it might not be genuine. At work, they accuse managers of "corporatespeak" and of saying the right things but not practicing what they preach.

Be direct and straightforward with Gen X employees. Get right to the point. Don't say, "I'd really appreciate it if you would…" when you mean, "Please do this now." Explain why. Expect questions, and give them short, honest, reasonable answers. Use e-mail when it's appropriate. Keep meetings to a minimum. And talk to them about benefits—what's in it for them?

20. Who is Generation Y?

The newest generation—born about 1980 to 2000—is sometimes called Generation Y. Others call them the Nintendo Generation, the Digital Generation, or Generation Next. Several thousand of them sent suggestions about what they want to be called to Peter Jennings at abcnews.com, and "Millennials" was the clear winner. They're a work in progress, so we're just beginning to get a handle on who they may become. Currently, it looks like they're collaborative, civic-minded, goal- and achievement-oriented, and sociable. Experts compare them to the World War II Generation. Since they tend to be more optimistic and altruistic than Generation Xers, they may be more attracted to careers in nursing. When it comes to the nursing shortage, the Millennials just may be that bright spot on the horizon.

BIBLIOGRAPHY

1. Abrams RB: A Nurse's Viewpoint. Healthleaders.com, December 5, 2000.
2. Bradford LJ, Raines C: Twentysomething: Managing and Motivating Today's New Workforce. New York, MasterMedia Limited, 1992.
3. Raines C, Hunt J: The Xers and The Boomers. Menlo Park, CA, Crisp Publications, 2000.
4. Raines C: Beyond Generation X. A Practical Guide for Managers. Menlo Park, CA, Crisp Publications, 1997.
5. Santos SR, Cox K: Workplace adjustment and intergenerational differences between Maturers, Boomers, and Xers. Nurs Econ 18(1):7–13, 2000.
6. Zemke R, Raines C, Filipczak B: Generations at Work: Managing the Clash of Veterans, Boomers, Xers, and Nexters in Your Workplace. New York, Amacom, Big Apple, 2000.

29. NEGOTIATION

Polly Gerber Zimmermann, RN, MS, MBA, CEN, and Camilla L. Jones, RN, BBA

Life does not consist of holding good cards but of playing a poor hand well.

Thomas Fuller

1. What is negotiation?

Negotiation is a process whereby two or more parties come together to discuss issues and compromise to meet synergetic goals and objectives. The most effective negotiation process provides a win-win solution for everyone.

2. Is networking the same as negotiation?

Networking is the process of aligning oneself with others to obtain information, ideas, advice, power, and influence. It has a long-term objective and requires sincere effort on the part of the parties to establish honest relationships with others. The most effective networking includes socialization and sharing of information, creating personal bonds between people.

Negotiation usually has a defined goal. During the networking process, the objective may be in the future, but the relationship is being developed now. Networking, therefore, enhances motivation for compromise during negotiation. It can provide a platform for information gathering and influence during the decision-making process.

3. Is consensus building the same as negotiation?

Consensus building requires networking skills and is probably the most effective form of negotiation. It is the process of informal meetings, discussion, and subsequent agreement on issues or decisions *on a personal level* prior to formal decision-making processes. The key to quick consensus is productive information flow, and the focus is on agreement, not method.

Consensus building is relatively new as a negotiating method in the United States. However, the Japanese are masters at this technique, as it is part of their life culture. There is a Japanese saying "nimuwashi" that translates as: if two people are stakeholders in a transaction, it is up to those two people to informally develop the consensus from the bottom up through interpersonal interaction.

4. How does consensus building help speed the negotiation process along?

Historically, Americans have used a "ready, fire, and aim" approach for decision processes. Problems inevitably develop because agreement has not been obtained from all stakeholders. In the Japanese "nimuwashi" model, all of the problems are considered prior to the final decision. From the outside world, it looks like no decision is being made, when in reality, a complete solution is being determined and agreed upon. This "ready, aim, fire" method improves the likelihood of approval and success dramatically because all parties agree and present the decision in a positive "can-do" format.

5. What are steps in consensus building?

- Include all stakeholders.
- Learn what the other parties want and need. Don't assume you know.
- Gather enough information.
- Discuss pros and cons.
- Begin informal consensus building.
- Continue to gather information and review options.
- Place final decision in writing for all parties to review.
- Confirm the agreement or make revisions prior to presentation

6. **What is involved in principled negotiation or negotiation by merit?**

Consensus is not always possible. Traditionally, we negotiate from a position of trying to meet a desired goal or objective. The classic book *Getting to Yes* advocates that managers negotiate on merit. The four basic points involved are

- Separate the people from the problem.
- Focus on interests, not positions.
- Generate a variety of possibilities before deciding what to do.
- Insist that the result be based on some objective standard.

7. **List some rules I need to know about negotiation.**

- Expect to gain something; expect to lose something.
- Realize you may have to bend in values as well as tangible goods. This doesn't mean that you give up your values, but rather that you allow the other person to keep his or her values as well.
- Negotiate for the long haul as well as for the immediate issue at hand. Go for a solution in which, ultimately, both parties can win.
- Understand that the objectives of all involved parties are both common and diverse.
- Realize that first offers are generally not accepted.
- Try to get the other side to make the first concession on a major issue.
- Get something in return for every concession.
- Keep negotiations as simple as possible.
- Expect some resistance.
- Consider third-party interests.
- Understand that the most important ingredients are often not the material elements, but the symbolic ones. People respond to understanding, acceptance, and respect.

8. **What are some techniques for negotiating?**

- Control the agenda and start with vital issues, rather than haggling on small issues.
- Always start with the affirmative side. Otherwise, you spend your time tending to negatives.
- Fix the burden of proof on the other side. However, make sure you go in loaded with information.
- Present your plans to get a "yes" response early.

9. **List some techniques I can use if things are really starting to go badly.**

- *Stall for time.* The best way is to change the subject, "Now getting back to the previous point of..."
- *Fall back on an "absent decision maker."* You can always say you need to "check this" before making a final decision.
- *Appeal to authority.*

10. **Talk about appeals to authority I can use.**

All of the following are a "higher" authority than your opinion or desire. Use:

- *Better numbers.* "Percentage-wise, this idea is stronger."
- *Printed evidence to back your case.* Have the related articles there.
- *Weight of dollars saved or lost.* People are influenced by large figures—"This will save $40,000."
- *Literally the weight (volume) of paper.* While saying something like "the computer printout doesn't support that position," hoist 5 pounds of printouts onto the table. (Who is going to read all of that to verify your statement?)
- *Legal considerations.* "This will cause lawsuits."
- *Regulatory/government considerations.* "This won't meet JCAHO's standards."
- *Historical relations.* "In the 5 years of working with you in this program...."

- *Future.* Cite future predictions, known facts (inflation), or novelty/being the first.
- *"Arguments of the crowd" (size).* "All of the other community hospitals are doing this."
- *Appeal to an expert.* The opinion of an expert is usually accepted as valid at face value.
- *Official organizations.* "The Emergency Nurses Association's position statement on this is...."

11. Isn't it better to use an objective outsider and go into arbitration?
Always try for a decision between the involved parties, rather than one imposed by outsiders. The negotiating parties have stronger motives than an arbitrator. The arbitrator may not decide as you thought!

12. What are "straw bosses" and how do they affect my success in negotiating?
All organizations have some form of "straw bosses." Straw bosses are the first-line leaders and, if not involved, can undermine your objective and cause it to fail. Straw boss leaders can help the manager speed up buy-in (and consensus) from staff if they are brought in and used to give and gather information. If the straw boss buys in, the rest of the staff will usually follow suit. The manager also has a perfect opportunity to empower people and motivate them by giving credit away, thereby increasing staff morale during decision-making processes.

13. What are some obstacles that can occur in negotiation?
Defensive posturing and territorialism are common obstacles. It may help to back up and reassess whether you have missed what the other party really wants. If recognition is an obstacle, a good manager will give up credit. Ultimately, the outcome is more important. Hold out a few compromises as "wild-cards" whenever possible in case they are needed at the end of the process to build consensus.

14. I'm going into this negotiation knowing I'm in a weaker position. Are there tips to use in this type of scenario?
- *Play for home-field advantage.*
- *Avoid defensiveness.* Don't complain, don't explain.
- *Never attack the stronger party on a personal level.*
- *Use deference and persistence.* Do favors for the other side. Concede certainties.
- *Establish your credibility.* Stress any affiliations you have.
- *Go prepared.* Privately construct a range of acceptable level of solutions. Anticipate the other party's questions and objections.
- *Protect your needs by giving away some items you would like to have but could get along without.* Split the issues and negotiate each one separately.
- *Present an avalanche of facts.* Control the evidence. Get help from others; bring along the expert or lawyer.
- *Offer them a surprise they will like.* Offer some variety.
- *Use time for your side.* Do small things first. Watch deadlines; decisions are often made right before them.

15. What can I expect to accomplish if I learn to negotiate well?
Negotiation is imperative to win-win interactions between management circles. Objectives can be met through other methods, including autocratic decision-making. However, "buy-in" is critical for employee endorsement and higher morale level, which improve worker productivity. Negotiation supports input and compromise between stakeholders.

16. Are there references that can help me with this?
Two classics are Roger Fisher and William Ury's *Getting to Yes* and Roger Fisher and Scott Brown's *Getting Together.*

BIBLIOGRAPHY

1. Brooks E, Odiorne GS: Managing by Negotiations. Malabar, FL, Krieger Publishing, 1984.
2. Fisher R, Ury W: Getting to Yes: Negotiating Agreement Without Giving In. New York, Penguin, 1981.
3. Fisher R, Brown S: Getting Together: Building Relationships as We Negotiate. New York, Penguin, 1988.
4. Jurrens WG: Junior Executive NEC: Interview. Austin, TX, 2001.
5. Moorehead G, Griffin RW: Organizational Behavior. Boston, Houghton Mifflin, 1995.
6. Strasen L: Key Business Skills for Nurse Managers. Philadelphia. J.B. Lippincott, 1987.

30. LABOR UNIONS

Robert W. Stein III, RN, BSN, MSHA, CHE

We all belong t' th' union when it come t' wantin' more money and less work.

Frank McKinney Hubbard ("Ken Hubbard")

1. I've never been a manager in a unionized facility before. What do I need to know about unions?

Union activity is guided primarily by the National Labor Relations Act and enforced through the National Labor Relations Board. Any interference, domination, discrimination, or refusal to bargain is considered to be an unfair labor practice by management. The five phases of unionization are organization, recognition, negotiation, administration, and decertification.

2. Tell me more about the first phase, organization.

You are first likely to hear of a unionization effort during organization. This is when informal "rumbling" of dissatisfaction among the workforce will be heard. The union organizers will be assessing employee interest in unionizing through informational meetings. Any organizing effort must occur in nonwork areas and on employees' own time.

The only action that management may take at this point is to quickly assess and address the needs of the employees that lead to their dissatisfaction. If the employees see that management is actively attempting to meet their needs, the organizing effort may fail. If dissatisfaction remains high and there continues to be sufficient interest in unionizing, the organizers will proceed to the recognition phase.

3. Describe the recognition phase.

In the recognition phase, organizers will begin passing out authorization cards for the employees to sign. Handing out authorization cards is solicitation and may be prohibited during work hours. Solicitation during nonwork hours such as breaks and meal periods is permitted.

Buttons and lapel pins supporting the unionization effort frequently appear during this phase. If your dress code prohibits these items, you may continue to enforce the dress code. If the dress code does not address buttons and lapel pins, you cannot arbitrarily decide that they are now prohibited.

Should the union receive authorization cards from 30% of the employee group, a vote will be scheduled. Management must post date, time, and location of the election. Any employees with supervisory responsibilities are considered management and are ineligible to vote in the election.

Should the union lose the election, it is prohibited from seeking certification from the same group of employees for a 12-month period. If the union wins the election, they will prepare to negotiate a contract with management.

4. What points does the union make to recruit nurses to join?

Union representatives discuss sharing power and having democracy. They often make the point that someone is fighting for you in an environment where consistency or fairness has been a problem. A union is presented as a way to take charge of the profession, particularly for working conditions and compensation. Union representatives cite other professions, such as teachers or lawyers, as using unions to gain benefits and respect.

5. What happens in the negotiation phase?

During the negotiation phase, teams consisting of representatives of the union and of management will meet to negotiate the terms of the contract. Once the negotiating teams agree on contract terms, the employee group must then ratify the contract before it becomes binding. After the represented employee group ratifies the contract, implementation or administration of the contract begins.

6. What occurs in the administrative phase?

In the administration phase, terms of the contract have been clearly defined and are enforced. The role of management is to clearly understand and abide by the terms of the contract. Any deviation from the terms of the contract can lead to a grievance hearing. Terms of the grievance procedure are usually included in the union contract.

7. What is a grievance procedure?

Grievances can be filed by the unionized employee against management for real or perceived violations of the union contract. This often occurs because the unionized employee is more motivated to understand the terms of the contract than is management. During a grievance proceeding, evidence and arguments are heard from both sides and a decision rendered as to how the contract addresses the situation at issue.

8. Tell me about the decertification phase.

The decertification phase occurs once the unionized employees decide they no longer wish to be represented by the union. Decertification works basically the same as the recognition phase. A decertification petition must be signed by 30% of the represented employees to bring it to an election. The represented employees vote and, if passed, the union is removed.

The role of management during the decertification phase is to continue to meet the needs of the employees. Small group meetings can further develop employee-management relationships. The decertification election is more likely to succeed if the employees have confidence in management and feel that they are trustworthy.

9. I don't want a union. What can I do to avoid having a union come in our institution?

The easiest way to avoid unionization efforts is to remove the need for the union. Meet the needs of your employees and treat them with fairness and respect. Basically, act as if you were operating under a union contract and you will eliminate any need for a union.

For instance, in one Chicago hospital, a nurse sought to bring in a union after some dissatisfying restructuring moves. Senior administration made some key changes before the union vote, including personnel changes and a "clinical governance" structure. The vote went against the union. Administration stated it showed the staff's confidence in the new mechanisms; the staff said they now believed administration was listening.

10. How do I work with the union we have in our hospital?

Research is mixed regarding productivity and satisfaction with a union. The point is that the union should never become the determinant in providing good care. Considerations include the following:
- *Know your contract.* It is mandatory reading.
- *Ensure consistency with your peers.* Unions tend to focus on any situation that one manager handles differently.
- *Keep the focus on patient care and good employee relationships.* It is possible to develop and obtain letters of agreement on key issues, such as maintaining competency, with the unions support.
- I*nvolve the union in the plan development, not just the implementation.* Being a partner from the beginning can help limit knee-jerk negativity.

BIBLIOGRAPHY

1. Greene J: Collective Threat. Hosp Health Networks 72(8):60, 1998.
2. Marriner-Tomey A: Guide to Nursing Management, 3rd ed. Mosby, St Louis, 1988, pp 316–324.
3. Zimmermann PG, Pierce B: Managers Forum: Unions and ED nurse managers. J Emerg Nurs 25(3):225–226, 1999.

V. Meeting Standards

31. LEGAL CONSIDERATIONS

Robert W. Stein III, RN, BSN, MSHA, CHE

The law is not an end in itself, nor does it provide ends. It is preeminently a means to serve what we think is right.

Justice William J. Brennan, Jr.

1. What is informed consent?

Informed consent has meant different things over the course of humankind. Physicians in Ancient Greece were considered all-knowing, and discussion with patients was discouraged beyond what was required to gain the patient's obedience. The use of manipulation and deceit were considered acceptable to that end. Up until the mid-20th century the law of assault and battery required only that the physician disclose the proposed treatment and gain permission of the patient.

In recent years, the fundamental right of self-determination has been recognized and requires the collaboration of the physician and patient. This right to self-determination was recently re-affirmed in the Patients Bill of Rights adopted by most health care facilities. This newer standard requires the disclosure of the following elements to be considered informed consent.
- Diagnosis
- Proposed treatment and probability of success
- Substantial risks and benefits of the proposed treatment
- Alternatives to the proposed treatment
- Substantial risks and benefits of alternative treatments
- Risk of doing nothing

2. You consistently refer to "physicians." Are only physicians responsible for informed consent?

The provider performing the treatment or procedure has the responsibility for obtaining informed consent. As director of the treatment plan, most often the providing physician in collaboration with the patient will have this responsibility. The teaching and counseling roles of the nurse will reinforce and augment the information provided to the patient, but nurses cannot assume the providing physicians' responsibility of informed consent.

3. What role, if any, does the nurse have in informed consent?

As educators and counselors, nurses teach and reinforce health care information that may be included in an informed consent. They are not responsible, however, for obtaining informed consent. Only the providing physician can obtain informed consent.

4. How do consent forms fit into informed consent?

Many health care facilities use consent forms to document that informed consent has been obtained. Nurses are frequently asked to complete and witness the patient's signature on these documents. The witnessing of a consent form is not the same as obtaining informed consent. Informed consent can be obtained only through a meaningful discussion between the patient and treating physician, leading to the acceptance of the proposed treatment by the patient.

5. Doesn't the "consent to treatment" signed upon admission into the hospital cover all procedures performed during the hospital stay?

An admission "consent to treatment" cannot replace informed consent because it does not include all the required elements as outlined in question 1. Additionally, informed consent can be obtained only through dialogue with the treating physician.

6. What about practicing procedures on the recently deceased? Some do not want to ask the families for fear of adding to their grief. Does consent need to be obtained from the next-of-kin? Is this practice even legal?

Practicing medical procedures on the recently deceased is probably the best way to teach health care providers. For example, learning endotracheal intubation on a plastic and latex mannequin has its value but cannot be compared with intubating a human being. The practice does, however, raise a number of significant legal and ethical issues. Frequently, hospital policy and procedure manuals do not offer guidance as to what is permissible when it comes to these areas.

There are no state or federal statutes that specifically address the practicing of medical procedures on the recently deceased. It is generally recognized that legally the deceased no longer have any right to privacy. As a result, the usual frameworks of autonomy and informed consent do not apply.

Florida, Georgia, and Michigan courts have ruled that any rights to privacy or property that belonged to the deceased cannot be claimed by the next-of-kin. The U.S. 6th Circuit Court of Appeals ruled slightly differently by asserting that the next-of-kin in fact did have a property interest in the deceased remains. They found that a hospital could be held liable if the procedures practiced on the newly deceased without consent caused the next-of-kin emotional distress. Also, most states have some statute prohibiting the mutilation of a corpse.

Research studies have shown that when consent to practice medical procedures on the recently deceased is sought, the majority of families give their permission. From an ethical perspective, this makes it difficult to argue that the educational value of such procedures outweighs any potential harm of practicing them without first obtaining the family's consent. (See also Chapter 35, Ethics.)

The practicing of medical procedures on the newly deceased, while not strictly illegal, may expose the facility to some liability if the procedures are done without consent from the next-of-kin. Procedures should be limited to those that are less disfiguring. For example, endotracheal intubation may be acceptable, whereas practicing a thoracotomy may not be.

Your local community standards and state laws will provide some of the legal and ethical answers about this practice in your locale. Hospital legal counsel, administration, risk management, ethics committee, and education department should evaluate their training needs and options, establish policies that include obtaining consent, and outline which procedures are considered acceptable.

7. What are advance directives?

Advance directives are a mechanism for individuals to formally declare their desires for health services in the event they are unable to provide or withhold informed consent because of their medical condition. For example, a patient with a terminal illness may request that his or her life not be artificially extended through intubation or other extraordinary measures. In essence, it is an informed refusal to consent signed in advance of its need. (See also Chapter 35, Ethics.)

8. What role does the nurse have with respect to advance directives?

Nursing needs to determine whether a patient has a completed advance directive. If a current advance directive exists, a copy should be placed in the patient's medical record and the physician informed of its existence. The physician will then write orders for "no intubation" or "no code" as per the patient's desire.

If no advance directive exists, information about it should be provided to the patient. Many hospitals have prepared booklets and fill-in-the-blank forms that can be provided to patients and their families upon request. There is no requirement for anyone to have an advance directive.

9. What should the nurse do if the patient suffers cardiac arrest before the physician orders a "no code" or whatever the advance directive indicates is the patient's desire?

Ethicists may have a different answer; however, legally the medical orders should be carried out as written. An exception to this, however, exists in some states. In some states an emergency medical system (EMS) "DNR" or "Do not resuscitate" form can be signed by a terminally ill patient and the physician. It specifically directs paramedics not to initiate cardiopulmonary resuscitation (CPR) or advanced life support measures. Frequently, emergency department staff are included in the definition of "emergency medical service (EMS) personnel" and may withhold CPR or advanced life support without any additional medical orders.

10. What if CPR or advanced life support measures are initiated before the existence of a signed DNR form is known?

Once CPR or advanced life support measures have been initiated, even if in error, only a physician may order that they be terminated.

11. What should the nurse do if the admitting physician refuses to write orders consistent with the patient's advance directive?

The conflict needs to be discussed between the physician, patient, and family. Nurses can help to bring these groups together and facilitate the discussion. If an acceptable agreement cannot be reached, the situation should be referred to the hospital ethics committee for review and recommendation. The patient may prefer to request a different physician whose beliefs about health care services to the terminally ill are more closely aligned with his or her own.

12. Does transfer to another facility require informed consent?

Transfer to another facility for ongoing care requires informed consent. As a medical treatment choice, the patient must be provided all the elements of informed consent (see question 1) and agree to the transfer prior to being transferred to another facility.

13. Are there any other special requirements before transferring a patient?

The federal Emergency Medical Transfer and Active Labor Act (EMTALA) has very specific requirements for transferring a patient with an emergency medical condition from one facility to another. If an emergency medical condition does not exist, the requirements under EMTALA will not apply. Initially written as an "anti-patient-dumping" statute, EMTALA applies to both insured and uninsured patients alike.

The act primarily affects the emergency department; however, the courts have ruled that the requirements of EMTALA apply to in-patients as well as patients in the emergency department and thus has implications for all nursing units. The requirements of EMTALA for general nursing units are summarized as follows:

- Informed consent: The meaningful dialogue between physician and patient must also include the benefits of transfer (e.g., higher level of care, additional available resources) and the risks of transfer (e.g., traffic accidents, equipment failure en route).
- Stabilization: Any and all resources ordinarily available to patients in the hospital must be used to stabilize the patient prior to transfer. If attempts at stabilization fail, then the physician must certify that the benefit of transfer outweighs the risk of transferring an unstable patient.
- Accepting physician: Before a transfer can occur, arrangement must be made with a physician at the receiving facility to accept responsibility for the continued care of the patient. The transferring and accepting physicians may one and the same, assuming he or she has admitting privileges at more than one facility.
- Accepting facility: Before a transfer can occur, the receiving facility must accept the patient, thus ensuring that resources will be available upon the arrival of the patient. Resources needed before the accepting facility can agree to receive the patient include bed availability and sufficient nursing staff to provide care to the patient.

As with any transfer of care, a complete report must be given to the nurse receiving the patient at the accepting facility, as well as any ambulance personnel involved in the transportation of the patient. A complete copy of the medical record, including any relevant radiologic studies, must accompany the patient to the accepting facility.

14. Under what circumstances can the nurse delegate tasks and procedures to unlicensed assistive personnel?

The nurse can delegate only those tasks and procedures that are within their knowledge, skill, and scope of responsibility. Before delegating to unlicensed assistive personnel, the nurse must determine that the unlicensed assistive personnel can properly and safely perform the delegated task or procedure. When delegating, the nurse must clearly communicate specific direction, potential for complication, and the expected result. The nurse must then provide the unlicensed assistive personnel with the appropriate level of supervision. Responsibility and accountability remain with the nurse and cannot be delegated with the task or procedure.

15. How do I determine whether a particular task or procedure can be appropriately delegated?

A task or procedure can be appropriately delegated if it requires no independent nursing judgments, assessments, complex observations, or critical decision-making. The task or procedure should be routine in nature, performed according to a standardized procedure, have predictable results, and the consequence of performing it improperly minimal. Delegated tasks or procedures must be within the training, skill, experience, and job description of the unlicensed assistive personnel. The National Council of State Boards of Nursing adopted the Five Rights of Delegation in 1995 to assist nurses in determining which tasks and procedures are appropriate for delegation to unlicensed assistive personnel. They are as follows:

- Right task: one that is delegatable to a specific patient.
- Right circumstances: appropriate patient setting, available resources, and other relevant factors considered.
- Right person: right person is delegating the right task to the right person to be performed on the right person.
- Right direction/communication: clear, concise description of the task, including its objective, limits, and expectations.
- Right supervision/evaluation: appropriate monitoring, evaluation, intervention as needed, and feedback.

16. Are there any tasks or procedures that are inappropriate for delegation?

Tasks or procedures that involve the nursing process are inappropriate for delegation. The nurse must perform assessment, problem identification, and outcome evaluation. Teaching, medication administration, triage, and the coordination and management of care are nursing functions that cannot be delegated.

17. As manager, am I responsible for the tasks or procedures that the nursing staff choose to delegate to unlicensed assistive personnel?

Yes. You are responsible for determining which tasks and procedures fall within the training, skill, experience, and job description of the unlicensed assistive personnel. The facility and/or state may also have rules or guidelines about what activities unlicensed assistive personnel can perform.

18. Are you saying that, as manager of my nursing unit, I am responsible for what the nursing staff delegates whether or not I am here to directly supervise them?

In a word, yes. As manager, you are responsible for determining which tasks and procedures fall within the training, skill, experience, and job description of the unlicensed assistive personnel. The role of the nurse manager in the supervision of unlicensed assistive personnel is summarized as follows:

- Define appropriate tasks or procedures for delegation to unlicensed assistive personnel through written job descriptions, policies, and records.
- Ensure that unlicensed assistive personnel have the necessary training, skill, and experience needed to competently perform those tasks or procedures deemed appropriate for delegation through performance appraisals, skill checklists, and in-service education.
- Communicate to the nursing staff the information they need to delegate appropriately through job descriptions, policies, protocols, and direction.

19. Is there a difference between the terms *negligence, professional negligence,* and *malpractice*?

There are several different types of negligence, but generally, negligence is the failure to exercise the degree of care that a reasonable person would exercise under the same or similar circumstances. Professional negligence or malpractice is the negligence of professionals in the performance of their duties, done intentionally, through carelessness, or through ignorance.

20. How is professional negligence or malpractice determined?

A claim of malpractice requires four elements to be successful. There must be a duty owed, a breach of the standard of care, damages, and causation. These terms are defined as follows:

- Duty: obligatory conduct owed by one person to another. In malpractice, this is determined by the existence of a nurse-patient relationship or physician-patient relationship.
- Breach of duty: failure to perform a duty owed another person or failure to exercise that care which a reasonable person would under the same or similar circumstances. The standards of care define what a reasonable professional would do in similar circumstances.
- Damages: an injury, harm, or loss.
- Causation: a direct cause-and-effect relationship between the breach of a standard of care and any damages suffered. A bad health care outcome by itself does not imply malpractice in claims of professional negligence. The damages must have occurred as a direct result of a breach of the standards of care.

21. Maybe an example would help clarify all this legal mumbo jumbo.

Sure, let's use delegation to unlicensed assistive personnel as an example. Assume that a nurse is assigned to a patient. The nurse has a duty to provide nursing care consistent with the standards of care owed to that patient. The nurse then inappropriately delegates a task or procedure to unlicensed assistive personnel, violating one of the Five Rights of Delegation. The nurse has now breached the standard of care. Assume now that the patient suffered an injury or damages as a direct result, meeting the criteria for causation. The four elements of negligence, duty, breach of the standard of care, damages, and causation have all been met. The nurse in this example could be found liable for malpractice.

22. You said there were other types of negligence. As a manager, do I need to know about them?

Under the doctrine of corporate negligence, the hospital or health care facility may be held liable separately for breach if its duties. As an employer, they have a duty to hire competent staff, to adequately supervise and monitor the employees, to provide adequate training and orientation, and to maintain appropriate policies and procedures. Breach of these duties that result in harm to a patient could be considered corporate negligence.

23. Can you give me an example of corporate negligence?

Sure. Let's use the same example as above. The facility has a duty to its patients by virtue of accepting them into their facility for care. The standards of care require job descriptions, policies, and procedures to be in place. Assume there was a lack of monitoring, supervision, or policies in place that allowed the inappropriate delegation to occur. The facility has now breached the standards of care. Since the patient suffered an injury—damages as a direct result—causation has been established. The facility could be found liable for corporate negligence.

24. Is the nurse manager always responsible for the neglectful conduct of the staff? I'm not sure I want this job anymore!

No. As long as you have provided the necessary framework or guidelines through job descriptions, policies, and procedures and adequately monitor and supervise your staff, you have met your duty. Generally, employees whose conduct extends beyond the scope of their job responsibilities or violates established procedures are liable for their own actions.

25. What do I need to know about sexual harassment?

Any complaint of sexual harassment must be taken seriously and requires your immediate action. It is a form of sex discrimination that violates Title VII of the Civil Rights Act of 1964. Consent to the unwelcome sexual conduct may explicitly or implicitly affect the victim's continued employment or unreasonably interfere with the person's ability to perform his or her job duties, or create an intimidating or hostile work environment. The harassment may be verbal or physical and can occur between any combination of the sexes. As a manager, your performance will be judged on how seriously you take and how swiftly you respond to the complaint.

26. What should I do if a staff member comes to me complaining that they are being sexually harassed?

Offer the employee reassurance that you will investigate and deal with the situation immediately. Facility policies differ, but you will want to involve administration, the human resources director, and/or the hospital risk manager. Ask for a full accounting of the events leading to the complaint, including any witnesses. Ask the employee to put the specific complaint in writing as well.

Until the investigation is completed, you should ensure that the people involved are not required to work together. If necessary, consider schedule changes or paid suspension until the matter is resolved.

Schedule a meeting with the accused person and present him or her with the allegations. Ask for and evaluate the person's explanation of the events leading to the complaint, including any witnesses. The accused person should also prepare a written response.

Meet individually with any witnesses named to collaborate or refute the allegation. If the allegation is believed to be true, swift termination of the harasser is in order. Should the complaint prove to be untrue, swift termination of the alleged victim is in order.

27. How do I protect myself against accusations of sexual harassment?

Assuming that you will not blatantly be harassing anyone, your best protection is in recognizing the diversity among the workforce. Sexual jokes, innuendoes, and touching can be interpreted in many different ways. Set a climate in your department in which verbal or physical conduct that could be considered sexual in nature is not accepted. Most certainly you will want to avoid any behavior that could be misinterpreted yourself.

28. Can I copyright a brochure I developed for my job?

As soon as a work is created, it has federal copyright protection. The public copyright notice consists of the word Copyright (or the abbreviation COPR) and © (the Universal Copyright convention symbol), followed by the name of the copyright owner and the year of first publication (e.g., Copyright © Stein 2001). This is differentiated from a trademark symbol ™, which is used to distinguish manufacturers' products and provide quality assurance. The symbol ® means that a trademark is federally registered. A trademark for services is usually indicated by SM (service mark).

Something you produce as part of your job responsibilities, assignments, or while at work is most likely classified as a "work made for hire." In these cases, the employer is considered the corporate copyright owner. Review your employer's policies regarding intellectual property for specific guidelines. However, many employers will give permission for you to use or display your creation in other settings. In addition, you can publish an article describing the created item, which then attributes it to you.

29. Why is that every time I ask our hospital's legal department a question, they always seem to be vague initially?

Most everyone has heard the joke that the lawyer learns to answer every question with "it depends." While it is humorous, there is some element of necessity there. Many legal issues of concern to nurse managers arise from federal regulations and rulings, thus providing the ability to answer some broad legal questions. But state and even local laws vary, so when a legal question arises, it is always best to consult your hospital attorney, who may need to research regional interpretations and applications.

BIBLIOGRAPHY

1. Bogart JB, et al (eds): Legal Nurse Consulting: Principles and Practice. New York, CRC Press, 1998, pp 70–72, 350–355.
2. Burns J, Reardon FE, Truog ED: Using newly deceased patients to teach resuscitation procedures. N Engl J Med 332:1446–1447, 1995.
3. Davis JH: Managers Ask and Answer: Copyright. J Emerg Nurs 24(3):273–274, 1998.
4. Emergency Nurses Association: Position Statement: The Use of the Newly Deceased Patient for Procedural Practice. Available at http://www.ena.org/services/posistate/2000/NewlyDeceased.htm (accessed September 2000).
5. EEOC: Facts about Sexual Harassment. Available at http://www.eeoc.gov/facts/fs-sex.html (accessed January 15, 1997).
6. Furrow BR, et al: Health Law, 2nd ed. St. Paul, MN, West Publishing, 1991, pp 321–323.
7. Miller GL: Frequently Asked Questions about the Emergency Medical Treatment and Active Labor Act (EMTALA). Available at http://www.emtala.com/ (accessed July 1, 2000).
8. National Council of State Boards of Nursing: Delegation: Concepts and Decision-Making Process: National Council Position Paper. Available at http://www.ncsbn.org/files/publications/positions/delegati.asp#references (accessed 1995).
9. Patton MJ: The standards for disclosure of risk in informed consent. J Legal Nurse Consult 11:(1):17–19, 2000.
10. Southwick AF, Slee DA: The Law of Hospital and Health Care Administration. Ann Arbor, MI, Health Administration Press, 1988, pp 350–353.
11. Whetter K: The Nuts and Bolts of Legal Nurse Consulting. Carlsbad, CA, Medical Legal Resources, 1994, pp 116–120.

32. REGULATORY ISSUES

Kathleen M. Ferriell, RN, MSN

In any organization, there are ropes to skip and ropes to know.

R. Ritti and G. Funkhouser

1. What is the JCAHO?

The Joint Commission on Accreditation of Healthcare Organizations (JCAHO) is an independent, non-profit organization that monitors compliance with mandatory standards regarding quality patient care. Health care organizations request and pay for the JCAHO review to credential that their organizations and facilities are meeting their national standards. The JCAHO reviews organizations at least on a scheduled triennial basis (laboratories are reviewed every 2 years) and may also review organizations unannounced.

Information, standards, and compliance measures are published in manuals available from the JCAHO or through the web site at *http://www.jcaho.org.*

You can also directly contact JCAHO with your specific questions. However, it can take up to several months for a response. (See also the chapter on quality management.)

2. Do you have suggestions on how to get ready for a JCAHO survey?

The best way to prepare is to always be ready with ongoing compliance. For a scheduled survey visit, remember that you eat an elephant one bite at a time. Break up the preparation for a scheduled JCAHO survey into "bites" as well. Some specific suggestions follow:
- Read the information provided, especially the JCAHO newsletter, in which hot topics are generally highlighted.
- Network with peers at other hospitals that were recently surveyed. The same hot topics are generally reviewed in each facility.
- Start *early* because there will be many last-minute problems that will be of higher priority than *your* last-minute problem.
- Verify that you have proper policies and procedures for each standard and data readily accessible to demonstrate your compliance.
- Review educational topics with staff, such as where the fire extinguisher is located, how to handle cultural diversity, and the hospital's mission. Surveyors will talk with staff to determine whether your facility "walks the talk."
- Develop checklists for each area or room to ensure that standards are maintained based on the specific function of and supplies in that area.

3. Describe what you mean by a "hot topic."

Within any year, there is a repetitive focus at most reviewed institutions on some universal topics. These are often based on sentinel events or publicized trends, such as pain relief. For example, a current hot topic emphasis is patient restraint. All areas using restraints or seclusion must meet the same requirements for documentation of need, consideration of alternatives, staff education, verification of competency, proper application, documentation of ongoing safe maintenance, and patient and family information. Other predicted areas of emphasis in the future include medication errors and staff competency (owing to the December 1999 Institute of Medicine [IOM] report of a possible 98,000 health care deaths per year from errors), staffing levels (owing to the nursing shortage and the large percent of sentinel events with a relationship to staffing), and disaster (bioterrorism) preparedness.

4. How will the surveyor determine compliance with a hot topic?

Commonly used approaches include randomly questioning staff ("Tell me how you would verify a patient's identity before administering a unit of blood"), reviewing random charts of clients who had this procedure, verifying documentation of staff education on the topic, or examining meeting minutes for inclusion of the topic. They may ask to review your incident reports for the past 3 months or your staffing schedule for a particular day. In addition, some surveyors chose to speak directly to current patients ("What did your nurse say to you about pain?"). One surveyor even asked the housekeeper, "What is your role in patient care?"

5. What is a "sentinel event"?

A sentinel event is defined as "an unexpected occurrence involving death or serious physical or physiological injury, or the risk thereof." Serious injury specifically includes the loss of limb or function. The phrase "or the risk thereof" includes any process variation for which a recurrence would carry a significant chance of a serious adverse outcome.

For an event to be classified as "sentinel," it must result in unanticipated death or major permanent loss of function and not be related to the natural course of the patient's illness. Examples include in-patient suicides, transfusion-related deaths, infant abductions, or surgery at the wrong site.

The JCAHO maintains a list of the top sentinel events. In 2000, the number one cause of sentinel events was the lack of or inadequate orientation, training, and education. If your hospital had a sentinel event, the JCAHO surveyor will want to see evidence of follow-up pursued to the point of identifying and rectifying the contributing factors and cause.

6. Describe how you use checklists for your preparation.

List essential aspects for each physical area. An out-patient examination area checklist might include the following:

- No unsecured medication is in the room.
- No prescription blanks are in the room.
- Needle boxes are present, correctly mounted, and less than half full.
- Equipment is clean and in working order and is checked according to procedure.
- No loose tape, papers, and so on are on the cart, floor, or counters.
- Staff is able to demonstrate safe use of the equipment.

The list would change for different locations so that one department may have eight to 10 different area checklists (e.g., nurses station, medication area, kitchen, treatment room). Many managers then assign responsibility for each list to a different staff member.

7. How do you prepare for the day of the visit?

Common advice includes the following:

- *Keep the day free from other commitments.* You must be available to respond when a surveyor asks for any documentation. For instance, every nursing department's continuing education record for the manager and its three most senior employees may be requested.
- *Stay close to the department.* The surveyor typically examines throughout the hospital, with stops at random departments. You should accompany the surveyor while in your department, prepared to answer department-specific questions. For instance, one surveyor asked the emergency department (ED) to explain their patient log and policy for handling drug samples.
- *Treat the surveyor with respect; rectify any problems immediately.* While in the department, deficiencies may be noted (e.g., alcohol wipe or linen on the floor) by you or the surveyor. Experienced managers relate that the best response is to just calmly take care of it right then. Never argue or become defensive.
- *Schedule your most experienced staff that day.* This is not the time to orient new employees or have a nervous new graduate stammering out an answer. One department was cited when the newer ED nurse shared with the surveyor that she still didn't feel comfortable.

• *Schedule extra staff.* Just because JCAHO is in the building doesn't keep "disasters" away, such as two cardiac arrests at the same time. You, and others, will not be as readily available to help out as you might at other times. You want to avoid having the appearance that your staff is frantically scrambling when the surveyor walks through.

8. Will I always know when a surveyor is arriving?

No. There is the "tip" that they typically come Tuesday through Thursday, during the day, to allow travel time for the surveyors during the business week. But there can be unannounced visits or visits at any hour. EDs also report that surveyors have reported to the ED triage area stating they have chest pain, and then noting how they were initially treated as a "patient" (stopping the staff before actual treatment was given).

9. What is ORYX?

ORYX is the name of the Joint Commission's initiative to integrate performance measures into the accreditation process. The ORYX initiative is a data-driven, continuous survey and accreditation process that complements JCAHO's standards-based assessment. JCAHO states that the use of outcomes-related data in accreditation activities serves as a greater stimulus for health care organizations to examine their processes of care and take action to improve the results of care.

Hospital, long-term care, network, laboratory, home care, and behavioral health care accreditation programs currently have performance measurement requirements under the ORYX initiative. Six clinical measures are chosen from a predetermined list of relevant measures, for which data is collected and reported on through their quality improvement processes. Failure to comply will result in a Type 1 recommendation.

10. What is a core measure set?

A core measure set is a unique grouping of performance measures that are selected because the grouping illustrates the care provided in a given area. JCAHO's plans call for identifying sets of core performance measures for each accreditation program in a staggered approach. Surveyors will then assess the health care organization's use of these in their performance improvement activities during the JCAHO on-site review process.

For hospitals, the four initial core measurement areas are acute myocardial infarction, heart failure, community-acquired pneumonia, and pregnancy and related conditions. Hospitals will begin collecting core measurement data for patient discharges beginning July 1, 2002. For more information, check the JCAHO's web site address *www.jcaho.org* (select "For Health Care Organizations and Professionals," and then ORYX).

11. What happens if your facility fails a JCAHO survey?

If the surveyors judge that you have failed to meet some standards, the hospital can choose to refute or appeal findings or to develop action plans to come into compliance. However, a JCAHO failure sends up a red flag to the other regulatory agencies, such as HCFA/CMMS and OSHA, and may trigger reviews by those agencies. JCAHO standards are generally mirrored in their standards.

"Type 1 Recommendation" is the most serious infraction, and multiple standards must be judged as such before your entire organization will be at risk for failure to meet accreditation. Losing accreditation doesn't happen after one survey, but only after failing to rectify deficiencies. But losing JCAHO accreditation does mean a potential loss of Medicare/Medicaid or other reimbursements.

12. Is JCAHO the only option?

Some states, such as New Hampshire, determine the requirements for accreditation and allow a choice between HCFA or JCAHO. Check with your state hospital association.

13. What is OSHA?

The Occupational Safety and Health Administration (OSHA) is a federal agency charged with the responsibility of providing workers safety from occupational injuries and illnesses. Workers may file complaints with OSHA if they feel their workplace is in violation of any safety standards.

Areas where OSHA currently focuses that affect health care organizations include sharps safety, blood/body fluid exposure, workplace violence, tuberculosis exposure, radiation exposure, and ergonomics. There are two arms of OSHA; one arm is for regulation and compliance and the other for training and consultation.

14. How do OSHA's requirements compare to all the other agencies' regulations and requirements?

Most of OSHA's requirements are mirrored in the JCAHO standards (see table below). If you are in compliance with JCAHO, you are likely in compliance with OSHA. OSHA is more specific regarding some issues, such as decontamination services, construction, and ergonomics. You must comply with the strictest interpretation of the standard anytime agencies differ.

OSHA Topics Compared with Joint Commission Standards

OSHA TOPICS	JOINT COMMISSION STANDARDS
Voluntary Protection Program (VPP)	EC1.1 and EC2.1: Safety Management HR.1, HR.3 and HR.4, EC2.8 PL1, PL2, PL3, PL3.3, PL4, and PL5
Ventilation	EC1.1, EC1.3, EC1.5, EC1.6, EC1.7, EC2.1, EC2.3, EC2.5, EC2.6, EC2.10.1, EC2.10.2, EC2.10.3, EC2.10.4, EC3.2.1, and EC2.7: Utilities Management
Information Management	EC4 IM Chapter HR4, HR4.2, HR4.3, and HR5 PL1, PL:2, PL3, PL3.3, PL4, and PL5
Patient Handling, Lifting, and Moving	PL3.32: Risk Management Data in Improving Organization Performance chapter
Safety and Health Programs	EC1.1, EC1.1.1, and EC2.1: Safety Management EC4.1–EC4.3
Workplace Violence	EC1.2 and EC2.8: Security
Laboratory and Hazcom	EC1.3 and EC2.8: Hazardous Materials and Waste
BBP, TB, and Legionella	IC1
ETO, H₂CO, and Glutaraldehyde	EC1.3, EC1.6, EC1.7 EC2.3, EC2.6, EC2.7, EC2.10.3, EC2.10.4
OSHA Record Keeping	IC3, EC1.1.1, EC1.3, EC1.7, EC2.3, EC2.7, EC2.10.4
Hazardous Drugs, Reproductive Hazards, and Anesthetic Gases	EC1.3, EC1.6, EC2.3, EC2.6, EC2.10.3 HR5
Walking and Working Surfaces	EC4, EC4.1, EC4.2
Fire Safety	EC1.5, EC2.8, EC2.9.1
Electrical Safety	EC1.7, EC2.8
Safety and Health Statistics MSDS and OSHA 200 Log	LD2.3 and LD2.7 EC2.3 and EC2.4

Table continued on following page

OSHA Topics Compared with Joint Commission Standards (Continued)

OSHA TOPICS	JOINT COMMISSION STANDARDS
Education/Professional Qualifications of Parties Responsible for the Safety and Health Program	LD2.8 EC2.8 HR4 and HR4.2

Note: All standards are from the Joint Commission's Comprehensive Accreditation Manual for Hospitals. Those labeled EC are from the Environment of Care chapter; IM refers to the Management of Information chapter; PI refers to the Improving Organization Performance chapter; those labeled IC are from the Surveillance, Prevention and Control of Infection chapter. HR = human resources, LD = leadership. Reprinted from the Joint Commission's 1997 Environment of Care Series, Issue 3, "OSHA and Environment of Care Compatibilities." For further information about this publication, please call Joint Commission customer service at 630/792-5800 and ask for publication Order Code PTSM-845.

15. Does OSHA schedule their inspections in advance?

Usually OSHA will not have notified you in advance about the visit, and by law no advance notice is required. But an inspection must be conducted "during regular working hours." However, a hospital's regular working hours could mean 3:00 AM.

Generally OSHA visits the workplace because of an accident, report of a catastrophe or fatality, or an employee complaint. An inspection can occur even if you believe there is no legitimacy to the complaint. OSHA inspected one company after an employee complained that another middle-aged male employee died from a heart attack while on the job. An inspection may also be a programmed inspection or the result of a concern of an "imminent danger."

16. What do I do if an OSHA inspector suddenly appears at my door?

- *Verify the inspector's credentials.* The inspector must present you with his or her identification. If there is doubt, call the area office to confirm identity.
- *Have an administrative representative accompany him or her on the inspection.*
- *Ask to see the inspection warrant, which will identify the scope of this inspection.* Although it is technically within your rights to refuse entry to an OSHA inspector without a warrant, it may not be in your facility's best interest to do so.
- *Continue status quo compliance with routine safety procedures.* If you observe any breaks in safety policies or procedures while you are with the inspector, immediately address them.

17. What will the OSHA inspector want to see?

Required documents and logs regarding areas of safety are usually reviewed. These can include material safety data sheets (MSDS), employee injury logs, safety inspections, and safety committee minutes. The work area will also probably be viewed for safety concerns. For more information, access the OSHA web site at *http://www.osha.gov/*.

18. What would it mean to my facility if we were cited for any OSHA violations?

It would mean that your facility would likely be fined or have criminal investigations initiated, or both, depending on the safety violation. The cost of fines can be significant for *each* described violation. The costs in community image, public relations, and worker morale could be of even greater significance. In addition, other agencies, such as JCAHO, could decide that these findings warrant their organization's own inspection.

19. What is NIOSH? How is it related to OSHA standards?

The National Institute for Occupational Safety and Health (NIOSH) is a federal agency of the Department of Health and Human Services (HHS). NIOSH's mission is to conduct research and make recommendations for improving safety and health in the occupational environment.

NIOSH can conduct workplace investigations and require that employers measure and report employee exposure to potentially hazardous materials. They may also require employers to provide medical examinations and tests to determine the incidence of occupational illness among employees. NIOSH may pay for these examinations if they are required for its research purposes.

NIOSH provides technical assistance to OSHA and makes recommendations to OSHA. Although these recommendations carry some weight, they are not binding, and NIOSH does not impose fines. However, OSHA may develop these recommendations into standards that can then have fines associated with them.

20. What role does HCFA/CMMS have in the regulation of health care facilities?

The Health Care Financing Administration (HCFA) administers Medicare, Medicaid, and the State Children's Health Insurance Program (SCHIP) for the federal government. It also performs quality-focused activities such as the regulation of laboratory testing (CLIA), review and certification of health care facilities (nursing homes, hospitals, intermediate care facilities for the mentally retarded, home health agencies), and development of coverage policies. In the summer of 2001, the organization's name became Centers for Medicare and Medicaid Services (CMMS) without any substantive organizational changes.

The agency has been in the spotlight lately because of hospital billing fraud and coding allegations. Managers and hospital billing departments must be aware of and comply with coding and coverage changes for the federally funded programs under HCFA/CMMS, such as APC (Ambulatory Payment Classifications).

21. How do the FDA and the Safe Medical Devices Act relate to hospitals?

Facilities that use drugs or medical devices (such as an infusion pump) are subject to Food and Drug Administration (FDA) inspection under the Safe Medical Devices Act of 1990. All patient incidents involving medical devices or drugs *must* be reported to the FDA. The two primary reasons that a hospital FDA visit occurs are to investigate a specific device-related problem and to conduct on-site audits for compliance with the user reporting requirements.

22. How do I report unsafe medical devices?

You must complete the FDA form and submit it to your FDA liaison. This person, designated by your facility, is usually the chief pharmacist or the risk manager. You also need to ensure that your report is filed through your regular occurrence/incident reporting system.

23. What will a FDA inspector want to view?

The inspection may include the reviewing and copying of records, including patient medical records. However, even though the FDA *must* have access to some records, any records provided the FDA could ultimately be available to the public through the Freedom of Information Act. Therefore, check with your legal counsel or medical records department for your hospital's procedure to handle any FDA requests for records.

24. Describe HEDIS.

The Health Plan Employer Data and Information Set (HEDIS) was developed by the National Committee for Quality Assurance and suggests performance indicators that can be used to assess the quality of managed care organizations. Organizations volunteer to participate and receive a "report card" from the more than 60 performance indicators.

25. Tell me about DOT urine collection for drug testing.

The procedure for the Department of Transportation (DOT) drug urine test collection must adhere to the new regulations that went into effect on August 1, 2001. There are now stricter requirements regarding collector training. For more information, contact *www. datia.org* or *www.drugtestingnews.com*.

Experts recommend always using an outside vendor or a select group of hospital personnel (such as designated laboratory staff) to do the procedures. This will help ensure a valid collection process that will stand up against legal challenges.

Private employers will sometimes contract with health care facilities to provide a urine drug testing service for their employees. Private employers are not subject to the same strict DOT drug testing regulations. However, most collectors use the same DOT collection procedures because they have proven to be the gold standard of the industry.

26. Is there one organization that will cover all the standards my organization is required to meet?

No. Although most of the national requirements are mirrored in the local and state requirements, your state standards may require more stringent criteria in some areas. Check with your state hospital association.

27. How can I know what my community, state, and national standards are?

Keep abreast of local developments through reading and checking with your hospital's legal counsel or risk manager. Network with peers in neighboring facilities to learn more about the community's applications of standards. In addition, your professional association can provide information.

BIBLIOGRAPHY

1. Briggs CW: How to Handle an OSHA Inspection. Shelton, CT, OSHA/Health Care, WEKA Publishing, 1996, pp 1–22.
2. ECRI: Responding to FDA inspections. Healthcare Risk Control 2(1):1–8, 1996.
3. Perry J: Legislating sharps safety. Nurs Manage 31:27–28, 2000.
4. Vogler S: Managers Forum: Feasibility of an ED DOT drug program. J Emerg Nurs 2001 [in press].

33. QUALITY MANAGEMENT AND PROCESS IMPROVEMENT

Steven A. Weinman, RN, BSN, CEN

Remember always that the recollection of quality remains long after the price is forgotten.

H. George Selfridge

1. What is quality management?

"Quality management, quality assurance, continuous quality improvement, total quality management...." Although the latest term changes, one word remains consistent: *quality*.

Quality is a characteristic that defines the value of a service or product. Although it is often perceived differently, quality can be defined and measured. Health care organizations place a great deal of emphasis on the ability to measure and compare quality. Even more important is that the patient demands better service and optimal clinical outcomes. These factors are among the leading driving forces behind the need to monitor clinical practice and effect changes when necessary. The Joint Commission on Accreditation of Healthcare Organizations (JCAHO) has embraced the principles of quality management as a major tool to be used by hospitals in their performance improvement efforts.

2. Why is quality management important?

Today's hospital environment is characterized by rapid patient turnover, decreased length of stay, expanded outpatient services, increased levels of severity, acuity, and nursing intensity, and an aging patient population with multiple needs.[6] Nurses are increasingly being judged, not just on individual knowledge and institutional capabilities for treating the ill and injured, but also on the ability to actively improve the quality of care and reduce errors with a decreasing number of resources.

As nurses, we cannot be content with providing patients with good care based on established standards. Quality management challenges us to continually evaluate our practice and seek opportunities to improve it.

3. What is the origin of quality management?

Quality management arose out of the careful and disciplined study of traditional management approaches by a group of innovative thinkers, including W. Edwards Deming, Joseph Juran, and Philip Crosby. Core to the values they believed was that the leadership of an organization must be committed to improvement; the top management must "walk the talk."

4. Is there a role for nursing in quality improvement?

Since the time of Florence Nightingale, nurses have been at the forefront of evaluating the quality of patient care. Florence set standards for patient care and gathered data to support her observations. The first nursing audit was developed in 1957 at Thayer Hospital in Maine. In 1967, evaluation of care was defined as one of the four functions of the nursing process.[9]

Nurses really began to take an active role in quality management activities in the 1970s. Nurses became pivotal in the creation and utilization of standardized methods to review the quality and effectiveness of nursing care. The American Nurses Association (ANA) first published *Standards for Nursing Practice* in 1973. Nursing specialty organizations soon followed suit, creating standards for specialty nurses that paralleled those of the ANA. Nurses are indeed essential to the process of quality management. For an example, see the chapter on one hospital's experience with care management.

5. What are the major components of quality management?

Traditionally, major components of a quality management system include standards that described quality, a system for collecting information about the degree of achievement of standards, and a system for acting to bring performance in line with those standards. From an operational standpoint, each department or service is assigned the responsibility for overseeing, monitoring, and evaluating its own performance.

6. What are the five key concepts of quality management?

Five key concepts that have been identified are (1) focus on the customer, (2) focus on the process, (3) use an analytical or scientific approach, (4) understand and reduce variation in processes, and (5) involve your staff.[4]

7. Tell me more about the first concept, focus on the customer.

To provide a quality service or product line, you must first identify the customer. The customer is that person who will benefit and receive the services you provide. In health care, the customers are not only the patients but also their significant others, the community, other hospitals or health care organizations, payers, physicians, and/or other departments within the hospital.

Customers are subdivided as internal or external. An internal customer is someone within the organization who uses your services. For example, the intensive care unit is an internal customer of the pharmacy. External customers are people using the services of a department who are not part of the organization. For example, the third-party payer is an external customer of the intensive care unit.

Having a customer focus means meeting or exceeding the customer's expectations for quality in the services you provide. To provide focus on the customer's needs, wants, and expectations, we need to first ask our customers to define their expectations. Once known, there is a need to collate these expectations and determine where to focus quality management initiatives.

8. Describe what is meant by the second concept, focus on the process.

Each process involves a series of steps or activities designed to achieve a specific outcome or goal. Every activity that nurses perform is part of a process. The process most familiar to clinical nurses is the nursing process.

Quality management focuses on improving processes. Quality is determined by what happens at every step, how the steps interact, and the process's design. Although an individual's skill and judgment may occasionally compromise quality, the majority of deviations are related to process problems. For example, a seasoned nurse may pick up on the signs of hyperkalemia, but the outcome would be affected if the laboratory is too slow in processing the blood specimen for a stat potassium level.

9. What is the difference between processes and systems?

A system is composed of many interrelated processes. Examples of hospital-based systems include registration, laboratory, and dietary. Each of these systems has many interrelated processes that contribute to the overall success of the system. Often, quality improvement efforts fail because the team will try to improve a system rather than a single process.

10. Tell me more about what you mean by the third concept, use of an analytical or scientific approach.

To effectively improve on a process problem, an analytical or scientific approach works best. This typically involves collecting data, reviewing the data, developing improvement actions based on the results of the review, and testing the developed actions.

An analytical or scientific approach means that the final plan for process improvement is not based on anecdotal information, feelings, or hunches. This allows for an informed, permanent solution rather than a "quick fix" or a "band-aid" for the problem. W. Edwards Deming's model titled Plan-Do-Check-Act Cycle (Walton ,1988) is a sample of a straight-forward problem-solving model.

11. List the steps of the Deming's Plan-Do-Check-Act Cycle.

The model is composed of four steps.

1. *Plan* change by studying a process, deciding what could improve it, and identifying data to help.

2. *Do* test the proposed change by implementing data simulation or a small-scale trial.

3. *Check* the effects by studying the results, modifying the planned change if necessary.

4. *Act* to improve the process by implementing change.

12. Describe the fourth concept, understand and reduce variation in processes.

Variation exists in all processes. To make the outcome of processes as predictable and consistent as possible, you must understand the sources of variation and reduce its effect on the process.

There are two types of variation. The first is special cause variation, which is variance from unpredictable causes (such as power failure). The second type of variation is common cause variation, which is variation that can be anticipated because of its inherent frequency. The goal is to minimize common cause variation.

Another method to minimize variation in a process is to limit the steps in that process. The more steps, the greater the chance for variation.

13. How do you accomplish the fifth concept, involve your staff?

No single person knows everything there is to know about all facets of a process. Involvement of all knowledgeable persons is the most effective method of process redesign. Involvement creates ownership and a desire to see the efforts succeed.

14. How do I go about choosing a quality improvement project?

Quality improvement projects should be well defined and involve a process (rather than a system). Initial common areas to review for potential quality improvement projects are compliance with regulatory guidelines, such as adherence to standard precautions, daily crash cart checks, or frequency of vital sign documentation during conscious sedation procedures.

15. What types of patient populations should be included in quality improvement initiatives?

Patient populations that need to be monitored as part of any quality improvement program include the following;

- Low-volume (i.e., infrequently performed procedure, such as postoperative lung transplant patient)
- High-risk (i.e., likely to have ominous consequences if anything goes wrong, such as a blood transfusion patient)
- Problem-prone (i.e., historically known to have a higher incidence of complications or irregularities, such as multiple procedures or intoxicated patients)

16. What is benchmarking?

Benchmarking, first conceptualized by Robert Camp at Xerox Corporation, is formally defined as "the continuous process of measuring products, services, and practices against a company's toughest competitors or those companies renowned as industry leaders."[1] A more practical definition for healthcare is "the search for an implementation of best practices."[7] Traditionally, managers have relied on data and trends collected internally to judge their quality. Benchmarking allows the establishment of practices based not only on internal data but also on the data of other institutions. It guides the setting of direction and goals for a department or organization.

17. Describe the types of benchmarking.

There are four type of benchmarking[2]:

1. *Internal:* Reviews basic similar internal functions that can serve as the baseline to begin to understand processes. For example, laboratory turn-around time is compared for the ED, ICU, and Med/Surg areas.

2. *Competitive:* Compares a work process with that of the best competitor in the industry. For example, the average drug-to-door time for thrombolytic administration is compared between your hospital's and the fastest in the country.

3. *Functional:* Compare a work process to that of a functional leader, often in a different industry. For example, the hospital comparing computerized physician order entry with the order entry process used in a restaurant or catalog company.

4. *Generic process:* Similar to functional; compare a key business process with a similar application in another business. For example, hospital bed assignment process is compared with the hotel industry occupancy reservation process.

18. How have health care organizations found their benchmarking data?

Health care managers cite three major sources:

• Comparing with local facilities of a similar size and patient population in the same geographic region.

• Performing a literature search.

• Using resources available from the facility and/or professional associations. Some examples are the American Heart Association, the Volunteer Hospital Association, the Institute for Health Care Improvement and the Health Care Advisory Board.

19. Tell me about other health care managers' experience with benchmarking.

Overall, most managers agree that benchmarking is useful when used as one, not the only, yardstick for making decisions. On the positive side, managers report that benchmarking has supported needed, realistic improvements, highlighted innovative ideas, and initiated collaborative networks. It worked best when limited to a specific area, such as thrombolytic drug administration time, rather than a general topic, such as improving customer satisfaction. And sometimes a perceived deficiency was actually found to be acceptable.

On the negative side, mangers report that it is not so helpful when applied to an area with high variation, such as staffing levels in an emergency department with seasonal fluctuations, or when there is no commitment from senior administration. Also, discretion is necessary in communicating the concept to staff. Announcing that the unit is "0.2 hours over the national length of stay" only frustrates staff, especially if they do not know how to control the discharge time.

20. I have heard that "retroactive chart audits" should not be used for quality improvement activities. Is this true?

The majority of quality improvement activities are based on a retrospective review of care provided. Critics have argued that retrospective audits measure only the "quality" of documentations and have questioned the relationship between the quality of documentation and the quality of care. To date, no evidence has been provided that support these claims.

Some departments have attempted to have staff perform prospective quality studies. These prospective studies have met with the criticism that they force the clinician to focus on the study. thus delaying patient care; that they are not completed as nurses try to balance their already limited time,;or that a Hawthorne effect will skew data collection.

Either way, the concept is to continually try to improve quality. It is never enough to simply record and note the findings without appropriate action.

21. How does quality improvement relate to patient satisfaction?

Assurance of quality standards is associated with customer satisfaction. Many quality improvement projects focus on customer service in that they emphasize the best ways to meet costumer needs. Consumer health care expectations have been influenced by growing pubic access to information, the media, rising costs, diminished resources, increasing technologic complexity, and ethical dilemmas. Customer dissatisfaction is not always an indicator of poor quality of care but it does reflect a failure in the system to meet consumer expectations and needs.

22. How can I increase my staff's compliance with carrying out unit-based quality improvement initiatives?

Staff compliance is a common problem. A key point is to convert staff to understanding its importance. Some approaches include the following:

- Have involvement in quality improvement as a component of the performance evaluation.
- Hold each staff member accountable for a certain monthly quality improvement activities.
- Parallel quality improvement data collection to other activities that are being monitored; use self-audits.
- Create (and reward) staff experts in this area.

23. Is forming a project team for quality the best approach?

It depends. Teams are rarely the most efficient or fastest way to achieve a goal, but they can provide staff buy-in.

If you are using teams, carefully design and establish the initial team. If the foundation is not correct, efforts to coach the team will be ineffective. Often a first order of business can be suggestions, with a group vote, on acceptable ground rules. You want a group that holds one another accountable rather than viewing themselves as individuals who are accountable only to the boss.

It is important to give the team a "good" goal. Using numbers alone is rarely motivating, even big ones such as "reduce medication errors by 50%." Avoid vague generalities, such as "improve patient care." The goal should have measurable results, make small wins possible along the way, and challenge the team to make a difference. Examples of a good goal might be to achieve 100% staff education on the new pain protocol with at least a 10% improvement in patient pain documentation in the next quarter, create a systematic process to improve inpatient education about diabetes, or develop and implement a community program for wearing bicycle helmets for injury prevention.

24. Are patient outcomes enhanced by a solid quality improvement program?

Yes. The aim of health care is to assist the patient in achieving the best possible health outcome in the most efficient manner. Outcomes are the effects that timely and accurate care has on the ability of the patient to make a maximal recovery. Negative outcomes include increased mortality, morbidity, readmission needs, complaints, and cost over-runs. Positive outcomes include physical, emotional, and psychosocial well-being; improved functional state; and overall satisfaction with health services provided. Many major consumers in the health care economy are choosing outcomes measurement as the best means of assessing the quality of health care they purchase.

25. Is the provision of continuing education beneficial in ensuring quality of care?

Maintaining the essential knowledge and skills is integral to the quality process. Deming dedicated two of his fourteen points of organizational transformation to increasing the knowledge base of a workforce. In nursing, standard continuing education is provided with clinical competence as the measurable outcome. The JCAHO requires that all staff, including temporary agency personnel, be given basic orientation and have verified competency.

26. Do critical pathways enhance quality of patient care?

The use of standardized, outcome-focused plans of care has taken the health care arena by storm. Clinical pathways (also called care maps or critical paths) have been shown to improve overall quality while decreasing resource utilization. Clinical pathways are interdisciplinary guidelines that serve to map the daily, appropriate actions for patients for many common patient diagnoses from admissions to discharge.

There are those who disagree with this approach. Critics call these pathways "cookbook medicine" and are fearful that deviation from these pathways will be used against them in legal proceedings. This untested belief has lad to a large number of institutions abandoning clinical pathways altogether.

27. What type of impact has the Joint Commission had on hospital quality improvement?

Possibly no organization has had a greater impact on quality management in health care than the JCAHO. Founded in 1951, it is a voluntary accreditation agency. Its primary mission is to improve the quality of care that health care organizations provide the public.

In the 50 years since its inception, JCAHO has continually evolved the processes by which it ensures that health care organizations provide optimal care. In 1995, JCAHO shifted its focus to patient-centered functions common to all organizations. The five patient-centered functions follow:
- Patient rights and organizational ethics
- Assessment of patients
- Care of patients
- Education
- Continuum of care

Nursing performance is evaluated within each of the functions. All aspects of care are expected to be multidisciplinary and intertwined between all of the functions. This is in contrast to previous JCAHO philosophy of evaluation based on clinical services or specialty areas (e.g., ICU, ED, OR). See also the chapter on regulatory agencies.

BIBLIOGRAPHY

1. Camp RC: Benchmarking: The Search for Industry Best Practices that Lead to Superior Performance. Milwaukee, WI, American Society for Quality Control, Quality Press, 1989.
2. Camp RC, Tweet AG: Benchmarking applied to healthcare. Jt Comm J Qual Improv 20:229–238, 1994.
3. Deming WE: Out of the Crisis, 2nd ed. Cambridge, MA, MIT Press, 2000.
4. Emergency Nurses Association: CQI: Building the Foundation. Des Plaines, IL, Emergency Nurses Association, 1994.
5. Fischetti M: Managers Forum: Making teams work. J Emerg Nurs 24(5):441, 1998.
6. Jones KR: Maintaining quality in a changing environment. Nurs Econ 9:159, 1991.
7. Mayer TA, Salluzzo R: Theory of continuous quality improvement. In Salluzzo R, Mayer TA, Strauss RW, et al (eds): Emergency Department Management. St. Louis, Mosby, 1997.
8. Walton M: Deming Management Method. New York, Dodd, Mead, and Co, 1988.
9. Yura H, Walsh MB: The Nursing Process: Assessing, Planning, Implementing, Evaluating, 5th ed. Norwalk, CT, Appleton & Lange, 1988.

34. CARE MANAGEMENT PROGRAM: ONE HOSPITAL'S SUCCESS

Karen Bry, RN, BA, and Susan Sim

The music has changed—so must the dance.

African proverb

1. Why was the Care Management Program developed?

The Care Management Program was developed in response to a focused review by a national consulting firm. Our institution was provided, at the close of the review, with large manuals outlining suggested process changes. The problem was that we did not believe the process fit our institution or would be helpful in solving any future problems. We did not reject the consultant's emphasis on data analysis, but were wary of their tendency to tie process design so tightly to external benchmarks.

Our goal in developing the Care Management Program at St. Anthony Hospital was to create a process that was grounded in data analysis and responsive to both internal and external benchmarks. But, it also needed to be practical and ultimately used as a standardized means of problem-solving hospital-wide.

2. Explain the difference between your Care Management Program and traditional quality assurance (QA), utilization review (UR), or performance improvement (PI) programs.

The Care Management Program was designed to integrate the core concepts of all three departments and programs. QA departments structure their process to monitor, maintain and enhance quality patient care. UR/case management focuses on appropriate resource utilization and cost containment and integrates quality standards to provide individualized plans of care. Performance improvement is a process whereby problems are evaluated using PI models of varying levels of complexity to guide the study process. The most widely used schema for performance improvement is probably Deming's PDCA:
- Plan: Plan the improvement
- Do: Collect the data
- Check: Analyze the data
- Act: Determine an action plan or re assess process

This process, like most performance improvement models, is designed to uncover problems and correct processes in a continuous manner.

3. What model was used for your Care Management Program?

We realized the interdependence of all three processes in the analysis and management of outcomes. Our plan was to pull all of these specialties under one umbrella, thereby integrating the fundamental concepts of each discipline. In doing, so we hoped not only to react to the latest crisis with a quick fix but also to identify the cause of a problem and develop a method of resolution that was systematic in nature and fit the culture of our institution.

The schematic of the St. Anthony Hospital Care Management Program model is as follows:
- Problem identification
- Delegate to a responsible party
- Data gathering
- Data analysis
- Standardized tool development

4. How do you identify the problem to focus on?

The source of the problems is often financial or quality-based. However, the problem can also be identified through internal or external benchmark variation, peer review organization findings, or simply problem patterns uncovered by observant employees.

5. Describe how you accomplish the second step, delegation to appropriate, responsible people.

It is critical that the right mix of people be involved in the data gathering/analysis and eventual resolution of the problem. It is important to formally assign the responsible party and schedule reporting on a timely basis. Executive levels of management should be involved when a problem is located in a specialty area.

6. How do you handle the third step, data gathering?

It is essential to have good, reliable data. Key sources include the following:

• Dependable financial data for utilization/cost analysis.
• Computerized information system for large volume of data to compare practice patterns to national benchmark averages.
• Internal quality indicators, such as pathway monitoring, for evaluating best practice compliance.
• Medical records retrospective chart review as a source of very detailed information that can be used in determining practice and utilization patterns.

Finally, an excellent source of data collection can be the very staff members who originally discovered the problem. Through concurrent chart review and data collection, our experience is that these employees can capture a surprisingly accurate real time picture of the identified problem.

7. Describe the fourth step, data analysis.

Statistical evidence must be sound and irrefutable to lay the foundation for future tools and change processes. Since data analysis is highly dependent upon the involved team's ability, we assign it to the members most expert in the problem area being evaluated. For example, length-of-stay data would be evaluated and interpreted by the utilization review staff while the quality assurance department analyzes best practice patterns and benchmarking.

Often the data analysis phase yields unexpected results. It is then the responsibility of the team to use their combined knowledge and experience to determine the real meaning of the data under study. Errors in the collection methods or statistical interpretation must be considered. We have had the data indicate, surprisingly, that the problem under study is less serious than originally thought and therefore requires no intervention.

8. Describe your final step, the standardized tool development.

The key to the Care Management Program success is the development of processes or tools that will resolve the problem in a systematic way. It must target the party or process responsible for the problem with a standardized solution.

Once the developed tool is in place, it serves to automatically guide the process away from former troubling patterns of practice and toward positive outcomes. It then becomes only a matter of intermittently verifying ongoing compliance.

9. How did you apply this process at your hospital?

Our early projects were resource utilization studies. Our goal was to determine the cost per case and determine length of stay (LOS) while monitoring quality of care and patient satisfaction. Later studies were designed to address other quality issues and other physician practice patterns.

We began by taking a hard look at a financial breakout that identified the hospital charges versus the actual hospital cost of each diagnosis-related group (DRG). We pursued why the costs of outlier DRGs were so expensive. The process involved extensive chart review, financial study of physician practice, and evaluation of hospital policy and procedures. The interesting aspect about this review was that each DRG outlier revealed a unique source for the cost overrun. The challenge became to track down a common denominator between the cases to help come up with a solution that fit the culture of our institution.

10. What determines whether a DRG is an "outlier"?

A DRG outlier status can be based on LOS or cost overrun issues. In either case, the determination of the outlier status is only the beginning of the evaluation process. Since most reimbursement is based solely on LOS, there is a great incentive for a hospital to meet that benchmark. However, it is not uncommon to have the DRG outlier fall out in both LOS and cost categories. This then requires analysis to evaluate and determine the patterns of practice that are contributing to the excessive LOS or cost overrun.

11. Can you illustrate an example of this type of outlier?

Our hospital encountered LOS and cost DRG outlier issues in both our pneumonia and sepsis patients. The typical population for both of these diagnostic categories is an older, sicker patient with multiple comorbidities. This clinical picture was supported in our chart review and utilization analysis. The problem was how to reign in high costs, knowing the treatment of these diseases in this population generally requires a long, expensive length of stay. Once again, it was impossible to just implement an industrial model and expect it to work, so we depended on our multidisciplinary team.

Utilization review examined the cause of the cost overrun. Analysis of each case by physician, length of stay, cost per case, and ancillary department usage was done for each patient with pneumonia and sepsis. The resulting data provided a means of comparing individual physician practice patterns to their peers and national benchmarks.

The most important link we were able to establish was that higher costs were directly related to pharmacy utilization and the overall length of stay. Although these findings are not especially profound, they were grounded in sound data and therefore formed the basis of our plan of action.

The study findings were presented to the physician staff in their monthly departmental Internal Medicine and Family Practice meetings. Actual peer comparisons were made available to the department chairman. The presentations explained the overall impact that each physician could make by containing length of stay and pharmacy charges on a case-by-case basis.

The pharmacy department then provided a brief summary of the most effective antibiotic coverage for treating sepsis and pneumonia. A physician formulary handout, along with an educational program, was developed by the pharmacy staff and presented at regular intervals to the residents and medical students in their orientations. Finally, the physicians were introduced to the on-site skilled nursing unit as an option for longer-term, lower-cost hospital stay.

Utilization review physicians now regularly review all pneumonia and sepsis admissions on day 5 of the hospitalization. They ensure that the antibiotic coverage and length of stay are within national best practice standards. This review helps identify problems early on and guides the attending physician in a realistic and timely discharge plan.

12. What do you mean when you say a solution must "fit the culture of your institution"?

We believe that although our problems are similar to those of other hospitals, our solutions have to be tailored specifically to our institution. For instance, our labor and delivery population LOS was high when compared to the national benchmark (which was less than 48 hours). We discovered that one of the reasons our length of stay was higher was because the pediatricians were reluctant to discharge the babies home any earlier. They were considering social issues related to poverty, parent education, and lack of community resources. Obviously, flow charts and process tools were of no value for this instance.

After consultation with the pediatric medical staff, it was decided that the best way to a solution in the short term was to be realistic and just allow the physicians to keep the patients hospitalized for those few extra hours beyond the national benchmark. The long-term solution became our current development of a outpatient newborn clinic. This clinic for infant follow-up provides a thorough newborn examination and addresses the social and educational needs of the family.

13. Is there any role for staff nurses in the resource utilization process?

The nurse's roles are many and instrumental in the early detection of problems. Often complaints are actually early indicators of process failure or system abuse.

This is well illustrated by the cost issues encountered in our in-patient psychiatric unit. The psychiatric case manager uncovered a pattern of overutilization with admission testing. Her observation revealed that psychiatrists automatically ordered "routine" admission laboratory tests regardless of the patient's need or history of having had the same test performed recently. It was a difficult issue to address because it involved changing the practice patterns for every psychiatrist on staff.

Our committee developed a set of preprinted admission orders that excluded the unnecessary or redundant testing. The nursing staff then implemented and monitored its use. With this simple design change, we were able to trim a projected $400.00 in charges per psychiatric patient admission. In this case, it was the nursing department that was in the best position to uncover the utilization issue and monitor the system to reverse the cost overruns.

It is important to note that we worked closely with the psychiatrists on this matter and never denied them the freedom to order any test they felt a patient might need. Our goal was to rid the routine admission orders independently of the patient's history or diagnosis.

Recent literature supports this key role of nursing involvement. Solberg found that, while physician opinion leaders are a useful vehicle for instituting change, the real instrument of behavioral change was delegating the new delivery system to the nursing staff.

14. Is there commonly such a close relationship between nursing and resource utilization?

There is frequently a close relationship between the two. The emergency department (ED) management of the appendectomy patient exemplifies how the nursing process is tied intricately to both the problems and the solutions of resource utilization.

The care management team identified appendectomy without complication as a cost outlier with the cost per case exceeding reimbursement by 38% annually. The challenge then became to define the specific reasons for the cost overruns. Through chart review, it was determined that our LOS was within the national benchmark average of 2.4 days. A regional comparison determined that our operating room charges were consistent with those of other area hospitals. Finally, a departmental charges breakdown revealed that ED ancillary testing was a major source of excessive utilization.

The question then became why this testing was done: for diagnostic or routine purposes? After a second chart review explored physician practice patterns, we found that much of the ED imaging and laboratory testing ordered was performed for preoperative purposes rather than the need to diagnose the appendicitis.

We met with the ED, anesthesia, and surgery department chairpersons. A consensus was reached that much of the routine ED preoperative testing, for this diagnosis, was unnecessary and should be eliminated, including the commonly ordered ultrasound exam. The elimination of routine preoperative type and screen, chest x-ray, PT/PTT, ECG for anyone under age 50, and ultrasonogram of the appendix represented a combined savings in charges of $624.00 per admission. We learned that having a discussion at the director level helped eliminate a lot of historical assumptions.

It is important to understand that the ordering patterns of the ED staff were done with good intentions. Usually the ED physician ordering the test, or the ED nurse automatically sending it, did so out of a desire to be thorough, to speed up the process, or to meet a presumed requirement.

15. Where there any "surprises" in your studies?

In-patient management of transient ischemic attack (TIA) was a major LOS outlier. A closer examination of the data revealed that an information systems error was responsible for adding days that contributed to the higher than average LOS. While we were grateful to have the aberrant LOS so easily explained, our chart review had uncovered some expensive physician management patterns.

The physician management pattern was costly because it involved a multisystem work-up. The diagnosis of TIA is really a diagnosis of exclusion. So the physicians would typically order cardiac, metabolic, and neurologic testing. Clearly, this comprehensive in-patient work-up reflected the physicians' concern for patient safety. The question became whether there was a way to reduce hospital costs yet still ensure a safe, comprehensive patient work-up. An extensive review of the literature provided assurance that it could be done.

The most common models present in the literature addressing the cost/utilization issue of TIA approached the problem by developing the work-up into distinct in-patient versus out-patient portions. The in-patient work-up involved a diagnostic screening for high-risk cardiac, metabolic, and neurologic disorders or events. When the events were ruled out, the patient was discharged and the low-risk screening was performed on an outpatient basis.

Our Medical Director and UR Director evaluated the model with input and approval from the Department of Neurology. All agreed that a systematic approach to TIA management would reduce in-patient testing while providing safe, quality care. A diagnostic algorithm was developed by the physicians, presented at departmental meetings, and then distributed to the general staff. The algorithm standardized the diagnostic approach and served as a guide to test sequencing.

16. What do you recommend for our hospital?

Our Care Management Program is an example of one hospital's success in resolving some internal issues of cost containment, resource utilization, and quality of care concerns. It became clear to us that a process was needed to define, examine, and resolve the problems.

We learned that this process must be simple, flexible, and grounded in data. The ultimate goal is to design a tool or device that would correct the problem in a standardized or systematic way. In each example, our process worked because it was practical and adaptable.

Another key to the success is team membership. Pull in senior management and physician directors into the process early on because they will be needed later to champion major system changes.

And don't fail to include all levels of employees. Some of our greatest successes sprang from observant nurses and diligent case managers.

BIBLIOGRAPHY

1. Brown RD Jr, et al: Transient ischemic attack and minor ischemic stroke: An algorithm for evaluation and treatment. Mayo Clinic Proc 69:1027–1028, 1994.
2. Deming WE: Out of the Crisis. Cambridge, MA, Massachusetts Institute of Technology, Center for Advanced Engineering Study, 1986.
3. Solberg LI: Guideline implementation: What the literature doesn't tell us. J Qual Improve 26(9):525–535, 2000.

35. ETHICS

Bernard Heilicser, DO, MS, FACEP

There is only one duty, only one safe course, and that is to try to be right.

Sir Winston Churchill

1. Why is nursing ethics more important now than ever before?

Nursing ethics has become an everyday issue in your professional and personal lives. You are called upon to be involved in decisions that require tremendous responsibility and wisdom in the care of patients, and in relationships with other health care professionals. It cannot be escaped. Ethical dilemmas are consistently presented in the media, and are ever-present in your practice. It is essential that you be aware of these dilemmas not only to help your patients but also to maintain your own professional and personal well-being.

2. What are these ethical dilemmas?

Nurses are the ones who really know their patients. They are, or should be, involved in discussions dealing with end-of-life decisions, informed consent and refusal, treatment futility, honest disclosure and truth telling, and allocation of resources. Being aware that a dilemma exists in the first place is even more important.

3. How do I know an ethical dilemma is present?

Basically, if the patient or family and health care team disagree or are in conflict, an ethical dilemma may be present. This can be related to aggressive treatment versus hospice care, what is perceived to be in the patient's best interest, withholding or withdrawal of life support, honest flow of information, and actual patient triage. However, if everyone is in agreement, this does not preclude the presence of an ethical dilemma. You must still answer: Is it moral?

4. What should nursing ethics do?

Nursing ethics should improve patient care. It should identify, analyze, and resolve ethical dilemmas. This is accomplished by the use of certain principles and by incorporating the patient's wishes, preferences, and values into the decision-making process. This mechanism will also help the entire health profession.

5. Name the four principles used in ethical analysis.

Autonomy, beneficence, nonmaleficence, and justice. These four principles help us to identify an ethical dilemma (when principles collide), analyze the dilemma (who has standing or rights in the situation), and resolve the dilemma (hopefully, an intelligent, reasoned and wise decision).

6. What is patient autonomy?

In a democracy, people have a right to "self-rule." The concept of autonomy has consistently been upheld by the courts. We must realize this and work with it (however frustrating it may be). Patients have rights. These rights, however, are predicated on the patient having decision-making capacity, competence as legally determined, noninterference with the rights of others and no intent to deliberately injure themselves or others.

Patient autonomy also involves the concepts of advance directives and informed consent. Patients should be free to make the medical decisions that involve their bodies. We can and should educate them and guide them but not coerce them in these decisions. Would we demand anything less if we were the patient?

7. Describe beneficence.

Beneficence means you want to contribute to the welfare of the patient. We know what's best! The term *paternalism* has been used to describe this (*parentalism* would be more gender neutral). Examples include a patient who refuses chemotherapy for a potentially curable condition, religious beliefs that prevent a patient from accepting a life-saving blood transfusion, or a patient with unstable angina who refuses hospital admission. In these types of scenarios, a patient can autonomously make a decision that would probably conflict with what we think is best for them. It is easy to see the potential dilemma in autonomy versus beneficence.

8. Why nonmaleficence?

What many consider the cardinal rule of medicine is related to the teachings of Hippocrates: "First, do no harm." Considering that most patients will get better in spite of us, then let's not mess things up by getting in the way. That is nonmaleficence.

The ethical dilemmas related to withholding or withdrawal of treatment or determination of quality of life are associated with nonmaleficence. Will your treatment decision burden the patient unnecessarily?

9. Is there justice?

The fourth principle used in medical ethics analysis is justice. How do we maintain fairness in patient care? How do we decide who gets what?

Do you have a responsibility to advocate for your patient at the bedside? Should this be left to legislative bodies to decide? Where does rationing fit in? Which patient is the most appropriate candidate for an organ transplant: an unemployed father of three, a homeless former nurse who has been dealt many of life's misfortunes, or the alcoholic politician? How do we make such a decision in the context of autonomy, beneficence, and nonmaleficence?

10. What is informed consent?

Informed consent should be obtained from the patient by the person who is going to do the procedure to them. That means nurses *witness* this process but do not obtain the consent. Essentially, informed consent requires that the patient know the following:
- What is being proposed
- Its expected benefits and known complications
- The available alternative treatments with benefits and complications
- The consequences of no treatment

Obviously, this requires decision-making capacity and the patient's being allowed to make his or her decision autonomously without pressure from family or friends. You should not do what you should not do.

11. How does informed refusal apply?

Remember autonomy! Patients have a right to refuse any medical modality. Consequently, they have the right of informed refusal. This certainly requires the same information that would be provided for informed consent. Keep in mind that all consents or refusals should be well documented.

12. Are you competent?

We often refer to patients as being either competent or incompetent to make decisions. This is incorrect. Competency is presumed (yes, even your supervisor is considered competent). It requires a judicial decision to determine incompetency. This is not a medical decision. And, if a patient is found to be incompetent, then someone needs to be appointed as a guardian for that individual. We do not determine competency.

13. Where does decision-making capacity fit in?

Decision-making capacity is a medical determination. It can be issue or decision specific. These are some of the parameters that help determine decision-making capacity:

- Does the patient understand what is going on?
- Does the patient appreciate the consequences of the decision?
- Is the patient able to repeat back to you a comprehension of the circumstances?
- Can the patient effectively weigh the information he or she has received and provide a logical reasoning for his or her answer? (Beware, beneficence!)

14. What if the patient lacks decision-making capacity? We are not talking about competency here.

Under the doctrine of implied consent, if patients present for treatment (on their own, by others, dragged in) they are our responsibility. If they lack decision-making capacity, it is "implied" that a prudent layperson would do the logical thing and "consent" for treatment. Consequently, if a medical standard of care applies, we are obligated to treat accordingly. Essentially, the loss of autonomy allows for our enhanced beneficence. We really need to be in touch with our prejudices to avoid abuse of this concept or to lose our objectivity and compassion.

15. What is an advance directive?

An advance directive provides a mechanism for patients to maintain autonomous beliefs when they lack decision-making capacity. These are essentially two types of written advance directives: a *living will* and a *durable power of attorney for health care.*

A living will usually requires that the patient lack decision-making capacity, be in a terminal or vegetative state with no hope for recovery, and have this documented by the attending physician. This would then allow for the withholding or withdrawal of life support. However, unless specifically indicated, withholding of artificial nutrition and hydration may not be permitted. This would obviously prolong the dying process.

A durable power of attorney for health care allows the patient to appoint an agent who is empowered to make all medical decisions on the patient's behalf when that patient lacks decision-making capacity. A qualifying medical condition need not be present. This does allow for the withholding or withdrawal of all medical modalities.

When an advance directive is not present (how many of you have one?), many states have developed Health Care Surrogate Acts, which legislatively delineate a surrogacy order for family or friends to be medical decision-makers for the patient. Various criteria may be needed for this to take effect. See also the legal chapter.

16. Is there a difference between withholding treatment and withdrawal of treatment?

Conceptually, there is no difference in withholding or withdrawal of treatment. If the appropriate legal criteria have been met (i.e., advance directive or surrogate act), then removal of life support is acceptable. Often, this can be emotionally troublesome for health care providers. But we must recognize this would be the patient or appropriate surrogate's legal right.

17. What is a good quality of life?

Often, in the health profession we see things that have great impact on ourselves. A devastating injury or illness will demonstrate our own fragility. We then say we would "never want to be like that." However, "like that" may be fully acceptable to that patient. Their quality of life may be meaningful and still comfortable.

What this means is that only the individual patient knows what is a good quality of life for himself or herself. Not the family, not the physician, not the nurse, and not the HMO gatekeeper. Only the patient knows. For a patient with a stroke or confined to a wheelchair, the ability to look at a garden or smile at his or her grandchildren may be a good quality of life.

18. What is futility?

Is there ever a time when medical treatment is worthless? How can we justify not providing a treatment to such a patient? This concept can be particularly difficult when dealing with a patient's family. Although we never want to take away hope, certain situations do present themselves as futile. Would you take the cachectic 85-year-old patient with metastatic liver cancer to the cardiac catheterization laboratory with a myocardial infarction? Medicine is not obligated to perform or provide treatment that is just not indicated.

Nurses speak with families about "what's going on and what can be done." Patients and families will talk to nurses more so than to their physicians. How will you respond? Being aware that a situation is futile (defined as 100% of all patients with this condition will have an unsuccessful outcome) will allow you to guide the patient and family through this tragic time.

We should not be asking what they want done but should be informing them what can be done. There is a fine line here, but offering a treatment that is not medically indicated does not benefit the patient or the family.

19. What should I do if I observe a blatant unethical clinical situation?

If the unthinkable happens, the nurse must intervene. Examples could be a physician preventing (rather than withholding or withdrawing) treatment (e.g., deliberately obstructing a tracheostomy tube on a patient) or mistreatment, such as a police officer violently, unnecessarily striking a patient. Direct confrontation could be attempted but may not be timely or physically safe. Similarly, contacting a supervisor or department chairperson afterward will not stop the unacceptable action now. The only definitive action to effectively stop the activity immediately is probably to call for security.

Taking dramatic action is not easy and could be professionally counterproductive (e.g., if the physician admits many patients to the institution). However, the nurse is the patient's best advocate and may need to exercise this responsibility. After all, you do have to look at yourself in the mirror the next day.

20. How should staff handle the unaccompanied minors that walk in to the emergency department (ED) for treatment?

I encourage a liberal interpretation of what the parent would want and what is in the child's best interest. The obvious guiding principle is that if it hurts, or appears limb or life threatening, then the initial treatment is begun. A clarifying thought I offer is to ask, "Would the parents be considered negligent if they did not seek treatment for this presenting condition?" If so, treat.

Most EDs have "war stories" of minors seeking care for an apparent insignificant complaint, only to find a more ominous condition. For instance, the "sore shoulder" is really a septic joint. At some level, minors sometimes sense they are ill, although they may lack the ability to precisely articulate their acuity.

21. After an unsuccessful cardiac arrest resuscitation, resident physicians will "practice" some skills, such as intubation, on the deceased person. Is this ethical?

Years ago this was a widely accepted practice, and some hospitals still allow it. The thought is that in special circumstances, such as remote rural areas, there are limited training opportunities. It is therefore better to "practice" on the newly deceased to limit error on the live, viable, future patients. These practitioners often assume it would be too upsetting to ask the family for permission.

However, I do not allow this practice without the consent of the newly deceased patient's family. This is also the position statement of the Emergency Nurses Association (ENA). Once an action is no longer for the promotion of *that* individual's good, the implied consent is gone. I believe that to continue on is an intrusion into that person's sacred sense of being. I find it interesting that most of those who advocate the right to practice tend to do only procedures the family would never know about, such as intubation, rather than invasive self-evident skills, such as an open thoracotomy. See also the legal chapter.

22. Drug representatives provide us with many free product-identifiable items, such as pens and notepads. Is this common practice advisable?

A revolution of this familiar practice may be painful. I urge consideration of three aspects as you make your decision.

1. *This is subliminal information.* Academic information about a product is important and necessary. However, "goodies" with the name of the product are almost always meant to be bribery. The drug company hopes the product's name will come to mind. Use this product and you will get a prize!

2. *Who pays for these things?* Is it not possible that the cost of advertising this way is added to the cost of the product? With all the talk of hardship for patients to afford their medication, is there something that is conceptually unethical going on?

3. *Drugs are the answer.* Beware of the sensory overload of messages telling us that drugs are our solutions. Do we not already too often fall into the mindset that there is a pill for everything?

I encourage actively thinking about alternatives. If the drug representative brings in bagels, why not share them with the patients and families in the waiting room? At least encourage thinking twice about what you are taking and from whom you are really taking it.

23. We encounter so many difficult ethical situations on our unit. How can I help staff deal with them?

I started an Advocacy Program for Ethics at our hospital that has been running for more than 7 years. This program educates trained nurse liaisons to work with staff directly on their unit as the ethical dilemma develops. Dissemination of knowledge through readily accessible staff resources empowers the nursing staff to deal with ethical dilemmas as they occur.

A volunteer group of nurses from areas that have a predisposition to ethical dilemmas (obstetrics, critical care, medical-surgical, ED) meet with the Director of Medical Ethics Program every other month for an hour to discuss approaches to ethical conflict resolution. This approach includes formal lectures and reviews of actual hospital cases. In addition, nurses can bring cases (with anonymity) to our Hospital Ethics Committee for retrospective review and discussion.

24. Do I, as a nurse, have any rights?

Absolutely! All health care providers have very important rights. Probably, the most significant is the right of conscience. If you are asked (or ordered) to do something that is medically or morally against your better judgment, you have the right to refuse. This can take the form of being ordered to give an inappropriate drug dose or something that will place your patient in jeopardy. A mechanism for this right should be in policy form within your institution. Recourse to a supervisor or administrator is the usual means.

You must always remember that the patient's bedside is not the place to make a political or religious statement. If your job description requires you to participate in an activity that you cannot accept on a personal level, then this should be discussed and clarified in advance. You should never be forced to violate your conscience, but patient care can never be a battleground for this conflict.

BIBLIOGRAPHY

1. Beauchamp T, Childress J: Principles of Biomedical Ethics, 3rd ed. New York, Oxford University Press, 1989.
2. Catalano J: Ethical and Legal Aspects of Nursing, 2nd ed. Springhouse, PA, Springhouse Corporation, 1995.
3. Emergency Nurses Association: Position Statement: The Use of the Newly Deceased Patient for Procedural Practice. Des Plaines, IL, Emergency Nurses Association, 1998.
4. Hebert P: Doing Right: A Practical Guide to Ethics for Medical Trainees and Physicians. Toronto, Oxford University Press, 1996.
5. Heilicser B: Managers Forum: Euthanasia. J Emerg Nurs [in press].
6. Heilicser B: Managers Forum: Practicing on the newly deceased. J Emerg Nurs 27(6):590, 2001.
7. Heilicser B: Managers Forum: Accepting drug-endorsed free products. J Emerg Nurs 27(4):383, 2001.
8. Heilicser B: Manager's Ask and Answer: Ethics advocacy. J Emerg Nurs 24(3):274, 1998.
9. Heilicser B: Manager's Ask and Answer: Unaccompanied minors: To treat or not to treat.J Emerg Nurs 24(2):188, 1998.

36. APPLYING RESEARCH IN PRACTICE

Teresa A. Savage, PhD, RN, and Laura A. Leigh, MBA, MSN, RN, CRRN

Statistics are like a bikini. What they reveal is suggestive, but what they conceal is vital.

Andrew Lang

1. How can a nurse manager use research?

Research can be used to evaluate and improve practices, to stimulate critical thinking, and to promote career growth in terms of professional development.

2. What preparation do nurse managers need to do research?

Having an inquisitive mind and a desire to discover is a great start. The fundamentals to conducting research are found in theory, research design and methodologies, statistics, and research ethics. Research design and methodologies include both quantitative and qualitative methods.

In most undergraduate nursing programs, students are given an introduction to research and are asked to critique research articles. In graduate programs, nurses learn the fundamentals and are expected to conduct a research project, often in conjunction with an experienced faculty member's project. At the doctoral level, nurses are prepared to conduct independent research, demonstrated by the completion of their doctoral thesis.

3. What is the difference between quality assurance/improvement projects and nursing research?

Quality assurance is the monitoring of a particular procedure or policy adherence. The intent is to determine whether the policy or procedure is being followed as written. Quality improvement examines the process and what can be improved in the process. The ultimate goal is to improve patient care. Research is a systematic investigation of a phenomenon to produce knowledge that can be generalized. In most research, a hypothesis is generated or tested.

4. Should the nurse manager change policies and procedures that are inconsistent with the latest research findings?

The nurse manager should ask the following questions:
- Do these research findings fit with our circumstances, our personnel, and our mission?
- What resources are needed to effect change?
- What are the drawbacks in adopting these research findings and changing our policy and/or procedure?
- Does the study have scientific merit?

5. What is evidence-based practice?

Evidence-based practice is nursing practice based on convincing data, relevant to the institution's specific situations and needs.

6. How is the evidence gathered?

There are numerous ways to gather evidence, through literature searches of research articles, case reports, and meta-analyses, as well as by conducting empirical research on the phenomenon of interest.

7. Who decides whether a practice should be changed?

The impetus for change can come from many places: clinicians, patients' comments/complaints, or adverse events. The ultimate decision rests with the chief nurse executive in the institution who oversees nursing practice.

8. What kind of educational preparation does a nurse manager's staff need to do clinical research?

In addition to the qualification already mentioned, nurses can use the nursing process (identify the problem, collect data, make a plan, implement, evaluate, and revise) as a template for the research process. Many institutions employ nurses with advanced education to facilitate clinical research by staff nurses.

At a minimum, before investing the time and energy in a clinical research project, a staff nurse should consult with an experienced researcher to review the plan for data collection and analysis (i.e., method). Otherwise, the nurse could find, after using valuable time and resources to complete the study, that the results are meaningless because an inappropriate method was used.

9. What kind of resources does a nurse manager's staff need to do clinical research?

To plan, conduct, or participate in the research, the nurse needs dedicated research time. Although many nurses are highly motivated to do research, their clinical responsibilities prevent them from spending time on research, unless they are relieved from direct care responsibilities. The proposal must be developed, reviewed by the institution's research review mechanism for scientific merit, then submitted to the Institutional Review Board. Upon approval, the nurse begins with recruitment (if applicable), consenting, data collection, analysis, and interpretation of data. Depending on the study, the nurse may need equipment, supplies, and communication support, such as phone, fax, postage, or e-mail. Consultation from a statistician or content expert may also be desirable.

10. What should the nurse manager consider when a staff member asks to do a study on a clinical problem?

The nurse manager should consider these questions:
• How pressing is this problem?
• Is it relevant to improving care?
• What is/will be the effect on the unit?
• What will the perspectives of patients or other staff be?
• What is/will be the effect on the staff member who wants to do the study? Will this be viewed as promoting professional growth, as a "reward," or as a way of appeasing a "complainer"?
• Has the study plan been reviewed by an experienced researcher for data collection and analysis (i.e., method)?

11. Why should the nurse manager have "participation in research" as an expectation of staff members in his or her unit?

If the department or unit is within an academic medical center, there is usually an expectation that clinical research will be conducted, and the staff nurses may expect to be involved in the research on varying levels. The nurses should be aware of any studies being conducted on their unit and the implications of the studies on patient care.

The nurses may be expected to participate in data collection when doing so can be incorporated in routine nursing care. Often specific members of the research team will be assigned to collect data that is beyond routine nursing care. However, the nurses on the unit should be aware of the study. Many institutions require that the study protocol be available on the unit for nurses to access and a copy of the signed consent form kept in a specific research file or in the patient's medical record.

12. What are the effects of having staff nurses participate in research?

Nurses' participation in research, either as data collectors or as principal investigators, can have positive and negative aspects. The nurse participating in research facilitates advances in knowledge, promotes the mission of the academic institution, enhances critical thinking, and challenges one to think beyond the task-work and day-to-day activities.

However, this participation can also take away from current duties and add to the stress the nurse may have of feeling overwhelmed by the workload. Often there is no tangible "reward" for the nurse's involvement in someone else's research, so nurses may feel their role in research will be not be recognized or acknowledged.

The nurse manager can negotiate with the principal investigator the terms of nursing recognition commensurate with their effort. The principal investigator may support a percentage of salary for a nurse to recruit or collect data; at a minimum, the nurses' efforts should be acknowledged in the research report and any publications.

13. What is an IRB?

An IRB, or institutional review board, is a group of scientific and nonscientific members who review research projects for the purpose of protecting human subjects who may participate in research. In response to abuses by researchers in the United States and elsewhere in the past, all federally funded research studies are mandated to be reviewed by a local committee. Although a study may not be funded by the federal government, the institution usually requires that all investigators submit their studies for review by their IRB.

Many institutions have two or more IRBs—one for biologic studies and one for behavioral studies. The committee must have scientific members who are qualified to review research projects, as well as nonscientific members, who may be faculty members from the academic institution or community members. It should have regular members who have expertise or specialized knowledge of conditions that are often the focus of study at that particular institution, such as cancer, psychiatric disorders, or pediatric disorders. Some health care systems use a free-standing IRB and do not have their own IRB.

14. What is the nurse manager's responsibility when research is being conducted on the unit (or with the patients the unit serves)?

The nurse manager should ensure that all staff be aware of the study being conducted on the unit. If the nurses are involved in the study, it may be required by the institution that the nurses complete an investigator training module so that they are aware of the ethical issues related to research. The Department of Health and Human Services provides a tutorial that nurses can complete online, or the institution's office of research administration (often called Office for Protection of Research Subjects) may have its own education requirements. The nurse manager should ensure that effective communication between the researcher and the nurses has occurred so that all parties are clear on the expectations.

15. What constitutes informed consent to participate in research?

According to the Federal Policy for the Protection of Human Subjects Title 45 CFR Part 46, 46.116, General Requirements for Informed Consent (1991), there are eight basic elements of informed consent. These involve the information's content, records, compensation, contact information, and alternatives.

16. What is essential participant information for the consent?

Potential subjects must be informed in a language that they understand that they are being invited to participate in a study. The information must include the following:

- The study's purpose
- The length of the requested participation
- What specific procedures the participants will be asked to perform
- Which procedures are considered experimental
- Anticipated risks or discomforts for participants
- Anticipated benefits for participation
- Alternatives to participation, if any
- Description of the measures to ensure confidentiality of the records
- Compensation and/or medical treatment if the subject is injured by participating in the research.

- A number to call if there are any questions about the study, and the IRB number for questions related to the rights of research subjects
- Reinforcement that participation is voluntary and the subject may withdraw at any time without any penalty or loss of benefits

16. Should the nurse manager's staff be expected to obtain consents for research from their patients and deliver direct patient care to them?

If the staff nurses have been trained to obtain informed consent and are willing, and this task has been negotiated between the researcher and the nurse manager, staff nurses may obtain informed consent for the study. If the nurses perceive that obtaining informed consent may interfere with the nurse-patient relationship, or that they perceive their role as direct care provider as unduly influential in the patient/subject's decision to participate, then another person may be more appropriate to obtain consents.

17. What should the nurse manager teach the staff to look for in protecting human subjects from research risks?

If the nurse has indications that the patient-subject lacks the capacity to consent or, if after giving consent, does not understand the study, the nurse is obligated to notify the researcher or the designated person on the research team. The nurse should be aware of the protocol and should notify the researcher if there is a deviation from the protocol.

For example, a patient on an oncology unit may have agreed to participate in a randomized clinical trial for an experimental drug. The patient tells the nurse that he is glad he came to this institution so he can get the experimental treatment for his cancer. The patient further explains that he went to a local hospital and they were only going to give him the standard treatment, but he wanted the experimental treatment since the odds of cure are better. The nurse questions whether the patient-subject understands the concept of randomization, and that he may be randomized to the group that receives the standard treatment. The patient-subject tells her that his doctor promised him he will get the experimental treatment and states he will not participate if he does not get the experimental treatment. Before giving this patient any study medication, the nurse contacts the researcher to clarify.

BIBLIOGRAPHY

1. Bliss DZ: It's not just research—It may be evidence. Nurs Res 49(6):301, 2000.
2. Department of Health and Human Services: Subpart A: Federal policy for the protection of human subjects. General requirements for informed consent. Fed Reg 56(117):28016–2801, 1991.
3. Mateo MA, Kirchhoff KT: Using and Conducting Nursing Research in the Clinical Setting, 2nd ed. Philadelphia, W. B. Saunders, 1999.
4. President's Commission for the Study of Ethical Problems in Medicine and Biomedical and Behavioral Research: Making Health Care Decisions: The Ethical and Legal Implications of Informed Consent in the Patient-Practitioner Relationship. Vol 1: Report. Washington DC, U. S. Government Printing Office, 1982.
5. Stetler CB, Brunnel M, Giuliano KK, et al: Evidence-based practice and the role of nursing leadership. J Nurs Admin 28(7/8):45–53, 1998.
6. Woods SS, Jensen LB, Schulz P, et al: Collaborative research: A community approach. Clin Nurse Special 14(1):13–16, 1998.

VI. Related Topics

37. MANAGING MULTIPLE DEPARTMENTS

Irene Louda, RN, BSN, MHA, CEN, CNA

Reason and judgment are the qualities of a leader.

Tacitus

1. Did you volunteer to be responsible for multiple departments?
I, as most managers, was asked to assume this role by the senior administration and have been doing it for more than 5 years. While people may debate whether it is the best structure for the most effective management, it is a growing trend.

2. What is key to managing multiple departments?
- *Hire good people.* Robert Half is quoted as saying, "There is something that is much more scarce, something rarer than ability. It is the ability to recognize ability."
- *Be considerate and appreciate your people.* Use "please" and "thank you" often.
- *Develop good computer skills and become proficient in communicating in ways other than face-to-face.*
- *Use management by walking around.* You must be comfortable with overseeing rather than doing. Occasionally walk through the departments to get a feel for the area and to see people face to face.
- *Come in during off hours sometimes.* Come in late or early so you can have contact with all staff. One manager comes in and walks around at 3:00 AM only about twice a year, but his visits are a department legend. Another calls in occasionally at 5:00 AM, when she first wakes up in the morning, to check with the night shift.
- *Check for any regional variations in the county or state laws if the facilities are in different geographic locations.*

3. Are you an expert in all the areas you manage?
The skill for a manager of multiple departments is management. It is not always necessary for the manager to have those areas' specific clinical or operational skills. Your goal is to select good staff and then let them do the day-to-day operations. As one multiple-department manager described it, "I'm the resources and process expert" and the staff are the "doing experts.".However, to maintain some skills and knowledge in my clinical expertise, I do continue to teach competencies.

4. How do you handle a situation in which a clinical decision is needed but you do not have the clinical expertise to make it?
Use input from multiple people. For instance, when hiring an x-ray technician, I have the head of the radiology department, and possibly another x-ray technician, assist in the interview. Some managers will have the departmental head/charge person perform the clinical hiring, decisions, and evaluations. Any technique-type radiology questions that arise are referred to the department supervisor.

I also use the expertise of the hospital's resources. For example, I noted that the emergency department (ED) was consistently missing an area of documentation. I referred it to the clinical nurse specialist (CNS) who reports to me, but also works with the information systems. She developed a change in the computerized chart to include this mandatory information.

5. How do you determine where to spend your time and energies when responsible for multiple departments?

The yearly budget divides my position's salary between the different departments. But in terms of actual time, it depends on the areas' needs. There are weekly, sometimes daily, fluctuations. I do recommend coordinating your office/paper work at one main location. Although I have an office at each facility, I do most of that type of work, including using the mailing address, at only the main one.

6. Should I spend one full day in each area or share the day between areas?

Don't feel you need to share every day with every department. It is easier to make at least a token appearance if the departments are physically in the same building. Many multiple-department managers find it makes a difference to the staff if they at least just walk through the department. But when the departments are in separate facilities, most managers find it more effective to spend the day at one location. I have designated days for each location, with one flexible day, to avoid a "ping-ponging" commute between locations.

Shape staff's expectations. Some staff enjoy autonomy, but others may be used to and want a more constant presence. You cannot be everywhere and do everything for everyone. Ask staff what they want or need most from you and focus on that.

7. How do you stay in touch?

A cell phone, beeper, and voice mail are invaluable. I require that each charge nurse and secretary file a shift report in the computer so I can then check what is happening no matter where I am. I also have the hospital network system on my home computer.

8. How do you make it to all the meetings?

First schedule in the meetings called by your superiors or other departments or those that are held on set days. Then schedule your department and leadership meetings around them. Our hospitals have many managers responsible for multiple departments, so there is frequent polling to find the most convenient time for the majority.

If I have two meetings that are scheduled by my superiors for the same time at two different locations, I ask my supervisors to prioritize or do that myself. In the end, you have to decide how you will control what you want done.

9. How can I coordinate the work between multiple, similar departments?

Use a leadership team with representation from every department. Have the agenda available ahead of time to aid prepared contributions. I use a scribe to have accurate minutes, and those who cannot attend are responsible for reading the minutes. One manager has a monthly team meeting for universal concerns and individual meetings on a biweekly basis.

Other managers describe breaking down traditional unit boundaries to delegate similar responsibilities, such as scheduling or process improvement, to staff for all the areas. He approached the care (and related work) from his ED, intensive care unit (ICU), and telemetry units as a continuum.

Most multiple-department managers find that it is essential to have permanent charge-level staff members. They assume a large amount of the responsibility for the day-to-day events while you work on the bigger picture.

10. I never seem to have the paperwork I need when I go to a different facility.

One manager carries an accordion file with sections for each hospital and the physicians. She files things as they come up and always carries the file with her.

Another manager always carries a sheet of paper with sections designated for the senior administrator, each area, and each charge nurse. She does ongoing logging of items as they come up. That way, when she meets with people, she has a consolidated list of the related issues raised by all three units. For more discussion on this topic, see the chapter on office organization.

11. How do you handle uniting two different units?

When I had two emergency departments in different states, I took the approach that everything would change rather than that one place would become more like the other. Together we were creating something different and brand new. All positions became temporary while people reapplied for the openings that now had different criteria and standards. Aspects that helped unite these groups included the following:
- Developing a mutual vision statement.
- Cross-training the junior and new staff for both units. (The senior staff's experience was needed at their original department.) Cross-training helps staffing needs and improves mutual understanding.
- Completing required educational classes together.

Many managers coming into a newly created multiple-department situation find it is important not to make decisions about major responsibility or requirements too soon. I spent the first year simply evaluating and listening until I was ready to develop and institute criteria that have been workable for the long haul.

12. How can I get my department to actually work together beyond a casual tolerance?

Try a team-building meeting. Staff from the departments participate in an activity to obtain a consensus for the top three concerns and goals for the following year. They can then volunteer to work on what they have identified as important. For more discussion on this concept, see the section on retreats.

Some managers have successfully used an "exchange program"in which nurses visit the other facility for the day. It helps to understand the differences. For instance, one unit realized the other unit was slower in answering the phone because they didn't have a unit secretary.

Others also use a mutual "newsletter" with related hospital, department, and personal news. Be aware, however, that these can take significant time to produce on a regular basis.

13. How do you get it all done?

You never really get everything done. If you did, you'd be out of job! Make priority lists and keep your eye on the goals. Realize that today it is expected that a manager role will consume a minimum of 50 hours a week. And do find time to still have fun.

BIBLIOGRAPHY

1. Zimmermann PG: Manager's Ask and Answer. J Emerg Nurs 23(6):636–637, 1997.
2. Zimmermann PG: Mangers Forum: Responsibility for multiple facilities. J Emerg Nurs 25(4):316–317, 1999.

38. MANAGING RENOVATION PROJECTS

Nancy Bonalumi, RN, MS, CEN

Business will be better or worse.

Calvin Coolidge

1. Our department has just received approval to renovate. Where do I begin?

The planning process for renovation or new construction begins with an analysis of your current and proposed use of the nursing unit. Will this unit be dedicated for a general population, or will there be a specialty focus such as cardiac, neurologic, pediatric or surgical? Specialization may have an impact on the unit's occupation rate, the average length of stay, and patient acuity.

The demographics of your community or service area must be analyzed. Review your source of admissions over the past 5 years. A zip code analysis of the previous year of patients who were admitted to your hospital will indicate where your patients come from geographically. The Finance department can furnish you with a payor mix report, which breaks down, by percentage, each source of reimbursement for patients who use your hospital.

Your local community planners should be asked about proposed development in your service area. A new 400-house residential development or an industrial park being built within your area will have a significant impact the utilization of your hospital.

The population growth rate of your community can be obtained from the city or county commissioner's office or your state's division of vital statistics, usually located within the Department of Public Health. Are there projected trends in your community's demographics that are going to affect your community over the next 5 to 20 years, such as a declining birth rate or increasing numbers of people over the age of 65?

Your state hospital association is also a source. Ask for population data as well as health care trends, such as managed care penetration rates, that could affect hospital usage.

2. How many beds do I need, and of what type?

Once your population analysis is complete, you can begin to identify the scope of service you should be providing. Length of stay statistics for your current unit will be useful if your population is not expected to change.

However, if the purpose of the renovation or new construction is to change the unit's scope of service, you will need to gather data to determine what the appropriate utilization rate will be. For example, if the unit is going to exclusively admit post-cardiac interventional patients, the number of procedures the cardiovascular department plans to do on a daily basis will provide you an estimate of your daily admission rate.

The medical records department can run a volume report of discharge diagnoses related to the unit. Review a year of data at a minimum. This will also support your decision-making on number and type of beds.

A common problem among those who have gone through this process is that space considerations were based on the current census rather than the projected growth. By the time they were done, they needed to think about renovation again!

3. How are the architect and builder selected for this project?

The process of selecting the architect and builder is usually led by your hospital's senior administration. The committee traditionally is composed of board members, senior administrators, and other key stakeholders within your organization. Express your interest in becoming a part of this process, especially if it is just your department that is being considered for construction and you want to have a voice in its development.

Depending on the scope of the project, the nurse manager may or may not be considered for membership in this selection committee. If you are not selected to be on this committee, identify a key supporter who can bring your thoughts to the selection process.

There are two phases for selecting any consultant or vendor for a project, including architects and builders. They are the request for information (RFI) and the request for proposal (RFP).

4. What is a request for information?

The RFI contains a brief overview of the project. A request for information will be sent to a number of companies. Some specific information about the project should be contained to help the vendor provide more than a generic response. The turnaround time for the vendors to reply is usually 3 to 5 weeks. Based on the responses, the number of potential candidates will be reduced. The selected companies will be asked to provide a request for proposal on this project.

5. How does the request for proposal differ from an RFI?

The information contained in the RFP is more detailed and focused. Ask the vendor to reply to specific questions that will assist in identifying which candidate has the best experience, talent, and process to make your renovation/construction project a success. Because of the detailed response the candidates must make, the response time can be up to 8 weeks. At that time, the finalists will be asked make a presentation to the hospital's facilities planning committee. The finalists should bring to their presentation drawings and photographs of other nursing units they have done.

6. Will there always be an RFI and an RFP process for a renovation/construction project?

In some circumstances, the former architect and builder of your present department may be invited to work again at the facility. Again, the final decision will usually be made at the Board of Director level because of the amount of money represented in a renovation project. However, this process may be done for certain aspects of the renovation, such as a new cardiac monitoring system.

7. How do I know what design features I should include in the renovated department?

Ask the architect for samples of work he or she has done on similar departments. Site visits to facilities similar to what you are planning can provide you with design idea and features that you may wish to include in your final design. Use professional networking opportunities to gather information via Internet listserves or web sites. Look in health care journals that run features on facility redesign and construction.

8. Are there special considerations I should make for staff comfort and safety?

Keep in mind that the average age of a registered nurse is now in the mid-40s. The aging workforce needs to be considered in the planning of a new department. Distances between frequently trafficked areas such as the clean and dirty utility rooms, medication prep areas, and nurse's stations should be kept at a minimum. Flooring, lighting and acoustic considerations should be identified to reduce fatigue and risk of error. Countertop height and furnishings will also affect staff comfort and safety.

9. There are so many details we discuss at each planning meeting. How can I remember them all?

Detailed minutes need to be taken at every meeting. The planning process will take anywhere from a few months to 2 years, depending on the size and scope of the project. Written notes are critical to capture the infinite details that are agreed upon by the planning team members. The minutes should be distributed to the attendees and key stakeholders after each meeting. The minutes become your assurance that what was agreed upon is what is built.

10. The first set of blueprints has arrived. What do all the symbols and markings mean?

Reading blueprints is not a skill you were taught in nursing school. Therefore, to ensure your comprehension and to be able to explain the drawings to your staff, you need to become skilled at interpreting blueprints.

Ask the architect to explain every symbol and marking on the drawing. Go through each room or area of your project so that you understand the size, configuration and features of each space. There are immovable objects that exist in any department (e.g., structural supports or conduits for electrical and heating and air conditioning). Despite the negative impact these objects may have on the aesthetics or functionality of your department, these permanent structures cannot be moved.

11. Are there other mandatory requirements besides support beams and conduits that I need to be aware of?

Local and state building code requirements will dictate how far any area in the department can be from an emergency exit. Corridor width is mandated to be a certain number of feet across. The location of fire extinguishers, fire alarm pull stations, and medical gas shut-off valves may also be prescribed by code.

These building code regulations will also place restrictions on the size of rooms. For example, an open cubicle with a curtain covering the front may be built as small as 8×10 feet, but any fully enclosed room may have a minimum requirement of 10×12 feet.

It is the responsibility of the architect or your facilities manager to be sure the plans meet all building code requirements. In most states, the blueprints must be approved by the state Department of Health or other regulatory agency before construction can commence. Any variation from the approved plan may need to go back through the approval process.

12. I can see how big the rooms look from the overhead view, but what will the finished rooms really look like?

Ask for elevations of the room layouts. As opposed to looking down on an area, as in a standard blueprint, elevation drawings provide a face-on view of the wall, counter, or cabinet. Elevation sketches provide greater conceptualization of how the finished room will appear.

13. How much storage space should I plan for?

You can never install enough storage space in any department. Ask the architect to include as many cabinets, closets, and storeroom spaces as the project will allow. A room can look very big when empty. However, once you place a patient bed, supplies or specialty equipment, such as cardiac monitors and IV pumps at the bedside, even a large room can seem cramped

Storerooms seem never to be built large enough. Make sure adequate shelving is planned for the amount of supplies such a room will hold. Consider installing pullout shelves or drawers under countertops. Under-counter cabinets often have much wasted space or are difficult to reach into for supplies or restocking. Any corner cabinet or shelf should have a turntable installed to maximize space utilization.

14. How can I be sure the design meets the needs of patients and staff?

Every set of blueprints should be posted in an area where all staff can view them and comment. Let them write on the drawings, making suggestions and proposing changes. Some of the best practical suggestions have come from staff, such as a work shelf by the medications or sinks in patient care areas. Return the marked-up prints to the architect to have the recommendations incorporated into the design.

You can also post the proposed plan in a prominent area of your department, such as a waiting room or near the nurse's station. Solicit feedback from physicians, patients, and visitors.

A focus group open to the public and led by your hospital planner, marketing department, or the architect may draw additional comments and suggestions. Your customers' satisfaction with the final product will be enhanced if they have a voice in the design phase.

15. What can I expect during the renovation phase of the project?

Renovation of your current space requires a great deal of planning to identify every phase of the project. Each phase may last a few weeks to several months and will have an impact on your department's every-day activities. You can expect noise, dust, and disruption every day. This is unsettling to both the patients and the staff.

Provide for patient comforts such as earplugs. Additionally, make extra efforts to maintain customer satisfaction by providing "inconvenience" gifts such a water bottles, tote bags, or other promotional items. A personal visit each day to patients, with an apology, may go a long way to keeping the dissatisfaction to a minimum.

Staff will need additional motivation and morale boosters during this time as well. Special events such as ice cream sundae days or inviting a massage therapist to the department for a few hours may improve spirits and relieve tension.

16. What have others learned that help with the renovation process?

- *Keep an ongoing list of flaws or things not completed as promised.* See the contractor foreman at least once a day on things that need follow-up.
- *Insist on heavy-duty cupboards and flooring.* If your architect is not familiar with health care facilities, he or she may want to use more attractive kitchen-type cabinets that wear out with heavy-duty use.
- *Realize the budget is affected well after the construction phase.* Major items are part of the project, but there will be items needing replacement or repair as a result of the renovation.
- *Keep change to a minimum during the move process.* Orient staff to any new equipment during construction so they are not adjusting to new machinery as well as location.
- *Be aware that staffing needs may change.* Depending on the size and configuration, a greater distance to central areas (e.g., dirty utility room, medications) may mean less efficiency over the course of the day. One in-patient unit reconfigured to have an additional unit secretary/greeter desk by the elevator. The only problem is they did not have any approved budgeted position to fill it.

17. The renovation is finally done. What should we expect for our volume?

Most emergency departments report about a 10% to 15% rise in patient volume during their "opening months." The percentage will depend on their current market share at the time. Generally, the surge tends to lessen after 90 days or so, but not always. Consultants attribute this rise to the marketing effort and the perception by the public that this site is now more current.

18. What do we do to celebrate?

Ask your marketing department to take photographs and develop a press release for local media outlets such as television and the newspaper. Develop a promotional campaign for the new unit, especially if the scope of services has changed or been upgraded. If possible, have an open house. Invite community leaders and hospital and physician staff to tour the renovated unit, and highlight the new features and services you now offer. Celebrate with your staff as you use the new space!

BIBLIOGRAPHY

Zimmermann PG: New/remodeled emergency department. J Emerg Nurs 26(3):254–258, 2000.

39. MANAGING YOUR CAREER

Jo Manion, RN, PhD(c), CNAA, FAAN

Think . . . Think about Appearance, Associations, Actions, Ambition, Accomplishment.

Thomas J. Watson

1. I have always believed that with my nursing credentials, I could find a job anywhere. Why do I need to manage my career?

If there is a lesson to be taken from the 1990s, it is that no one's job or position is protected in any organization. Job security, as we once understood it, is gone. This is hard to believe while we are in the midst of yet another nursing shortage. But just because there are jobs does not mean they are jobs you would want.

Instead, each of us needs to accept responsibility for our own career, consider ourselves as free agents, and continually look for ways to increase our repertoire of skills and abilities. Then, if the unexpected happens, you will have options to consider. There are few more negative work experiences than feeling trapped in a position with limited and undesirable options.

2. As a nurse, I have always worked as an employee for someone else. What do you mean by free agent?

Free agent refers more to a mindset than an employment status. Free agents recognize that the organization does not "owe" them beyond the basic employee-employer relationship. It simply means that rather than depending on your organization to "look out for you," you take complete responsibility for your continued employability. In other words, you
- stay abreast of changes in your field
- update your skills and competencies continually
- obtain the education and experiences you need for continuing development
- have a keen understanding of your worth in the market place

3. What are the best ways to increase my continued employability?

The first step is to accept that you alone are responsible for the progression of your career. Additionally, there are several key skills to master. These include continued learning (including technology skills), articulation of your strengths and abilities, and development and maintenance of a solid network of contacts.

4. I'm so overwhelmed with work and things change so rapidly, I'm afraid I am falling behind. How can I remain current?

This is an almost universal experience, which doesn't make this problem any easier to solve. Many of us allow ourselves be overwhelmed and immobilized by the sheer magnitude of the task.

The real key to success here is to do *something*. It may not seem like a lot, but even reading a couple of articles a week can make a surprising impact over a year's time. Subscribe to a couple of basic journals, perhaps one in management and one in your clinical specialty. Many times your medical library staff is happy to circulate new issues of journals to managers before the issue is shelved. Or they may be willing to make copies of pertinent articles for you.

I have found it best to set a goal for myself. For instance, I will read two professional articles a week or one professionally stimulating book a month. With a simple commitment such as this, you will be further ahead than most of the people you know.

5. Do you have suggestions other than reading for staying current?

In today's world there are endless opportunities for continued learning.

- The Internet provides unlimited access (including approved continuing education courses).
- Continuing education programs offer timely topics.
- Travel provides opportunities to learn about practices elsewhere.
- Involvement in your community connects you with others.
- Talk with a traveling nurse and ask about his or her experiences in different parts of the country.
- Participate in professional organizations' programs (e.g., AONE, Sigma Theta Tau, ENA).

Simple, friendly questions that demonstrate your enthusiasm and curiosity can elicit a wealth of ideas, experiences, and glimpses into other worlds. These are just a few ideas and ways of expanding our knowledge base beyond our own, sometimes narrow, experiences.

6. I rose through the ranks and now fear I'm losing my clinical skills. How do others deal with this?

A common way many managers deal with this is to schedule time to work clinically. It doesn't have to be one day a week. Even a shift a month is useful in keeping these skills sharp.

The most important key to making this happen is to schedule it. If you always wait for a day that isn't too busy, or doesn't include any scheduled meetings, it's never going to happen. If you put this time on your schedule, you may need to change it (but only for a very good reason, and after at least some resistance), but it is more likely to be rescheduled. And don't be "on call" for administration issues. If they could cover for you if you were out of the building at a meeting, they could cover while you work a clinical shift.

Working clinically doesn't mean you must assume a charge nurse role. It can be a wonderful experience to simply take an assignment. And, it does not have to be the toughest assignment. In the same way your staff members would be unable to completely fill your shoes in your absence, you may not be as good clinically as your best staff nurse is. Be okay with this, and let your staff know as well. I think it discounts their skills and abilities if you assume you can just step in and be the #1 clinical nurse when you do it so seldom.

Some nurse managers feel too exposed to work clinically in their own department. Perhaps their skills are decidedly rusty, they are afraid they will "lose face" (or the staff's confidence), or their staff has exceedingly high expectations. Therefore, they periodically work clinically in other departments or facilities. This can meet your need of remaining clinically sharp, but you will lose the benefit of having your staff actually see put your clinical expertise to work!

7. What's the difference between a CV (curriculum vitae) and a resume?

Both are tools through which you present yourself to others with the intent of highlighting your accomplishments and achievements. Each is appropriate in different situations.

The primary focus of the resume is to outline your employment experience and it is used when you apply for a job. It is usually shorter than a CV; many experts suggest a maximum length of two to four pages. In fact, the shorter the better. This is based on the assumption that in normal situations, the person reading the resume has received many (sometimes hundreds). The resume is used to just do an initial "sort through" to determine which candidates meet the qualifications and are interesting enough to bring in for an interview.

A curriculum vitae is an expanded document that includes much of the same information but is meant to illustrate the depth of your professional activities and contributions. It is often used in academic settings and its focus is on education and credentials attained. Honors, awards, publications, and professional involvement are major components of this document. There are many excellent sources available in your library or through bookstores if you need help in creating either of these documents.

8. What is a career portfolio?

You will begin hearing more about this concept in the near future. Some hospitals use it as part of their clinical ladder. And some states are actually considering a requirement that all nurses maintain a career portfolio.

It is basically a comprehensive packet of information, according to Frank Shaffer, RN, PhD. It is completed by the nurse and "details the current state of his/her practice, background, skills, expertise and perhaps most importantly, a working plan for professional growth." Journalists, advertising executives, and architects are just a few examples of groups of professionals who use a career portfolio to showcase their work.

9. How does a career portfolio compare to a resume or CV?

The career portfolio is a broader, more expansive "packet" or document. In addition to the resume or CV, it includes the following:

- A capsule-like description of your career and your envisioned future
- Career goals and objectives
- Employment history (including job descriptions and performance appraisals)
- Educational history (including academic transcripts)
- Clinical validations (competency assessments, certifications)
- Health records
- References and recommendations (including personal letters commending your work)
- Formal recognitions and awards
- Involvement in community affairs
- Publications
- Presentations
- Research/grant projects

In addition to the statement of the facts, the portfolio includes illustrations of the quality of your work. The key point to remember is that you want to show progressive and varied experiences and skills.

10. What do you mean by illustrations of your work?

Examples of items commonly included are the actual articles published, brochures written, or project documents that illustrate your involvement. For example, if you served on a committee that wrote and presented a report to administration about a key organizational issue, you may include some artifact from the work that demonstrates your contribution (e.g., a new procedure, patient education pamphlet, or the publicity for a community event coordinated by the team). An artist does not prove their expertise by only stating, "I paint." Similarly, through a portfolio, professional nurses can display their capabilities and accomplishments.

Compiling your career portfolio is a major investment in time, but it pays off in the future. Once developed, it is easily kept updated. While you often uniquely tailor what you include for each situation, it allows you to rapidly respond to any new opportunity. And it is wonderfully affirming. Even the most accomplished of us rarely takes the time to sit down and reflect on all that has gone into our career.

11. Why do I need to spend time developing a network?

Credentials and experience are important. However, all of us can use help at times. Each of us is surrounded by a vast web of human resources, people who would be happy to lend a hand, share helpful information, or just pass our name along.

The best networks are formed when you see it as an opportunity to share your skills and expertise with others as well. Give-and-take is the fuel that keeps a network healthy. Exchanges at a certain point in time are not always equal. In other words, this time you may need something from your network member.

12. Where do I start if I want to strengthen my current network?

It is very effective to simply review what you are already doing and make some changes there. For instance, when you go to professional meetings, do you come in at the last minute and leave as soon as the meeting is over because you are busy? At break do you look for people you know so you can feel comfortable as you catch up with them? You get the drift here!

Recognize that an important part of attending any professional meeting is the networking opportunities it provides. Allow some extra time and promise yourself you will reconnect with people you haven't seen in a long time rather than hanging out with those closest to you.

Introduce yourself to people you haven't met before and engage them in conversation. This forces you to broaden your horizons.

13. Easy for you to say! I'm not gregarious by nature. What can I do to make mingling with others more comfortable?

First, take a good, honest look at what you have to offer others. Change your mindset so you see yourself as someone not only capable of sharing a good idea or two but also in whom other people would be interested.

Stock up on some small talk related to nursing or the group you are with. This is where reading one or two articles a week is helpful. "Did you see what is happening with the new surgical procedures?" Or, "What is this obsession people have with *Survivor*?" Toastmasters International (1-800-993-7732) provides practical experience in becoming conversant with anyone about anything.

Get the nurse you just met to tell you about his work. What is the department like? What does he like about it? Gentle, interested questioning combined with honest, considerate listening is one of the most wonderful gifts you can give another.

14. I am just not comfortable asking for help. Any tips for me?

Asking for help is easier if you also offer it unreservedly. Elizabeth Bibesco is credited with noting: "Blessed are those who give without remembering and take without forgetting." I think this should be our motto. There are a couple of rules of network etiquette I use that make it more comfortable for me to ask for help when I need it.

- Don't take it personally if someone cannot help me this time. Even another name is useful.
- Be businesslike in my approach, that is, brief, direct, and to the point. Then I don't feel like my request is an imposition.
- Think through what it is I want and pick the right people for what I am seeking.
- Take advice that is given, although I may modify it. Follow-up on leads. It's upsetting to spend time helping a colleague only to find later that your suggestion was simply ignored.
- Give the original supporter feedback. It is just simple courtesy, even if you only let him or her know that the discussion helped clarify your thinking.
- Pay for any involved expense, such as long-distance telephone call or lunch.
- Stay in contact with people even when you don't need anything. If the only time someone hears from you is when you need something, the relationship will soon wither and die.

When I keep these few "rules" in mind, it makes it easier to ask for what I need.

15. I am feeling very frustrated in my organization. I can't seem to get things accomplished. How do I know when it's time to move on?

This is a challenging question. You are really the only person who can answer it for yourself. You don't want to give it up too early when success may be just around the corner. On the other hand, it does you no good, nor the others with whom you work, if you stay in a malignant or toxic work environment where you feel unable to make beneficial changes.

The judgment to make this decision is often hard-won as a result of painful experiences throughout our career. In other words, sometimes you will leave too soon, sometimes you will stay too long. It is difficult, if not impossible, to get it just right. Basically, I think it's time to leave when you no longer feel that you are making an effective contribution or it is simply too costly (e.g., loss of reputation, emotional or psychological pain, decreasing opportunities) for you to remain.

To me, the most important step is an accurate assessment of your situation. A conversation with your supervisor is in order. Assertive feedback about the situation is crucial. This means an objective statement of facts: here is what I have tried, this is what has happened (or, more to the point, what hasn't happened), and a calm statement about your conclusion that it may be time for you to move on is appropriate. The response to this may vary from assurances of future changes, commiseration, positive feedback on your contributions, or even agreement. If your supervisor requests time to make some changes, you may choose to wait. However, if nothing seems to have changed in what you believe is a reasonable time period, it's time to be more forceful in your assertion. "Two months ago we talked and I have seen no changes. It is time for me to move."

If, in your judgment, the situation is so toxic that it feels unsafe to be honest with your supervisor, you may choose to do no more than simply position yourself as well as you can for leaving. In one instance, I obtained references from my supervisor to update my placement bureau file, found another job, and then talked with her about my leaving. I chose this way of handling it because I had observed her sabotage and vindictiveness on previous occasions.

16. My job feels like it has become a dead-end. I'm feeling bored and need some new challenges. Is it time for me to leave?

Perhaps, but perhaps not. There is plenty of meaningful and challenging work out there and it is important to continually develop your skills. However, don't be too sure that you have to leave your current job to find challenge or stimulation.

There are at least two approaches I would recommend. The first is to take a hard look at the work making up your day. Consider delegating some of the routine, less challenging responsibilities to others on your staff. What is "old hat" to you may provide variation, development opportunities, and challenges to others. And teaching others and watching them grow and become stronger brings its own form of excitement.

Second, seek opportunities outside your core position. Let other people in the organization know that you are looking for ways to develop new skills. Accept a new and challenging committee appointment. Offer to research a pressing issue. Become involved in community activities. Teach a course. Try your hand at publishing an article. Sometimes comfort and familiarity in a certain position gives us the opportunity to use it as a springboard. And, later, you can remind yourself to be careful of what you ask for in the future!

17. I've decided to leave my present job. How do I exit graciously?

Decide the best time to go public. Once your planned departure is known, there is a loss of effectiveness in finishing up projects. And avoid taking on extra projects now out of guilt from past underachievements.

Anticipate the inevitable question, "Why?" from others. Keep your answer brief. Focus on the new opportunity without gloating or comparing jobs. Avoid complaining. Your goal is to protect your reputation and leave people feeling good about your time there.

Schedule a transition plan. Discuss constructively what worked and what didn't work. Your last impression will be a good one if you make life easier for others when you leave.

Anticipate emotions in your colleagues. Some coworkers may distance themselves because they feel abandoned. Take them to lunch and let them see you can still have a relationship.

Respond appropriately to your own emotions. You may feel down. The temptation is to drag through the last 2 weeks, which leaves an unfavorable last impression. Act upbeat and work hard through the last day. And don't keep second-guessing yourself about this choice. Pre-move jitters are natural: remind yourself why you decided to take the new job.

BIBLIOGRAPHY

1. Bridges W: Creating You & Company. Cambridge, MA, Perseus Books, 1997.
2. Brooks B, Barrett S, Zimmermann PG: Beyond your resume: A nurse's professional "portfolio." J Emerg Nursing 24(6):555–557, 1998.

3. Gould SB, Weiner KJ, Levin BR: Free Agents: People and Organizations Creating a New Working Community. San Francisco, Jossey-Bass Publishers, 1997.
4. Hakin C: We Are All Self-Employed. San Francisco, Berrett-Koehler, 1999.
5. MacKay H: Dig Your Well Before You Are Thirsty: The Only Networking Book You'll Ever Need. New York, Currency/Doubleday, 1997.
6. Mandell T. Power Schmoozing: The New Etiquette for Social and Business Success. New York, McGraw-Hill, 1996.
7. Manion J: Enhancing career marketability through intrapreneurship. Nurs Admin Q 25(2):5–10, 2001.
8. Manion J: From Management to Leadership: Interpersonal Skills for Success in Health Care. Chicago, AHA Press, 1998.
9. Noer DM: Breaking Free: A Prescription for Personal and Organizational Change. San Francisco, Jossey-Bass Publishers, 1997.
10. Shaffer F: Developing your career portfolio. Presentation at the Staffing Crisis: Nurse/Patient Ratio Conference in Washington, DC, July 24, 2000.
11. Williams AG, Hall KJ: Creating Your Career Portfolio. Upper Saddle River, NJ, Prentice-Hall, 1997.

40. WELCOMING THE FUTURE

Linda S. Smith, MS, DSN, RN

A vision is not a vision unless it says yes to some ideas and no to others. It inspires people and is a reason to get out of bed in the morning and come to work.

George Pinchot III

1. Why is planning for the future important?

The future will require new resources and ideas with little room for the old "business as usual" paradigms. Through our collective forward momentum, health care will progress in this century. Thus, as nurse leaders, we determine our future by welcoming it.

2. Within the next decade, how will management-related communication change?

- *Electronic documentation with networked templates.* This will replace slow, difficult, cumbersome pen and paper formats. Evaluations will be word-processed records.
- *Data will be categorized at the individual and aggregate levels.* This will allow managers to easily archive and change data as well as identify trends, problems, and solutions. Access will be controlled by appropriate "need to know"' access codes.
- *E-mail will become THE communication vehicle.* This can facilitate information gathering from a larger pool of resources. For example, through e-mail tracking, you could discover information on who, when, where, and outcomes for a new medical device you are considering.

It will also facilitate staff communication, including the ability to collect a snapshot picture through a poll. It is predicted that e-mail will replace the telephone and fax as the primary means of physician communication with patients or insurers.

3. Tell me more about patient e-mail communication with health care providers.

Already there are pilot programs in which patients with stable health problems e-mail their physician. Based on this e-mail questionnaire, a nurse or physician either triages the patient for an office visit, returns the e-mail with self-care advice, or faxes a prescription. The patient's health plan is automatically billed for a $20 Internet consultation. The system is predicted to reduce unnecessary office visits by 20%.

4. What changes will take place in the area of information dissemination?

It will become increasingly easy to target announcements to appropriate staff pools, with their electronic reception noted. This will help eliminate incomplete information, the management time for individual face-to-face dissemination, or the "I didn't know" excuses. This electronic information dissemination shortens the change process.

5. What will be my own personal relationship with technology?

Since World War II, society has associated technology with progress. Our lives have been more comfortable, easier, and interesting because of such innovations as the dishwasher, television, and calculator. This trend will continue.

In the future, new technology will be introduced at an ever-increasing rate. Computers will continue to be smaller and faster. Technical competence in interpersonal communication and data management will grow increasingly important and facilitate a manager's rapid response to change.

What is important is that technology implementation be formulated, implemented, and evaluated with this question in mind: How will this technology increase the efficiency and effectiveness of our nursing care? Worthwhile innovations are about providing new access and connections that improve us as social, thoughtful, professional beings (Naisbitt, 2000).

6. Which computer skills will be essential for management and staff?

It has been noted that health care providers are lagging behind in their personal use of technology. One study of San Francisco nurse practitioners found that computers were mostly used to obtain client records or Internet searches. A Harris Pool found that only 13% of American physicians have ever used e-mail to communicate with their patients, and this proportion has stayed the same the past 2 years. Needed computer skills include the following:

- Alpha-numeric touch typing and keyboarding abilities
- Software utilization skills (including office tools, word processing, Lotus Notes, e-mail)
- Power Point skills for presentations
- Internet search and use
- E-commerce for ordering/distributing supplies

7. Which electronic documentation system will be most accepted by staff and most useful to me?

Electronic health care documentation is fast becoming standard procedure worldwide. On-line documentation will increasingly integrate a legally defensible, yet intuitively easy, charting-by-exception format with check boxes. This allows for improved data capture with trends demonstrated, with a reduction of duplication and errors.

However, not all systems are equally useful and accepted by nurses. The goal is easily accessible online systems that replace at least 90% of current paper charting and documentation. Inclusion of the following features is suggested:

- Capability to store digitalized pictures (e.g., wounds, injuries) as part of the permanent record
- Check-lists and prompts that give direction (e.g., forgotten or incorrect entries)
- Use of common, universal language and standards
- User-friendly features (e.g., intuitive movement between screens, appropriate help menus)

8. How will the world wide web (Internet) affect my work and life?

- *Education.* Nursing skills are perishable. The Internet will be able to implement worldwide staff development programs and requirements.
- *Standard of care dissemination and application.* Acceptable care standards will become national and international, rather than limited to just the regional location. Awareness of these standards will become the normal legal expectation.
- *Information sharing.* Information will include topics from clinical pathways to medication side effects to the latest health care research. Already government sources, such as the Centers for Disease Control (CDC), disseminate web-based data.
- *Reporting mechanism.* Direct online submission of confidential data such as adverse events from faulty medical devices or medication errors is now possible but will become ever more popular with busy nurse leaders. The more rapidly reported data from these online documents will facilitate improved Food and Drug Administration (FDA) information gathering and dissemination.

9. Which Internet resources will be most helpful to me as I implement nationally recognized, current care standards?

Some of the best sites for the nurse manager will continue to be government and health care organization-sponsored descriptions of current health care research, including how that research applies to clinical outcomes. Clinical practice guidelines and clinical pathways, developed at the federal level, are important ingredients for any care conference, policy, or program. Some of these are

www.ahcpr.gov: A government site that includes clinical practice guidelines and clinical pathways.

http://www.nih.gov/ninr: Current and future nursing research priorities.
www.guidelines.gov: This is the web site for the national guideline clearinghouse.
www.metacrawler.com: An excellent search engine that combines many search engines
into one. Use this site when you are looking for information but do not know the web address.
www.seniors.gov: Exceptional web site listing many senior-related links.
http://igm.nlm.nih.gov: Grateful med site with multiple links and important content.
www.ncsbn.org/public/regulation/boards_of_nursing_board.htm: Complete and current
listing of all boards of nursing. These boards have web sites from which you may download
current nurse practice standards.

10. Why would a health care facility need networked information systems?
    Networked information provides instant access to relevant data. Health care managers share
their information, such as minutes, schedules, or reports, by placing them on the network system.
It saves time, prevents loss of valuable information, and promotes collaborative strategies.
    Consider data group files as giant stew pots and the search engine software as a strainer.
When asked, the search engine will sort or strain the networked information. Data search and
retrieval tools do already exist, but it is predicted they will become more refined and powerful.
    For example, an infection control committee documents meeting reports on the network
server. All year, members have discussed issues concerning enteral feedings. Those meeting
minutes can be searched with the key word "enteral feeding," with all discussion sections identified, retrieved, reorganized, and refiled as a separate document. Additional facility resources
could be searched, such as minutes from the ethics committee, staff development, risk management, or even client records. There is a great advantage to having all of the data at hand during
accreditation visits, new enteral feeding evaluations, or staff competency assessments.

11. How would this relate to supplies?
    Medical supplies can quickly and easily be identified, charged, ordered, and restocked.
Incompatibles, product recalls, and expiration dates for these devices are instantly obvious.
Product information dissemination could include the FDA approved use of the product.
    For example, a nurse scans the IV bar code and client ID as the fluid is being hung and in-
stantly a charge is made and the IV administration is documented. This device will facilitate inventory management, allowing just-in-time ordering for inventory reduction and price controls.

12. Which electronic innovations will be more common for me and for my facility?
    Computerized systems will be enmeshed into every aspect of the health care business,
with faster access and better information. A few of the electronic innovations predicted to
become common within the next decade follow:
    • Streaming video with ability to broadcast on the Internet.
    • Wireless cell phones that download video. Nurses can watch live action (a clinical case,
      a new procedure, a conference) by using small handheld cell phones. Electronic diagno-
      sis and treatment will occur.
    • Mini-computers with special functionality to act as audio players or cell phones.
    • Digital cameras with full motion video that can be uploaded into client records or net-
      work systems. For instance, a nurse could assess a client's wound with palm-sized cam-
      eras, send images to a consultant, and receive real-time advice.
    • Digitalized documentation. This device could be designed as a hand-held clipboard
      (with bar code reader) capable of receiving spoken or written data and of saving the
      data onto a network server.

13. Tell me more about the use of digitalized documentation supporting error-free care.
    • *Prescription writing.* Handheld computers are now being used for electronic prescrib-
      ing or accessing drug information. Computer order entry will increasingly replace
      handwritten medication prescriptions. In hospitals, this system has been shown to reduce

50% to 80% of preventable medication errors. This is because it reduces poor legibility and has built-in safety checks for dose, allergies, drug interactions, and certain laboratory values.

• *Medication administration.* The nurse scans the client and medication bar codes. Automatic built-in checks and safeguards immediately tell the nurse key information such as the patient is allergic, wrong time, or the laboratory results contradict administration (e.g., heparin). If there is no problem, one additional click indicates actual administration. This device will save time as well as errors.

• *Resource information.* Personal digital assistants (PDA)—portable technology such as Palm Pilots—allow continually updated instant access to chart records and reference material.

14. Why will the process of mentoring carry greater importance in the future?

In the 21st century, leadership roles will become more complex and require greater clinical and cultural competence. Staff will need additional support because of rapid changes in the way nurses communicate, document, and intervene. Mentoring is the single easiest way to ensure facility achievement. It is the greatest gift nursing leaders can give to the profession.

15. How will staff development change?

In the future, we will have a focused and prioritized process of continuing education. Electronically stored and retrieved data will facilitate a defense or an awareness of a need for training.

16. What is outcomes-based research? Why will it be important for my unit's future?

Outcomes research is a multidisciplinary investigation of relationships among care processes, client characteristics, care costs, and outcomes of client satisfaction, health, and clinical status. It includes original data collection processes or large, existing data files to facilitate the best health care practice at the organization, family, and community levels.

To perform outcomes-based research, managers need to ask the following questions:
• How much measurement and reporting do we need?
• How much measurement and reporting can we afford (financial and human costs)
• What data can we collect and have access to?
• What data should we collect?
• Of existing data, what can we use and to what purpose?

17. In the future, how will systems management theory help managers deliver quality, efficient, and effective care?

Systems theory is a holistic way of viewing health care. Rather than thinking linearly, systems theory looks at the whole. Each system and subsystem affects and connects with all other systems. Identified client problems stem from system interdependence, not just one person or piece.

The future finds us needing to define new organizations. For example, health care organizations, such as home care and acute care, must network together to form single entities to improve efficiency and effectiveness. Implications for a systems approach to nursing leadership include the following:
• Knowledgeable, creative, self-directed, and empowered staff
• Proactive leadership that develops partnerships with internal and external customers
• Health promotion and illness prevention
• Fully informed, well educated, and supported clients
• Continuous assessment, evaluation of customer needs, expectations, care outcomes

18. What are predicted to be the top 10 issues in the near future?

Author, editor, and speaker Leah Curtain predicts the following:
• *Upsizing the system* (planning for the future rather than surviving the moment)
• *Hiring and developing nurse managers* (recovering from the managerial downsizing of the 1990s)

- *Reforming human resources* (better benefits and pay for all health care professionals)
- *Moving services back inside* (consolidating locations will use limited staffing resources better)
- *Private sector muscle* (demands of the major employers will be heard)
- *New regulations and legislation* (staffing ratios and maximum hours are in the forefront as union activity grows)
- *Reduced government reimbursement*
- *Health Insurance Portability and Accountability Act (HIPAA)* compliance (its effects are predicted to reverberate throughout health care)
- *Measuring and ensuring staff competence* (beyond traditional knowledge, skills, credentials, and experience; effects of fatigue and contingency staffing will be included)
- *Patient safety* (The Institute of Medicine [IOM] report has politicians demanding changes for safety)

19. What are other predicted health care trends?

Forecasts aren't always accurate. For instance, in the early 1960s, it was predicted everyone in America would be bowling at least 2 hours per week by now, which hasn't quite come true. Nonetheless, some predictions are
- Growth of health care services in the home
- Emphasis on prevention and promoting healthy lifestyles
- Strained health care services from baby boomer's chronic illnesses' complications
- Increased incidence of type II diabetes and infectious organisms with antibiotic resistance
- Increased attention to women's health issues (breast cancer, osteoporosis)
- New ethical dilemmas related to research and evolving DNA and genetic possibilities
- Ethnic awareness in health care services, including bilingual caregivers
- Geriatric issues, including a focus on Alzheimer's disease prevention and care
- Travel medicine
- Bioterrorism, including public health and facility readiness, staff education

20. How will quality leadership move nursing and health care forward?

Quality nursing leadership creates internal and external organizational climates that enhance and develop our profession. Using a systems theory framework, we will create more effective and efficient approaches to health care that keep customers in close view. With the help of technology, we will measure and report our work so that workloads are appropriate, nurse-client ratios adequate, and nursing's value enhanced. Through this research, we will attract new members and funding. Through networking and collaboration, we will generate reformed nursing practice standards. Communication between and among all nurses of all nations is the answer to the professional and personal challenges we face in the 21st century.

BIBLIOGRAPHY

1. Curtain L: Healthcare's top 10 issues for 2001. CurtinCalls 3(3):1,2, 2001.
2. Darbyshire P: User-friendliness of computerized information systems. Comput Nurs 18:93–99, 2000.
3. Houston S, Flescher R: Outcomes management in women's health. J Obstet Gynecol Neonatal Nurs 26:342–350, 1997.
4. Issel LM, Anderson RA: Take charge: Managing six transformations in health care delivery. Nurs Econ 14:78–85, 1996.
5. Jennings BM: Evaluating outcomes versus "McAnswers"—where are we going? Outcomes Manag Nurs Pract 3:144–146, 1999.
6. Maljanian R: Supporting nurses in their quest for evidence-based practice: Research utilization and conduct. Outcomes Manag Nurs Pract 4:155–158, 2000.
7. Naisbitt J: An interview with John Naisbitt: A 20th century forecast of 21st century healthcare trends. Health Care Finan Manag 54(2):28–31, 2000.
8. Smith LS, McAllister LE, Crawford CS: Mentoring benefits and issues for public health nurses. Public Health Nurs 18:101–107, 2001.

41. BEEN THERE, DONE THAT

Nothing can take the place of practical experience out in the world.

A. B. Zu Tavern

THE EMPLOYEE WHO WAS EXCESSIVELY "ILL"

Scenario

I was the new manager for the department. The staff had been resistant to, or at least hesitant about, a managerial change. One long-term employee, Sue*, immediately started a pattern of frequently calling in sick—12 times in the first 3 months! And she was often tardy on the other days.

When I confronted Sue about her attendance, she boldly proclaimed, "I'm your best worker and you know it. I can't help it if I am sick." The other staff were aware of her attendance, closely watching how I would handle this response.

Development

Sue never brought a physician's statement indicating a medical condition for her absences. When offered, she indicated that she did not need to take a leave of absence to deal with the causes of her frequent illnesses.

I proceeded to activate the disciplinary action. Sue only became firmer in her position. She went around telling other staff how cruel and cold the new manager was.

Sue eventually resigned when she realized I was actually going to go through with all of the disciplinary process. However, she first told everyone that the reason for her resignation was that the new management had given her so much stress that it had made her ill.

Comment

Exceptions, without justification, cannot be tolerated. It will bring down the morale of the department to see the "law breakers win," so to speak. This is particularly true when beginning in a new position, and some staff choose to test you.

This employee had a satisfactory attendance record before I came. I had no reason to believe that this involved an addiction, child care problem, or some other social issue that may have warranted the use of an employee assistance program.

Sometimes employees seem to want to leave and can't bring themselves to do it. I personally have seen this occur more in long-term employees who have a lot to lose (e.g., benefits, seniority). They will then "act out" in an objectionable manner that they know will force the termination (and their own decision).

THE EMPLOYEE WITH AN UNSATISFACTORY TRANSFER

Scenario

Hilga* had 2 years' registered nurse experience and was an in-house transfer from a surgical floor to our emergency department (ED). Her manager indicated that she was an adequate performer. It quickly became apparent that her ED orientation was not going well. Her preceptor started complaining immediately that she was "lackadaisical" and not learning anything she taught her.

Hilga had a strong ethnic personality, with some unusual traits. For instance, she would always eat six raw apples on each shift while openly criticizing the other staff for their eating habits. She called off "sick," requesting sick pay, for a day that she wasn't even scheduled to work. The preceptor did have a reputation as a complainer. I wondered if it was just a personality incongruence.

Development

I met with Hilga and the preceptor individually and together. Hilga thought there were no problems except that the night staff nurses were not helping her. I assigned her to the day shift for the 2 weeks and solicited another experienced preceptor's opinion.

Several day shift nurses indicated that they were surprised at Hilga's lack of basic nursing knowledge. For instance, she couldn't understand the difference between the concepts of cardiac "sounds" and cardiac "rhythm" and "rate." The term "odd" was repeatedly used.

There was no evidence of Hilga accepting any responsibility to rectify her deficiencies. She never read any of the provided literature. Instead, she intensified her complaints about the staff "not being willing to teach."

I decided Hilga was not successfully progressing in her orientation and probationary period. I thought I was being kind by describing it as "not yet being ready in her career development for the variety, acuity, flexibility, and complexity of the ED patient population." I assumed she would accept that there were problems too.

Instead, she was furious. She told everyone and anyone (who would listen) how the ED had "lured" her into this staff position and then refused to help her make the transition.

Hilga did obtain a transfer to the hospital's telemetry unit on the night shift. Two months later, she was found snorting cocaine in the staff bathroom while her patient was in cardiac arrest.

Comment

At the time I missed signs that could have indicated Hilga had a drug abuse impairment. Since then I have become more knowledgeable and perceptive about these signs and symptoms. But, even though I didn't know why at the time, the decision is still the same.

The bottom line for an orientation is always determining whether the nurse successfully meets the orientation's progression goals. In the end, a manager must require that each nurse be consistently competent. It was an uncomfortable, hard position to maintain when the individual vehemently disagrees, is an inconsistent performer, and insists that only one more chance is needed.

Afterward, through the grapevine, I learned that there had been problems with Hilga in her initial unit and her manager was eager to get rid of her. Two lessons I learned from this experience are to trust my gut when I sense something is wrong and not to blindly trust every reference.

THE ASSISTANT MANAGER WHO WAS NOT HANDLING THE RESPONSIBILITIES

Scenario

I was the newly appointed clinical director, coming from within the ranks. A popular older nurse, Maria*, had served as one of the two departments' "assistant director" for years. She viewed it as her privileged right because of her seniority but had never fulfilled any specific additional duties. It was rumored that she was offended that the clinical director position had not been offered to her (even though she did not apply). Maria assumed she would keep this assistive position, which paid an additional hourly rate.

Development

I initially clarified in my own mind what I wanted to accomplish and how much of that I could realistically do myself. I knew I would need two effective assistant managers. I developed a list of responsibilities and met with both assistants. Each chose what they would like to do among the mapped-out responsibilities. The newly developed assistant management evaluation criteria were also shared. It mainly consisted of management, not clinical, responsibilities.

The other assistant began performing her responsibilities, but Maria did nothing except her same level of clinical work. I started weekly meetings with Maria to get and to give feedback. There was no change. After 3 months, I clearly indicated that she was not fulfilling the defined duties of the assistant manager position and her upcoming annual evaluation would not be satisfactory unless changes were made.

The following week Maria informed me that she had decided she didn't want the extra responsibility and resigned from the position. She stayed, with a satisfactory performance, as a clinical staff nurse.

Comments

This nurse came from a culture that traditionally honors loyalty and seniority. It is difficult to prevent hard feelings when one views a title as an earned right. The key was to keep the focus on the discrepancies from the job description, rather than at a personal level. It made the deficiencies apparent but also gave her a way to save face.

THE CHRONICALLY TARDY EMPLOYEE

Scenario

One of the assistive personnel had a long-standing reputation for his chronic tardiness. The previous manager had never dealt with the issue. While Bill* was popular, it had even become a unit joke. Staff nurses held a daily pool to guess how late Bill would be. He was even told about it, with a promise that he'd be the winner if he was on time, but there still was no change.

Development

I was the new manager, promoted from within. About the time I began my role, a new, strict hospital-wide attendance policy went into effect. Time clocks were installed. Accruing 12 tardies within 12 consecutive months was automatic termination. The hospital had a pending lawsuit regarding this issue; institutional compliance was mandatory.

I repeatedly explained the policy and consequences to the staff. I told them I had no choice (citing the higher authority). I personally used authoritarian presence, while encouraging Bill's friends to use peer pressure.

His wife became pregnant with twins. I tried exhorting him: "Don't make me fire you! Do you want to be unemployed with two new babies?"

I eventually offered to change Bill's start time and he readily agreed. This worked for 2 weeks, and then he was just as late for his new start time. I started disciplinary procedures.

A game began. He meticulously tracked his tardiness and was on time—until the last month of the cycle was dropped. This allowed him one more tardy allowance, which he then immediately took!

He was eventually terminated for his tardiness. A year later his best friend told me he had a factory job and loved it.

Comment

My naivete made me believe I would change people's behavior. Looking back, I think this is a classic case of someone who was unhappy in this type of work and could not bring himself to leave (probably because of his seniority and benefits). His manipulative calendar game showed me he could change the behavior if he wanted to. But, by his being tardy, the decision was made for him.

After this experience I became more detached with mandatory policy enforcement. I present it but accept, in the end, that only that person can effect how he or she will respond.

* All names have been changed.

INDEX

Page numbers in **boldface type** indicate complete chapters.

Marketing, 4 P's of, 80–81
Markets, expansion of, 80
Market segmentation, 81
Maslow, Abraham, 64, 103, 139
Massachusetts Nurses Association, 161
Material safety data sheets (MSDS), 184
MBTI (Myers-Briggs Type Indicator), 38–39
McGregor, Douglas, 138
Mead, Margaret, 145
Meal periods, labor union solicitation during, 171
Medicaid, administration of, 185
Medical devices, unsafe, 185
Medical procedures, practiced on newly deceased patients, 174, 201
Medical records
 confidentiality of, 18, 77
 electronic, 133–134
 release of, to new insurance providers, 77
Medicare, administration of, 185
Medicare beneficiaries, hospitalization rate of, 74
Medication errors
 as Joint Commission of Accreditation of Healthcare Organizations' "hot topic," 180
 prevention of, 222–223
Mediocrity, of employees, 149
Meetings
 agenda of, 25
 decision making in, 143
 effective, 25–26
 management of, **25–30**
 for management of change, 36
 minutes of, 28
 for multiple-department management, 208, 209
 by new managers, 4–5
 for renovation project planning, 211
 scheduling of, 25, 208
 with supervisors, 4
Memo writing, 17
Men, as registered nurses, 156
Menninger, William, 103
Mentoring
 of charge nurses, 134–135
 as clinical ladder program component, 126, 127, 128
 of culturally diverse employees, 158
 evaluative criteria for, 128
 future importance of, 223
 of Generation X employees, 165
 of new graduate nurses, 93, 94
 as staff retention factor, 89
Merit, as basis for negotiation, 168
"Millennials," 166
Minors, unaccompanied, emergency treatment for, 201
Minutes, of meetings, 28
Mission, differentiated from purpose and vision, 32
Mission statements, 32, 78, 81
 application to management responsibilities, 33
 goals and objectives of, 32–33
3M Meeting Network, 26
Mobile entertainment fun centers, for pediatric patients, 40

Moore-Ede, Martin, 108–109
Morale, improvement of, 40
Morbidity rate, of patients, effect of registered nursing staff levels on, 51–52
Mortality rate, of patients, effect of registered nursing staff levels on, 51
Motivation
 for overworking, 23
 professional, evaluation of, 99
 of staff, **138–144**
 color coding-based classification of, 39
 definition of, 138
 by leaders, 8–9, 137
 as management trait, 8–9
 of mediocre employees, 149
 as ongoing process, 144
Motivational theory, 138–139
Moving ahead average (MAA), 50
MSDS (material safety data sheets), 184
Multiple departments, management of, **207–209**
"Musterbating," 20
Mutual non-disparagement, 150
Myers-Briggs Type Indicator (MBTI), 38–39

NAFTA (North American Free Trade Agreement) visas, 85
Narcotic addiction, signs and symptoms of, 153
National Committee for Quality Assurance, 185
National Council of State Boards of Nursing, Five Rights of Delegation of, 176, 177
National Institute for Occupational Safety and Health (NIOSH), 184–185
National Labor Relations Board, 171
National Sight-Saving Month, 81
NCH (nursing care hours), 49, 53, 55
Needs
 of employees, 139, 142
 hierarchy of, 64, 103, 139
Negativity, of staff members, 40, 146, 147
Negligence, 177
 corporate, 177–178
 nurse manager's responsibility for, 178
 professional, 177
Negotiation, **167–170**
 in budgeting, 58
 consensus building in, 167
 definition of, 167
 differentiated from networking, 167
 effective, 62
 failure of, 62
 obstacles to, 169
 in organizational culture, 61
 principled/by merit, 168
 rules for, 168
 techniques for, 168–169
 in unionization, 171–172
Networked information systems, 222
Networking, 216–217
 definition of, 61
 differentiated from negotiation, 167
 implication for conflict resolution, 66